Questions and Answers in

Pathology

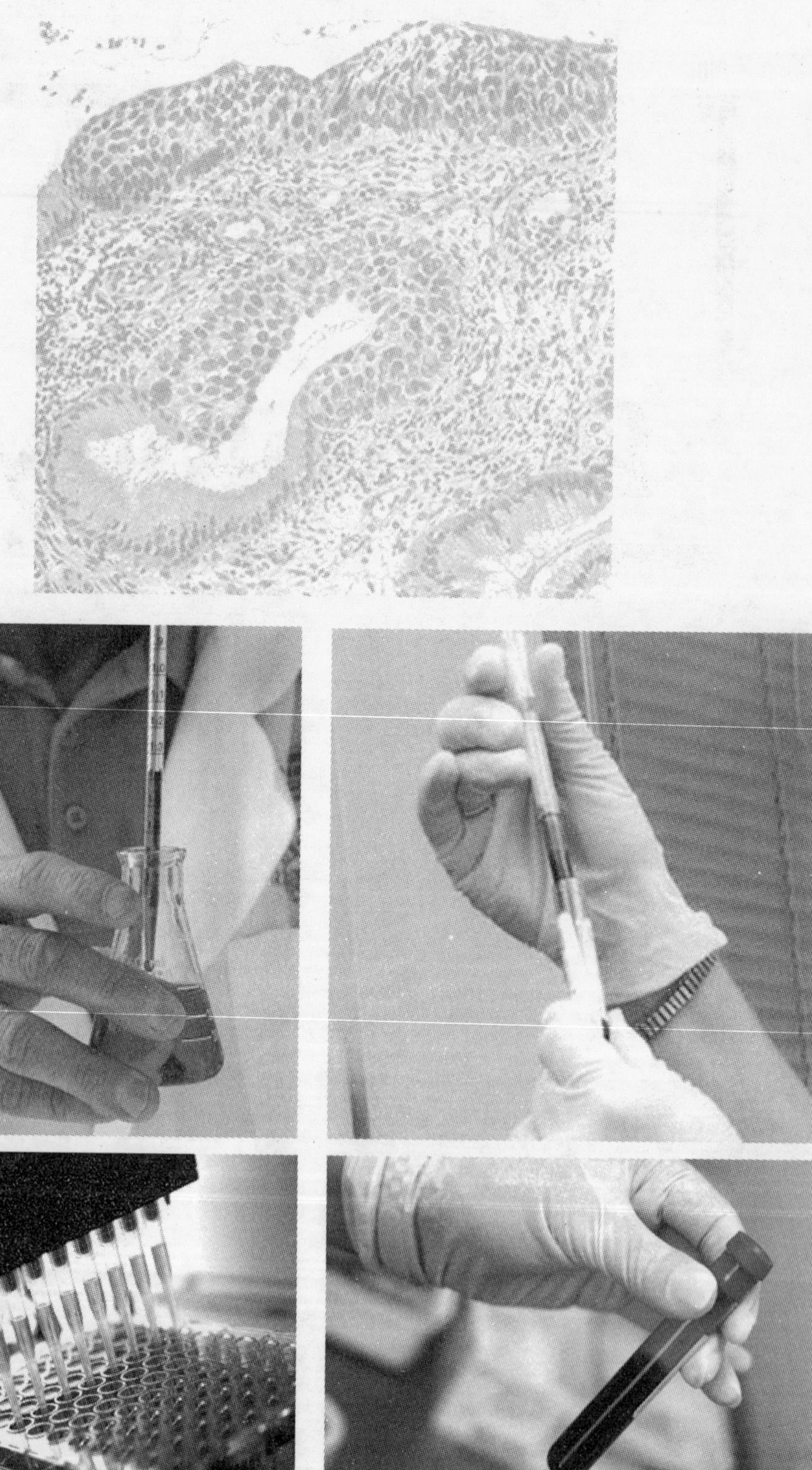

Questions and Answers in Pathology

Ashraf Mohammad
Diplomate of the American Board of Pathology

Professor and Head
Department of Pathology
Kathmandu University School of Medical Sciences
Nepal

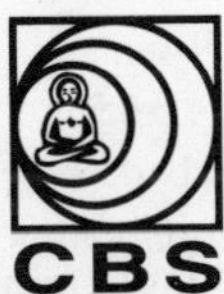

CBS Publishers and Distributors Pvt Ltd
New Delhi • Bangalore • Pune • Cochin • Chennai

- This book is not a medical treatment or a management guide and should not be used for that purpose.
- The two purposes of this book as stated in the Preface are: (1) To enable medical students to prepare for viva voce examination easily and pass it well by answering questions clearly, comfortably and confidently; answer short-answer, long-answer and multiple-choice questions intelligently and excellently in the theory examinations; and (2) for the students to get a solid foundation of good understanding of pathology to enable them to understand clinical medicine subjects well.
- It has been published in good faith that the material provided by the author is a presentation of existing knowledge in a simple, easy-to-understand format, without any claim to have discovered any new knowledge.
- Every effort has been made to ensure accuracy of material but the publisher, printer and author will not be held responsible for any inadvertent error(s).

ISBN : 978-81-239-1857-0

First Edition : 2010
Reprint : 2012

Published by Satish Kumar Jain and produced by V.K. Jain for
CBS Publishers & Distributors Pvt. Ltd.,
CBS Plaza, 4819/XI Prahlad Street, 24 Ansari Road, Daryaganj,
New Delhi - 110002, India. • Website: www.cbspd.com
e-mail: delhi@cbspd.com, cbspubs@airtelmail.in
Ph.: 23289259, 23266861, 23266867 • Fax: 011-23243014

Branches:

- ***Bengaluru:*** Seema House, 2975, 17th Cross, K.R. Road, Bansankari 2nd Stage, Bengaluru - 560070
  • Ph.: +91-80-26771678/79 • Fax: +91-80-26771680
  • E-mail: cbsbng@gmail.com, bangalore@cbspd.com
- ***Pune:*** Bhuruk Prestige, Sr. No. 52/12/2+1+3/2, Narhe, Haveli (Near Katraj-Dehu Road By-pass), Pune - 411051
  • Ph.: +91-20-64704058/59, 32342277 • E-mail: pune@cbspd.com
- ***Kochi:*** 36/14, Kalluvilakam, Lissie Hospital Road, Kochi - 682018, Kerala • Ph.: +91-484-4059061-65
  • Fax: +91-484-4059065 • E-mail: cochin@cbspd.com
- ***Chennai:*** 20, West Park Road, Shenoy Nagar, Chennai - 600030
  Ph.: +91-44-26260666, 26208620 • Fax: +91-44-42032115
  • E-mail: chennai@cbspd.com

Printed at :
India Binding House, Noida (UP)

to

our God, without whose will;
sweet memory of my beloved mom, without whose love;
my dedicated wife Shilu, without whose support;
my lovely niece Sofia [Graduate of The University of California, Berkeley, USA in 2006 with a BA in Economics, a BA in South Asian Studies, and a minor in Business Administration] without whose enthusiasm;
all my sincere students, without whose regular requests for my lecture notes;
and all the brilliant authors mentioned and not mentioned in the resources, without copious information from whose scholarly works;
this book would not have been possible.

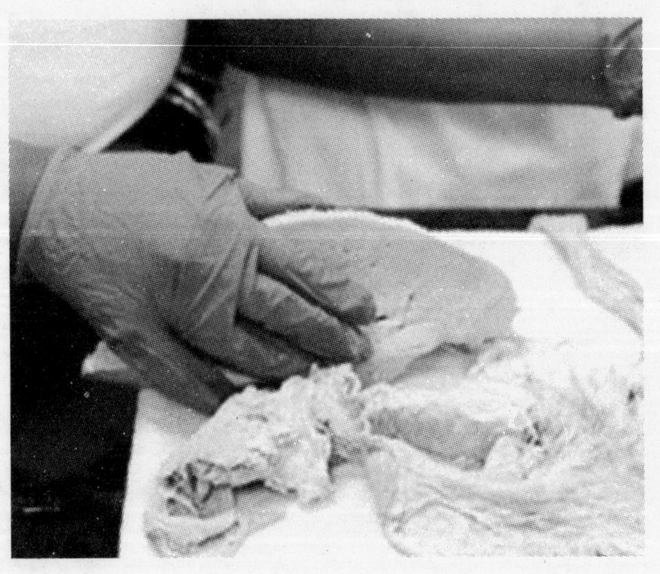

Preface

Pathology is the easiest subject in the entire medical curriculum. However, many students find it the most difficult subject. This poses double problem for them: First, they dread the examinations in pathology; and second, lack of good understanding of pathology makes it very difficult for them to understand clinical subjects such as medicine, surgery, obstetrics and gynecology, pediatrics, etc. because understanding pathology is the prerequisite to understanding clinical medicine subjects. As Sir William Osler said: "As is one's pathology so is one's clinical medicine".

Therefore, this book has been written in a very simple, easy-to-understand language with the two purposes in mind: First, to enable medical students to prepare for viva voce examination easily and pass it well by answering the questions clearly, comfortably and confidently; and, to answer short-answer, long-answer and multiple-choice questions intelligently and excellently in the theory examinations. Second, for the students to have a solid foundation of a good understanding of pathology to enable them to understand clinical medicine subjects well. The author is confident that this book will fulfill both these purposes.

Pathology is the easiest subject because there are only a few fundamental facts which apply to almost all the diseases of the mankind. Once the students have a good grasp of these fundamental facts, they will have no difficulty in understanding all the diseases that afflict the mankind and thereby make it easy for them to understand various clinical subjects easily.

Towards this aim, this book has been divided into two parts—Section 1: General Pathology and Section 2: Systemic Pathology. The basic facts are explained in very simple language in Section 1 in 7 chapters. These facts are then applied to the diseases of all the systems of our body in the subsequent 11 chapters in Section 2.

For an easy grasp, *overview* is given in the beginning of each chapter. For focused attention, pertinent facts are highlighted by *italics* or **bold** print.

Furthermore, for easy memorization; and, for quick review of the selected significant facts and various favorite questions of the examiners, mnemonics, definitions and notes are given as *pathology pearls* in the Appendices.

Hope, this book will not only help the students in their learning and preparing for the various examinations during their medical career; but also make them happy to have fond memories of their medical college days.

Suggestions for improvement in the future editions will be genuinely appreciated. Please send them to the author by e-mail: profmashraf@gmail.com.

Dr. Ashraf Mohammad

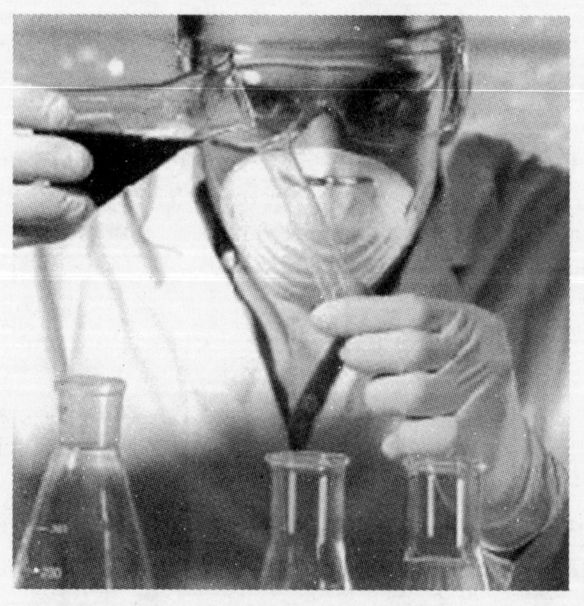

Abbreviations

DEF	Definition
DES	Description
CLASSI	Classification
ETIO	Etiology
PATHOG	Pathogenesis
PATHOPHY	Pathophysiology
MORPHO	Morphology
MICRO	Microscopy
LM	Light Microscopy
IM	Immunofluorescence Microscopy
EM	Electron Microscopy
C/Fs	Clinical Features
S/S	Symptoms and Signs
COMPLI	Complications
DIAG	Diagnosis
D/D	Differential Diagnosis
TRT	Treatment
PROG	Prognosis
HISTO	Histology
CSF	Cerebrospinal Fluid
LAB	Laboratory

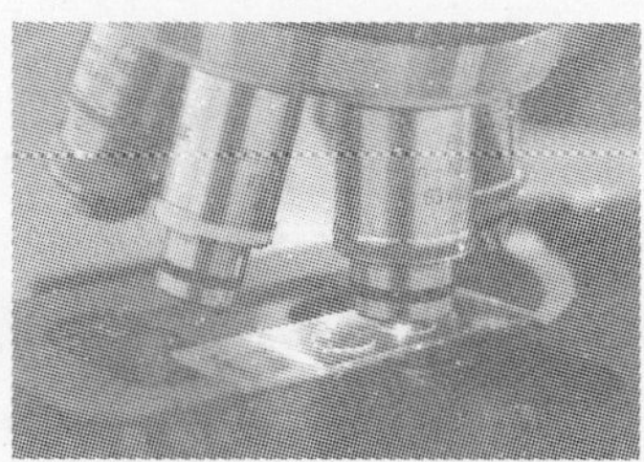

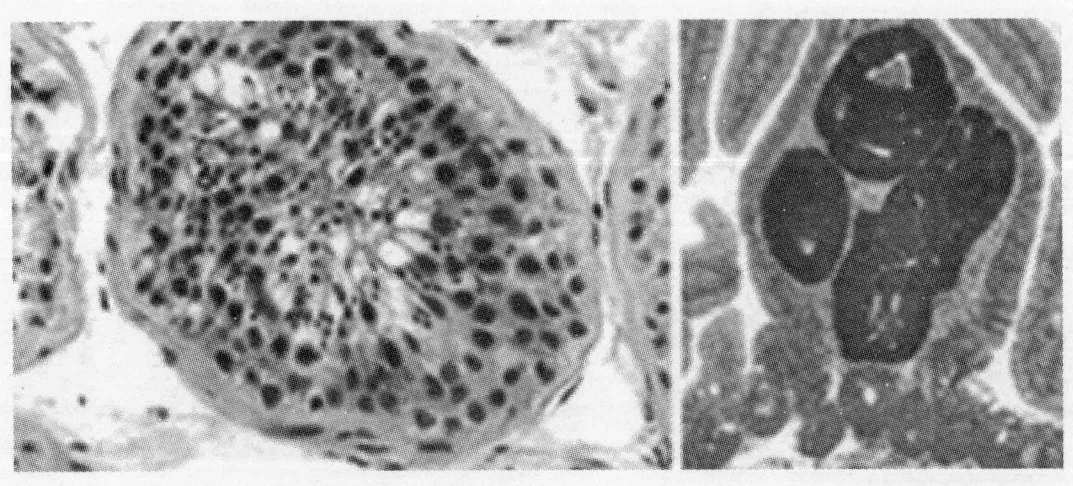

Acknowledgement

I am very thankful indeed to the publishers CBS P&D for their willingness to publish this book under their august banner and for doing an exceptional job of it. Any inadvertent errors are not of the publisher; but, of the author.

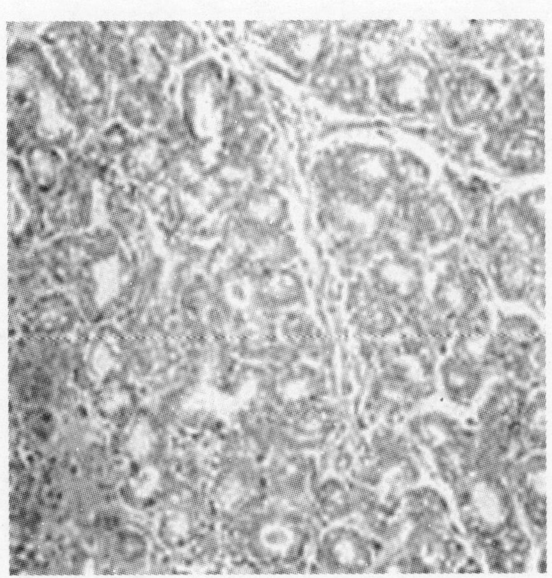

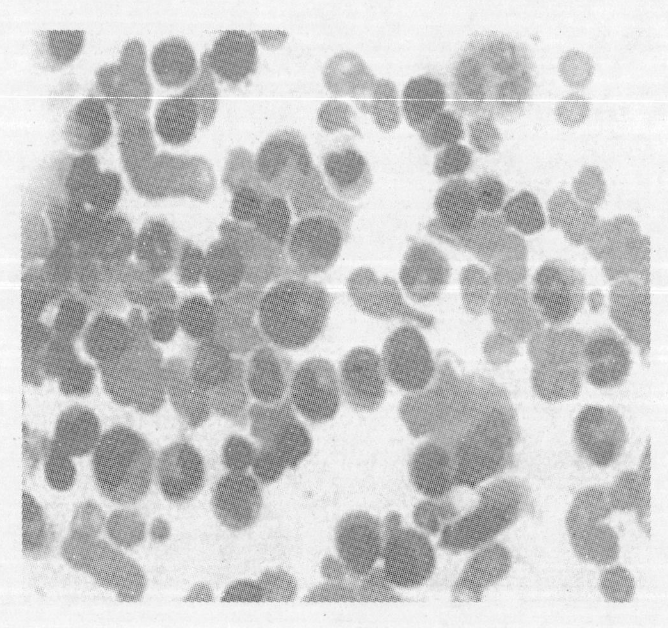

Contents

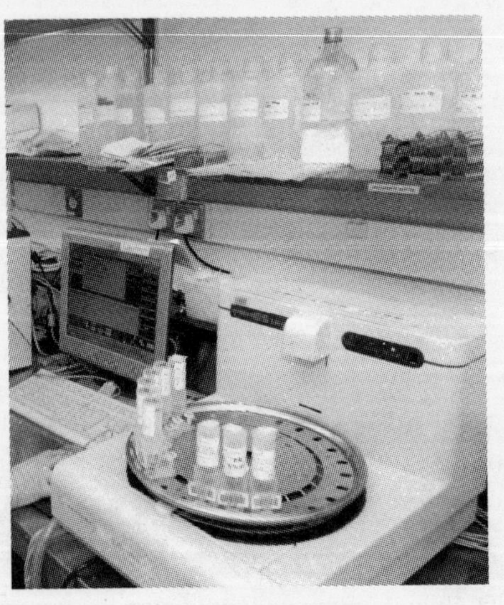

Section 1
General Pathology

1

Cell Injury

OVERVIEW

1. Responses of cells to injuries.
2. Sources, causes and mechanisms of injuries.
3. Important components of cells in injury.
4. Intra/extracellular depositions.

Injuries/diseases of our body begin at the cellular level.

Cells respond to injuries in the order of possibility by staying the same **(homeostasis)**, **adapting (atrophy, hypertrophy, hyperplasia, metaplasia)**, sustaining **reversible injury** (increased water or fat collection in the cell), sustaining **irreversible injury and dying**, or **becoming neoplastic**. After death the tissues in living body develop changes **(necrosis: coagulative, liquefactive, caseous, fibrinoid)**. In our body there is also provision for a way of death of cells where they do not undergo necrosis **(apoptosis)**.

Sources of our diseases are **hereditary** or **environmental**. *Causes are* **physical, chemical, microbiological**. *Mechanisms are* **direct actions** by these causes or **reactions** by our body.

Important components of cells in injury are the functions and structure of cell membranes, mitochondria, endoplasmic reticulum, lysosomes, cytoskeleton and nucleus. Ultimately, severe cell membrane damage causes death of the cell. The structure and functions of the cell and its components are linked together and injury to either one may occur first leading to injury to the other.

Understanding *cytoskeletons has significance as* knowledge of intracytoplasmic inclusions in hepatocytes **(Mallory's body)**; as **neurofibrillary tangles** in neurons in Alzheimer's diseases; as functional deficiencies in **Chediak-Higashi syndrome** and **Kartagener's syndrome** with susceptibility to infections; as therapeutic application in the treatment of gout; as diagnostic application in the differential diagnosis of anaplastic neoplasms.

Under certain circumstances different substances collect inside the cells and tissues such as water, different types of fats, carbohydrates, proteins, and minerals:

Water collects in the cells due to failure of sodium pump making the cells appear **cloudy** or **vacuolated.**

Cholesterol collects in the cells (macrophages, smooth muscle cells of arteries) in **atherosclerosis**; in hyperlipidemia in mesenchymal cells and macrophages **(xanthomas)**.

Glycogen collects in various hereditary glycogen storage diseases. Various sphingolipids and mucopolysaccharides collect in different lysosomal storage diseases.

Various proteins collect inside the cell such as synthesized immunoglobulins in plasma cells **(Russell bodies)**.

Amyloid, derived from different sources, collects outside the cells in different parenchymal and mesenchymal tissues in different conditions such as multiple myeloma, Waldenström's macroglobulinemia, chronic inflammatory diseases, neoplastic diseases, Alzheimer's diseases, medullary carcinoma of the thyroid, type II diabetes mellitus, old age. Amyloid causes injury by causing pressure atrophy to adjacent cells when deposited in interstitial tissue or when deposited in the wall of a blood vessel by narrowing the lumen leading to decreased blood flow or by causing increased permeability in glomerular capillaries resulting in albuminuria.

Calcium, with normal serum calcium **(dystrophic)**, collects outside cells in degenerated/dead tissues, e.g. in atheromas, overdamaged heart valves, caseous tuberculous lymph nodes; and in hypercalcemia **(metastatic)**, e.g. in kidneys causing kidney stones **(nephrolithiasis)** (when in the collecting system) and **nephrocalcinosis** (when in the interstitial tissue).

Iron collects in various cells and tissues of our body [without tissue damage **(hemosiderosis)** and with tissue damage **(hemochromatosis)**, e.g. in liver causing cirrhosis, in heart causing heart failure, in skin causing bronze color, in pancreas causing diabetes with bronze color of skin called **bronze diabetes**].

Copper collects in hepatocytes, Descemet's membrane in the limbus of cornea **(Kayser-Fleischer rings)** and basal ganglia of the brain, mainly in the globus pallidus and putamen (together called lentiform nucleus) in Wilson's disease **(hepatolenticular degeneration)**.

1. What is a cell? How is it related to tissues, organs and organ system of our body?

Ans. Cell is the **unit** of our body. Many cells together make **tissues**. Many tissues together make an **organ**. Many organs involved in similar function in our body make **organ system**.

2. What are the main parts of the cell?

Ans. Cell membrane, cytoplasm, cytoskeleton, mitochondria, RER (rough endoplasmic reticulum), SER (smooth endoplasmic reticulum), Golgi apparatus, lysosomes, proteasomes, nucleus and nucleolus (within the nucleus).

Nucleus has DNA and RNA (deoxyribonucleic and ribonucleic acids respectively). These being acids take basic stain (hematoxylin) and appear blue with H&E (hematoxylin and eosin stain). Cytoplasm is basic in its contents and, therefore, takes acid stain (eosin) and appears pink. Approximately 1% DNA is in the cytoplasm giving it a bluish tinge. The applied aspects of this information/knowledge are:

1. In injured cells there is loss of RNA (bluish tinge) from the cytoplasm thereby making it appear more pinkish (eosinophilic), i.e. an injured cell appears more pinkish.
2. Generally neoplastic cells are fast dividing cells requiring more DNA in their nuclei, making them appear more bluish (hyperchromatic—hyper = more, chromatic = color), i.e. neoplastic cells have hyperchromatic nuclei.

3. What are the responses/reactions of the cell to injury?

Ans. Responses/reactions of the cell to injury are:

1. *First*, the cell tries and stays the same by maintaining its internal and external environment unchanged. This is called **homeostasis**.
2. *Second*, if it cannot maintain homeostasis, it **adapts (adjusts)** in response to the injury.

   The adaptations are:

   a. Atrophy.

   b. Hypertrophy.

   c. Hyperplasia.

   d. Metaplasia.
3. *Third*, if it cannot survive with adaptation, it gets **reversible injury**.

   The reversible injuries are:

   a. Water accumulation (hydropic change).

   b. Fat accumulation (steatosis).
4. *Fourth*, if the injury is severe or prolonged, the **injury becomes irreversible**. Irreversible injury, if it is fatal, leads to changes in the living tissue called **necrosis**.

Types of necrosis are:

1. Coagulation.
2. Liquefaction.
3. Caseation.
4. Fibrinoid.

Irreversible, non-fatal injury to the genetic apparatus leads to **neoplasia**.

4. What are the sources of cell injury?

Ans. 1. Hereditary.

2. Environmental.

5. What are the environmental causes of cell injury?

Ans. 1. Chemical.

2. Physical.
3. Microbiological.

6. What are the mechanisms of cell injury?

Ans. 1. By the actions of the cause of injury.

2. By the reactions of our body.

7. What are the chemical causes of cell injury?

Ans. 1. Oxygen-related:

   a. Low oxygen (hypoxia).
   b. Oxygen under high pressure/in high concentration (100%).
   c. Free radical oxygen and other free radicals.

2. Ischemia and reperfusion.
3. Immunologic/inflammatory events.
4. Various natural, man-made and body-made chemicals.
5. Nutritional.

8. What is the pathogenesis of cell injury?

Ans. The injury can cause damage to either the function first or the structure first. Functions and structures are interrelated and damage to one causes damage to the other.

Example of function lost first: Cyanide inactivates cytochrome oxidase in mitochondria stopping aerobic respiration and ATP generation, leading to failure of sodium pump causing sodium and water entry into cell making cell swell up and break.

Examples of structure lost first:

1. *Free radicals:* Injure membranes by lipid peroxidation: Due to injury to SER membrane, metabolic function suffers. Due to injury to RER membrane and resultant separation of ribosomes, synthesis of enzymes and formation of structural protein suffer.
2. *Bacterial toxins:* Phospholipases break cell membrane phospholipids.
3. *Inflammatory events:* Certain inflammations activate complements and generate (C5b-C9, MAC$^-$, the membrane attack complex) and recruit cytotoxic lymphocytes, which are directly injurious to cell membranes.
4. *Chemicals:* Mercuric chloride, antineoplastics, antibiotics bind to sulfhydryl group of cell membrane and cause increased permeability.
5. *Injury to mitochondria:* Increased calcium, lipid breakdown products, free radicals, decreased ATP hypoxia, etc. cause injury to its inner and/or outer membrane making them more permeable. Inner membrane is made more permeable by punching of pores in them which are called mitochondrial permeability transition (MPT), which interfaces in ATP generation. More permeability of the outer membrane leads to leaking of cytochrome *c* and promoting apoptosis.

Critical intracellular functional/structural systems affected are:

1. Structure of membranes of the cell and intracellular organelles.
2. Mitrochondrial function of aerobic respiration with ATP generation.
3. Endoplasmic reticulum and ribosomal function of structural and functional (enzymes) protein synthesis.
4. Nuclear structure and functions of:
   a. Structural and functional (enzymes) protein synthesis.
   b. Growth-regulating protein synthesis may result in abnormal growth **(neoplasm)**.
   c. Cellular division—mitosis and meiosis.

9. What is hypoxia?

Ans. Hypoxia is decrease in oxygen. (Hypo = low; Oxia = oxygen).

10. What are the causes of hypoxia?

Ans. *The main cause of hypoxia is:* Ischemia (decreased blood supply).

Other causes of hypoxia are:

1. Decreased oxygen in the atmosphere (high altitude, smoke, air pollution, etc.).
2. Decreased intake of oxygen by our body from the atmosphere, e.g. due to various thoracic diseases or diseases of the CNS, which control our body's respiration.
3. Various upper and lower respiratory tract diseases (epiglottitis, croup, chronic bronchitis, emphysema, asthma, pneumonia, etc.).

5. Decreased oxygen-carrying capacity of the blood (anemia, hemoglobinopathies, carbon monoxide poisoning, etc.).
6. Decreased circulation of the blood (congestive cardiac failure).
7. Impaired utilization of oxygen by the cell due to the poisoning of enzymes of oxidative phosphorylation, e.g. cyanide poisoning.

11. How does hypoxia cause cell injury?

Ans. Oxygen is necessary for the synthesis of ATP (adenosine triphosphate) by the mitochondria. ATP is the source of energy by which all the normal structures of the cells are maintained and all the functions of the cells are carried out. Lack of oxygen leads to lack of ATP production. This leads to:

1. Sodium pump failure with influx of sodium and water inside the cell **(hydropic change)**, which causes cellular swelling, loss of microvilli, blebs formation, ER swelling, myelin figures formation.
2. Calcium homeostasis failure.
3. Mitochondrial injury.
4. Endoplasmic reticulum injury with detachment of ribosomes from the RER leading to decreased protein synthesis causing triglyceride deposition inside the cell **(fatty change)**. If oxygen supply is improved, these changes will reverse and cell will become normal again.

   But, if oxygen supply is not improved then due to anaerobic glycolysis with acidosis **irreversible changes will occur** consisting of breakage of lysosomes with release of lysosomal enzymes causing damage to nuclear and cell membranes and **death of cell**. Thus, loss of energy-producing ATP with subsequent failure of sodium pump and influx of sodium and calcium into the cell and cell membrane injury are the most crucial events causing cell death due to ischemia/hypoxia.

For treatment purposes, it is important to note that tolerance for hypoxia varies according to the type of cell, e.g. epidermal and connective tissue cells can tolerate hypoxia for a few hours, CNS cells for a few minutes, myocardial cells for approximately one hour. Therefore, in case of myocardial infarction the first one hour is called the **window of opportunity** to give the patient treatment to lyse the thrombus within the coronary artery to prevent necrosis of the myocardial cells.

12. What is the injury from high concentration / high pressure oxygen?

Ans. When given to premature babies it causes **retrolental fibroplasia** and **blindness**.

13. What are free radicals? How do free radicals cause cell injury?

Ans. Free radicals are high-energy atoms, molecules, or group of molecules with single unpaired electron in their outermost orbit. Therefore, they are "free" to give or take an electron. In our cells these are mostly produced from oxygen as follows: Oxygen is essential for life. ATP is formed by reducing molecular oxygen to form water. This is done by addition of 4 electrons to oxygen by the mitochondrial electron transport system. Approximately 98% oxygen which enters mitochondria is thus reduced to water. 2% of the oxygen accepts less than 4 electrons due to "leaks" in the mitochondrial electron transport system with formation of free radicals. These are **superoxide (O^-)** and **hydroxyl radical (OH^-). Hydrogen peroxide (H_2O_2)** is also formed, which is not a free radical, but it has the potential to generate OH^-. Free radicals are unstable and decay spontaneously without causing any injury. The rate of decay is increased by protective enzymes in our body, e.g. superoxide dismutase **(SODs)**, glutathione peroxidase **(GSH)**, **Catalase**, and also by **antioxidants (vitamin C** and **E)**. But, when production of these free radicals is increased, e.g. from neutrophils during inflammation, UV light, X-rays, chemicals, oxygen toxicity, radiation, reperfusion injury, etc. they cannot be neutralized and cause injury to the cell by injuring the cellular lipids, proteins and DNA, respectively leading to:

1. Damage to membranes of the cell and to its organelles.
2. Damage to:
   a. Structure (polypeptide fragmentation) and
   b. Function (enzymatic degradation) of the cell.
3. Death or malignant transformation of cells.

14. How does sodium pump failure causes injury to the cell?

Ans. Sodium pump keeps the excess sodium out of the cell. Failure of the sodium pump leads to influx of the sodium into the cell. Due to osmosis together with the sodium extra water also comes inside the cell and makes the cell swell **(hydropic swelling** or **vacuolar degeneration)**.

15. How does calcium homeostasis failure cause injury to the cell?

Ans. Calcium homeostasis failure leads to influx of calcium inside the cell. This leads to activation of:

1. **Phospholipases** with damage to various cell membranes.
2. **Proteases** with damage to various structural and functional proteins.
3. **ATPase** with reduction of ATP.
4. **Endonucleases** with damage to the DNA.

16. How does anaerobic glycolysis cause injury to the cell?

Ans. Anaerobic glycolysis causes decreased production of ATP and changes the intracellular pH from neutral to acidic leading to detachment of ribosomes from the rough endoplasmic reticulum (RER) with reduction in the synthesis of structural and functional (enzymes) proteins. Further reduction in pH causes breakdown of lysosomes with release of lysosomal enzymes into the cytoplasm with irreversible injury to various structures of the cell.

17. What is ischemia? What are the causes of ischemia? How do ischemia and reperfusion cause cell injury?

Ans. Ischemia is reduced blood supply to an organ or part of the body. (Greek-Isch = restriction, hemia = blood, restricted blood supply). *Some of the common causes of ischemia are:* Low blood volume (due to hemorrhage, dehydration), decreased circulation, e.g. congestive cardiac failure (CCF), or thickening of the blood vessels (atherosclerosis), blockage of the blood vessels either internal, e.g. thrombosis, embolism or external from compression from various causes such as mass of a neoplasm or inflammatory mass or torsion of an organ, etc.

Ischemia causes cell injury by:

1. Hypoxia—**Ischemia is the most important cause of hypoxia**.
2. Ischemia not only causes hypoxia (where glycolytic generation of energy can continue) but interferes in anaerobic glycolysis by depriving the delivery of substrates for glycolysis and removal of metabolites. Thus, ischemia injures tissues faster than hypoxia.

Reperfusion causes cell injury by: **Increased calcium** and increased oxygen-derived **free radicals** which cause damage to cell membrane and to mitochondria.

18. How do chemicals-toxins cause cell injury?

Ans. These cause injuries either directly or indirectly by free radicals.

Direct injury: For example, cyanide inactivates cytochrome oxidase in mitochondria stopping aerobic respiration and ATP generation causing failure of sodium pump leading to sodium and water entry into cell making cell swell up and rupture.

Indirect injury by free radicals: For example, CCl_4 can change to free radical CCl_3, which damages the RER membrane causing separation of ribosomes leading to decreased apoprotein synthesis and its availability to bind with triglyceride to form lipoprotein for exit from the hepatocytes resulting in accumulation of triglyceride inside the hepatocytes.

19. What are physical causes of cell injury?

Ans. These are mechanical, thermal (high or low), electrical, radiation, atmospheric pressure changes (described in detail in Chapter 7).

20. What are infectious causes of cell injury?

Ans. These are prions, viruses, bacteria, fungi, protozoa and helminths. Various diseases caused by them are described in the pertinent system in Section 2.

21. What are cytoskeletal structures? What are the normal cytoskeletal structures and their functions?

Ans. *Cytoskeletal structures are:*

1. Thin actin filaments (5 nm).
2. Intermediate filaments (10 nm).
3. Thick myosin filaments (15 nm).
4. Microtubules (20 nm).

Cytoskeletal functions are:

1. Facilitating locomotion of cell.
2. Facilitating fusion of phagosome with lysosomes to form **phagolysosome**.
3. Facilitating motility of sperms.
4. Facilitating intracellular movements of molecules and signals.
5. Facilitating in maintaining integrity and polarity of cells.
6. Facilitating mitotic spindle formation during cell division.

22. What are the applied aspects of cytoskeleton in medicine?

Ans. There are various applied aspects of cytoskeleton in medicine. These are:

1. Intermediate filaments collect in some conditions such as in alcoholic liver disease as pink (eosinophilic) intracytoplasmic inclusions called **alcoholic hyaline** or **Mallory's body**.
2. Microtubules appear as **neurofibrillary tangles in the brain in Alzheimer's disease**.
3. Defective microtubule polymerization causes delayed or decreased fusion of lysosomes with phagosomes resulting in impaired destruction of phagocytosed bacteria, e.g. in **Chediak-Higashi syndrome**.
4. Defective microtubule organization causes immobilization of cilia of the respiratory epithelium resulting in impaired clearance of inhaled bacteria and chronic infections and defect in motility of sperms resulting in sterility, e.g. in **immotile cilia syndrome (Kartagener's syndrome)**.
5. Defective cytoskeleton function of leukocytes causes their impaired chemotactic movement. During infection, this results in decreased body's defense. This property is utilized therapeutically in **gout** as follows: In gout, the injury is caused by movement of macrophages towards the urate crystals and attempts to phagocytose them with release of inflammatory mediators from macrophages and proteases causing tissue/joint injury. Drug, e.g. **colchicine** is useful in treatment of gout as this prevents microtubule polymerization with consequent decrease in chemotaxis and attempted phagocytosis of urate crystals, thereby reducing the untoward effect of damage to tissues/joints.
6. Another therapeutic application of microtubules function is in treatment of cancers by decreasing the division and thus proliferation of cancer cells: Microtubules form mitotic spindle for cell division. Hence, certain drugs which bind to microtubules, e.g. vinca alkaloids, hinder mitotic spindle formation resulting in decrease in cell proliferation.

7. Composition of intermediate filaments is different in different cells as follows: **Keratin** in epithelial cells, **vimentin** in mesenchymal cells, **desmin** in muscle cells, **glial acidic fibrillary protein** in glial cells. Antibodies against these are used to diagnose tumors arising from these cells.

23. What is adaptation? What are the types of adaptations?

Ans. Normally, the cells stay the same and do not change. Under certain circumstances (stimuli)—physiologic or pathologic, in order to meet the functional demand or stay alive, the cells adjust by some change. This phenomenon is known as adaptation. According to the circumstances (stimuli), these adaptations are of the following 4 types:

a. Atrophy
b. Hypertrophy.
c. Hyperplasia
d. Metaplasia.

24. What is atrophy? What are its causes? What is its pathogenesis? What is the morphology?

Ans. Atrophy is **decrease in the size** of cell and the organ. Causes include:

1. Decreased workload, disuse.
2. Loss of innervation.
3. Loss of endocrine stimulation, e.g. menopause.
4. Decreased blood supply.
5. Decreased nutrition.
6. Aging.
7. Unknown.

MORPHO: GROSS: Organ is smaller in size.

25. What is hypertrophy? What are its causes?

Ans. Hypertrophy is the **increase in the size** of organ or tissue due to increase in the size of cells. Causes include:

1. Hormonal stimulation, e.g. uterus during pregnancy (also there is hyperplasia).
2. Increased workload, e.g. skeletal muscle hypertrophy in weight lifter or manual laborer. Cardiac muscle hypertrophy in people with chronic hypertension.

26. What is hyperplasia? What are its types?

Ans. Hyperplasia is increase in the size of the organ due to **increase in the number** of cells.

ETIO: 1. *Endocrine stimulation,* e.g.

a. Proliferation of female breast at puberty and during pregnancy.

b. Enlargement of uterus during pregnancy (this is due to both increase in size and number of cells).
c. Prostatic hyperplasia after middle age.
d. *Endometrial hyperplasia:* This is due to increase in estrogen stimulation. When this increased estrogen stimulation returns to normal hyperplasia disappears. (This is the difference between hyperplasia and neoplasia. In neoplasia the growth of the cells continues even after the cessation of the stimulus).

2. *Compensatory hyperplasia:* Seen in healing and repair.

27. What is metaplasia? Give some examples of metaplasia.

Ans. Metaplasia is a change where instead of the cell type normally found in a given location another cell type is produced in order to cope better with the injury. Like hyperplasia, metaplasia is also reversible, i.e. when the stimulus/injury which caused the metaplasia is removed the metaplasia reverts back to normal. But, if injury continues metaplasia can progress to neoplasia, e.g. adenocarcinoma in Barrett esophagus. Examples of metaplasia are:

1. Replacement of normal ciliated columnar epithelial cells of the trachea and bronchi by the stratified squamous epithelial cells (squamous metaplasia).
2. Replacement of the normal columnar epithelial cells of the uterine cervix by the stratified squamous epithelial cells (squamous metaplasia).
3. Replacement of the normal transitional epithelial cells of the urinary bladder mucosa by the stratified squamous epithelial cells (squamous metaplasia).
4. Replacement of the normal stratified squamous epithelial cells of the lower esophagus by the gastric columnar epithelial cells (columnar metaplasia—**Barrett esophagus**).
5. Replacement of the soft tissue by cartilage or bone at the site of the injury (osseous metaplasia).
6. Proliferation of the hematopoietic tissue in the liver or spleen (myeloid metaplasia).
7. *Vitamin A deficiency:* Replacement of glandular epithelium of the conjunctiva and upper respiratory tract and transitional epithelium of the urinary tract by squamous epithelium (squamous metaplasia).

28. What are reversible cell injuries?

Ans. When the injury is mild or limited this causes reversible injury to the cell. These are:

A. *Collection of increased **water** in the cell:*

1. *Cloudy swelling:* Due to failure of cell's sodium pump, increased sodium enters into the cell together with iso-osmotically increased water. This is commonly seen in hepatocytes, cells of the convoluted tubules of kidneys and myocardial cells.
2. *Hydropic deg (vacuolar degeneration):* This is severe form of cloudy swelling. Water collects in the mitochondria, ER, Golgi. This is seen in hypokalemia

(due to severe vomiting/diarrhea). (K is drawn out of cells and replaced by Na + water). Also, this is seen in severe bacterial infections.

B. *Collection of increased* **FAT (mainly triglycerides)** *in the cell:* Seen in liver cells (most common), heart, skeletal muscle, kidney tubule cells. Caused by **ethyl alcohol (commonest),** CCl_4, severe infection, prolonged anemia, toxemia of pregnancy, malnutrition, obesity, diabetes mellitus. *This is due to:*

1. Increased triglyceride coming into liver cells (hepatocytes) because of increased production of fatty acids or release of fatty acids from the peripheral stores **(obesity, starvation, diabetes mellitus)**.
2. Decreased triglyceride moving out of the liver cells (hepatocytes) due to decreased apoprotein synthesis **(CCl_4 poisoning** and **protein malnutrition)**. (Triglyceride combines with apoprotein to form lipoproteins to be released from the hepatocytes).
3. Decreased utilization of the fatty acids (from which triglycerides are formed) in the liver cells due to decreased phospholipid synthesis, or decreased oxidation of fatty acids into ketone bodies and CO_2 **(hypoxia, anemia). Hypoxia** and **alcohol** inhibit fatty acid breakdown.

29. What are irreversible injuries?

Ans. If the injury is severe or prolonged, then the **injury becomes irreversible**. Fatal irreversible injury leads to changes in the living tissue called **necrosis**. Non-fatal irreversible injury to the genetic apparatus leads to **neoplasia**.

30. What injury to the cell causes death of the cell?

Ans. Severe injury to the structure and function of the **cell membrane** causes death of the cell.

31. What is necrosis?

Ans. When the injury is severe or continuous it causes irreversible injury to the cell ending in **cell death**. The morphologic changes which occur after cell death in living tissue and organs is called **necrosis**. Based on the cause of injury, the organ or tissue injured necrosis is basically of 4 types:

1. Coagulation.
2. Liquefaction.
3. Caseation.
4. Fibrinoid.

Two processes cause the basic morphologic changes of necrosis:

a. Denaturation of proteins.

b. Enzymatic digestion of organelles and other cytoplasmic parts.

Change in the cytoplasm consists of cytoplasm becoming more pink (eosinophilic) in color due to denaturation of protein and loss of ribosomes.

Changes in the nuclei give definite indication of death of a cell. In chronological order these are:

a. *Pyknosis:* Nucleus becomes small and dark blue in color.

b. *Karyorrhexis:* Nucleus breaks up into small pieces.

c. *Karyolysis:* Nucleus dissolves and completely disappears.

Changes in tissues/types of necrois: Changes in the tissue depend upon the **4 types of necrosis** which are:

1. **Coagulative necrosis:** Commonly seen in heart, kidney, liver. Usual cause is cutoff of the blood supply to the organ. Morphologic features in this type of necrosis are as follows: The main feature is that in early stages there is general preservation of the architecture of the tissue (because the enzymes are also inactivated) with cells having no nuclei and cytoplasm becoming dark pink in color.
2. **Liquefactive necrosis:** Commonly seen in abscess, brain. In the brain the usual cause is cutoff of the blood supply to the brain. Morphologic features in this type of necrosis are as follows: The tissue architecture is destroyed with liquefaction and softening of the tissue. This happens due to autolysis of the cells due to release of lysosomal enzymes. In the abscess, this happens due to release of proteolytic enzymes released from dead neutrophils.

   Gangrene: It is ischemic, **coagulation type** of necrosis mainly involving limbs and bowel.

   - *Wet gangrene:* When there is secondary bacterial infection with liquefaction.
   - *Dry gangrene:* When there is no secondary infection, no liquefaction, but drying of the tissue.
3. **Caseous necrosis:** Caseous necrosis has partly features of both coagulative and liquefactive necrosis. It is seen in granulomatous inflammation of tuberculosis and some fungal infections. On gross examination, the tissue appears cheesy (caseous). On microscopic examination tissue appears pinkish and structureless.
4. **Fibrinoid necrosis:** Commonly seen in **malignant hypertension** and autoimmune diseases such as **SLE** (systemic lupus erythematosus), **PAN** (polyarteritis nodosa), rheumatic fever. On gross examination, homogenous pink fibrin-like material is seen deposited in the media of the blood vessels in SLE, PAN and within the **Aschoff body** in rheumatic carditis.

   Gummatous necrosis: This is not a distinct type of necrosis. Gummatous necrosis is seen in granulomatous inflammation of tertiary syphilis. On gross examination the tissue appears gum-like (gummatous).

   Fat necrosis: This is not a distinct type of necrosis. Commonly seen in pancreas due to acute pancreatitis because of release of lipolytic enzymes from the injured pancreas. Lipolytic enzymes (lipase) break down triglycerides in the fat cells to fatty acids, which act with calcium ion to form calcium soaps. On gross examination the calcium soaps appear chalk-white in color.

32. What are the outcomes of necrosis?

Ans. *Outcomes of necrosis are:*

1. Complete restitution by regeneration, e.g. following necrosis in liver or kidneys.
2. Repair by fibrosis, e.g. following necrosis of myocardium.
3. Resorption of necrotic tissue with liquefaction, e.g. following necrosis in brain, or abscess formation in any tissue.
4. Pathologic calcification (normocalcemic-dystrophic).

33. What are the applied aspects in clinical medicine of the liberated enzymes from the irreversibly injured different cells of our body?

Ans. *Increased serum levels of enzymes help in diagnosis of several conditions, for example:*

1. From the broken RBCs LDH is liberated. Its increased serum level helps in the diagnosis of hemolytic anemia.
2. From damaged hepatocytes AST and ALT are liberated. Increased serum levels of these help in the diagnosis of liver injuries, e.g. hepatitis.
3. CK, CK-MB and cardiac troponin I (cTnI) are liberated from the damaged myocardial cells. Their increased serum levels help in the diagnosis of acute myocardial infarction.
4. From skeletal muscles CK-MM is liberated. Its increased serum level helps in the diagnosis of skeletal muscle disorder, e.g. Duchenne muscular dystrophy

34. What is apoptosis?

Ans. It is programmed death of single or small group of cells. The purpose of this way of cell death is to selectively remove unwanted cells without disturbing the surrounding cells.

35. What are some of the genes of apoptosis?

Ans. BCL-2 and BCL-X_L—These decrease apoptosis. BAD and BAX—These increase apoptosis.

36. What happens in dysregulation of apoptosis?

Ans. Decreased apoptosis leads to: Cancer and autoimmune disease. Increased apoptosis leads to: AIDs, neurodegenerative diseases, ischemic injuries.

37. Apoptosis is seen in what conditions?

Ans. It is seen in both **physiologic** and **pathologic** conditions, such as:

A. Physiologic:

1. Removal of cells during development of embryo, e.g. formation of kidneys, fingers, toes, etc.

2. In endometrium during menstruation.
3. Turnover of intestinal cells.
4. Thymus cells, which are auto-reactive in order to inducc self-tolerance.

B. Pathologic:

1. In viral hepatitis, dead liver cells become nuclear eosinophilic rounded bodies (apoptotic **Councilman bodies**).
2. In lichen planus, dead basal cells of skin are shed into papillary dermis **(colloid** or **Civatte bodies)**.
3. Death of tumor cells.
4. Cell death by cytotoxic T lymphocytes.

38. What are the differences between necrosis and apoptosis?

Ans. These are:

1. Cell size is enlarged in necrosis. Reduced in apoptosis
2. Nucleus shows pyknosis, karyorrhexis, karyolysis in necrosis. Fragmentation in apoptosis.
3. Plasma membrane is broken in necrosis. Intact in apoptosis.
4. Cell contents are enzymatically digested in necrosis. Intact in apoptosis.
5. DNA breaks randomly in necrosis. In nucleosome-sized fragment in apoptosis.
6. Inflammation in adjacent area is present in necrosis. Absent in apoptosis.

39. What is hyaline/hyalinization?

Ans. Hyalos = glass. Hyaline = glassy. When appearance of cell or tissue looks glassy it is called hyalinized and the process as hyalinization. Examples are: Alcohol hyaline in liver cells **(Mallory's body)**, **Russell bodies** in plasma cells, viral inclusions in cells, **Crooke's hyalinization** of corticotroph cells in pituitary gland in hypercortisolism, proximal kidney tubule cells in proteinuria, hyaline arteriolosclerosis in mild hypertension, hyaline membranes lining the alveoli in hyaline membrane diseases (infant respiratory distress syndrome) and adult respiratory distress syndrome.

40. What are some of the different substances that collect in the cell and/or in the tissues?

Ans.

1. Watcr.
2. Fat, mainly triglyceride.
3. Fat, mainly cholesterol.
4. Protein, amyloid.
5. Protein, albumin.
6. Protein, immunoglobulin.
7. Carbohydrate, glycogen.

8. Mineral, calcium.
9. Mineral, copper.
10. Mineral, iron.

41. What is cholesterol deposition?

Ans. Cholesterol accumulates in macrophages and smooth muscle cells and extracellular in cleft-like shape in atherosclerosis. Also, in hyperlipidemia in mesenchymal cells and macrophages **(xanthomas)**.

42. What is amyloid deposition?

Ans. Described in Chapter 2.

43. What is pathological calcification?

Ans. *DEF:* Abnormal deposition of calcium in tissues.
Types: It is of 2 types:
1. Dystrophic **(normocalcemic)**.
2. Metastatic **(hypercalcemic)**.

44. What is dystrophic calcification (normocalcemic calcification)?

Ans. *DEF:* When calcium deposition occurs in dead or dying tissue. It may occur despite normal serum levels of calcium.
Sites: 1. Atheromas.
2. Damaged heart valves.
3. Damaged muscle with calcification followed by ossification **(myositis ossificans)**.
4. Caseous tuberculous lymph node.
MORPHO: GROSS: White, granular deposits. *MICRO:* Intracellular or extracellular appears bluish in color by H and E stain.

45. What is metastatic calcification (hypercalcemic calcification)?

Ans. *DEF:* When calcium deposition occurs in normal tissue due to hypercalcemia.
ETIO:
1. *Hyperparathyroidism:* Primary or secondary with renal failure.
2. Bone tumors, e.g. multiple myeloma.
3. Increased intake.
4. Sarcoidosis.

MORPHO: May occur anywhere in the body, but mainly affects lungs, kidneys, interstitial tissues of blood vessels and gastric mucosa. Appearance grossly and microscopically is similar to as seen in dystrophic calcification. *C/Fs:* Usually none. But, extensive deposition in the lungs may cause respiratory failure and deposits in the kidneys **nephrolithiasis** and **nephrocalcinosis**, which may result in renal failure.

46. In what condition copper deposition is seen in tissue?

Ans. In **Wilson's disease (hepatolenticular degeneration)**. Described in detail in Chapter 11.

47. In what conditions increased iron deposition is seen?

Ans. Hemosiderin is produced in the body from the breakdown of hemoglobin. Its excess deposition in cells and tissues is seen in:

1. Hemosiderosis.
2. Hemochromatosis.

1. *Hemosiderosis:* Seen in increased iron intake, decreased utilization, increased hemolysis, multiple blood transfusions. In hemosiderosis the tissue structure is **not** damaged and its function is not impaired.
2. *Hemochromatosis:* More deposition of iron than seen in hemosiderosis with destruction of tissue and impairment of its function, e.g. in liver with cirrhosis, in heart with heart failure, in skin with bronze discoloration, in pancreas with diabetes mellitus (called **bronze diabetes** because skin is bronze in color). Inherited as autosomal recessive or acquired (*see* chapter 11 for more details).

2 Inflammation and Repair

OVERVIEW

1. Definition and types of inflammation.
2. Acute inflammation, its phases and participants.
3. Chronic inflammation, granulomatous inflammation (type of chronic inflammation).
4. *Repair:* Definitions, cell cycle, growth factors, steps in repair/healing, factors which delay/ hinder healing, complications in wound-healing.

Inflammation is the reaction of vascularized tissue in a multicellular organism to local injury (physical, chemical, microbiological) or in response to necrotic or neoplastic tissue or immunologic reactions of our body. It is a protective reaction. However, during the process the reaction which destroys the invading elements also can and does, in various instances, cause injuries to our own body tissues. Inflammation can be acute or chronic.

Acute inflammation starts early and usually ends early. It has two phases:

1. *Vascular phase* by which blood vessels at the site of injury dilate, become more permeable and deliver increased amount of fluid, chemicals and cells and
2. *Cellular phase* by which defensive cells reach the site of injury to free the body of the offensive agent.

These two phases are facilitated by certain chemicals. This process causes **swelling (tumor), redness (rubor), heat (calor), pain (dolor)** and **loss of function (functio laesa)** of the tissue/organ affected.

Chronic inflammation is prolonged (lasting weeks to years), main participating cells are different than those of acute inflammation; there is tissue destruction and simultaneous repair. A specific type of chronic inflammation is **granulomatous inflammation** seen in specific situations.

Repair of injured tissue is done by our body by:

1. Regeneration of original cells of the injured tissue/organ or
2. Replacement by fibrous connective tissue depending on various factors, e.g. type and extent of injury, health of the body to handle the injury, type of cells/ tissue/organ injured.

Various growth factors help in wound-healing.

Certain factors hinder wound-healing, e.g. persistent infection, impaired circulation, reaction to debris, metabolic disorders, malnutrition, immunodeficiency, other debilitating conditions or diseases, etc.

Wound-healing process can develop some complications, e.g. deficient scar formation, excessive formation of repair components, contracture formation.

1. What is the definition of inflammation?

Ans. *DEF:* Inflammation is the reaction of vascularized tissue in a multicellular organism to local injury.

2. What are the causes of inflammation?

Ans. 1. Physical.
2. Chemical.
3. Microbiological.
4. Response to necrotic or neoplastic tissue or immunologic reactions of our body.

3. What is the purpose of inflammation in our body?

Ans. Its purpose is to protect and defend our body from harmful agents, to limit their spread in our body, to neutralize toxins and to clear-up damaged tissue for our body to be able to heal the injury.

4. What are the harmful effects of inflammation?

Ans. Just like flame of fire can protect us from predators by keeping them away from us but it can also burn us; inflammation can protect our body from offending agents but it can also hurt our body by causing injury to not only the offending agents; but, also our body.

5. What are the types of inflammation?

Ans. 1. Acute.
2. Chronic (granulomatous inflammation is a type of chronic inflammation).

6. What is the definition of acute inflammation?

Ans. *DEF:* It is early response to injury lasting a short duration. Its main cell is polymorphonuclear leukocyte (PMN). It is characterized by **calor (heat), dolor (pain), rubor (redness), tumor (swelling)** and **functio laesa (loss of function)**.

7. What are the main participants of acute inflammation in our body?

Ans. 1. Certain blood vessels.
2. Certain cells.
3. Certain chemical mediators.

8. What are the phases of acute inflammation?

Ans. 1. Vascular phase.
2. Cellular phase.

9. What is the vascular phase of acute inflammation?

Ans. It mainly consists of:

1. Dilatation of arterioles and capillaries
2. Increased permeability of venules.

Dilatation causes increased amount of blood in the area **(hyperemia)** and slowing of flow resulting in increased hydrostatic pressure causing fluid to leak out into tissue (**transudate**, which is poor in cells and proteins with low specific gravity <1.012). Increased permeability leads to leakage of fluid (**exudate**, which is rich in cells and proteins with specific gravity >1.020). Hyperemia makes the area red **(rubor)** and warm **(calor)**, leakage of fluid makes the area swollen **(tumor)**, swelling causes irritation of the local nerve endings leading to pain **(dolor)**. Pain causes inability to work with the affected part of the body—loss of function **(functio laesa)**.

10. What is the cellular phase of acute inflammation?

Ans. **First line of defense is neutrophils**, which come out of the blood vessels and combat the offending substance in the tissue. *This happens in following steps:*

1. **Margination:** This is due to slowing of the circulation.
2. Loose adhesion **(rolling)**, firm adhesion **(adhesion)** of white blood cells to the endothelial cells followed by actively moving out of the white blood cells from the blood vessels **(transmigration)**.
3. Moving of the white blood cells towards the offending agent **(chemotaxis)**.
4. Engulfing of the offending agent by the white blood cells **(phagocytosis)**.
5. Digestion of the offending agent by the white blood cells.

11. How are the cellular events facilitated?

Ans. *These events are facilitated as follows:*

1. *Margination due to slowing of blood flow whereby:* Centrally flowing white cells fall to the margin by **laws of physics**.
2. *Loose adhesion, firm adhesion and transmigration by:* Adhesion molecules on white blood cells (e.g. **integrins, selectins)** and on endothelial cells (e.g. **E-selectin, P-selectin)**.
3. *Chemotaxis by:* **C5a** (a complement activated fragment), **leukotrine B4** (an arachidonic acid metabolite of the lipooxygenase pathway), **interleukin-8** (IL8-a chemokine).
4. *Phagocytosis by:* **Opsonins** (**IgG** by its Fc fragment and complement fragment **C3b**).
5. *Digestion by:*

   A. *Oxygen-dependent killing:* By **oxidative burst** involving increased consumption of oxygen with production of free radical oxygen during activation of NADPH (Nicotinamide adenine dinucleotide phosphate) oxidase. Free oxygen radical is converted to H_2O_2. H_2O_2 is converted to HOCl by MPO (myeloperoxidase) from white cell lysosomal granules in the presence of chloride ion. **HOCl kills the bacteria by denaturing its proteins similar to high heat.**

B. *Oxygen-independent killing:* By lysozyme, defensin, etc.

12. What are the harmful effects to our body from the cellular events of acute inflammation?

Ans. Leukocytes release into surrounding tissue lysosomal enzymes, proteases, free oxygen radicals, products of arachidonic acid metabolism (prostaglandins and leukotrienes) which cause tissue damage and can also lead to chronic inflammation. However, antiproteases and alpha 1-antitrypsin inhibit these. Therefore, in condition with **alpha 1-antitrypsin deficiency** proteases damage our body tissues without any restraint.

13. What are the participants of chemical mediators of acute inflammation?

Ans. 1. Vasoactive amines (histamine from basophils, mast cells and platelets and serotonin–5 hydroxytryptamine–5HT from platelets).

2. *Arachidonic acid metabolites of cyclooxygenase pathway:* Prostaglandins (PGD2, PGE2, PGF2), prostacyclin (PGI2), thromboxane A2 (TXA2) and of *lipoxygenase pathway*: Leukotriene B4, leukotrienes C4, D4, E4.
3. Nitric oxide (NO).
4. Cytokines (interleukins IL-1 to IL-15, chemokines, e.g. IL-8, tumor necrosis factor—TNF, interferons IFN alpha, beta, transforming growth factor—TGF alpha, beta, colony stimulating factors—CSFs).
5. Kinins, e.g. bradykinin.
6. Fibrinolytic proteins, e.g. plasmin.
7. Complements.
8. Platelet-activating factor—PAF.

Function-wise these are as follows:

A. *Those acting on blood vessels:*

a. Dilate:
1. Histamine
2. Serotonin (5-hydroxytryptamine, 5HT)
3. Prostacyclin (PGI2), prostaglandins (PGD2, PGE2, PGF2).
4. Nitric oxide (NO).
5. PAF.

b. *Increase permeability of blood vessels:*
1. Histamine
2. Serotonin (5-hydroxytryptamine 5HT)
3. Bradykinin
4. C3a, C4a, C5a
5. Leukotrienes (C4, D4, E4)
6. PAF

B. *Those acting on leukocytes:*

a. Chemotaxis:

1. Leukotriene B4.
2. C5a.
3. Chemokines (IL-8).
4. PAF.
5. Bacterial products.

b. Phagocytosis:

1. C3b.
2. IgG.

14. What are vasoactive amines?

Ans. These are histamine and serotonin (5-hydroxytryptamine, 5HT). Histamine is from mast cells, basophils and platelets and 5HT from platelets. These are released in response to mechanical stimuli, anaphylotoxins formed from complements (C3a, C4a, C5a), some neuropeptides, and interaction of antigen with IgE bound to plasma membrane of mast cells. Both of these cause vasodilation and increased permeability.

15. What is the complement system?

Ans. Complement system consists of a group of at least 30 plasma proteins (C1 to C9). These are formed in the liver. They are the primary, primitive and powerful defense system of our body. They are called complement because they help antibodies **(complementary to antibodies)** to kill organisms which invade our body. They exist in inactive state in the blood. They get activated upon certain stimulus. The **key step in this activation process is activation of C3 to form C3 convertase**. This is done by following paths:

a. *Alternative pathway (non-specific pathway):* This is evolutionary older path. This path is taken during acute inflammation. This is activated by toxins, enzymes, foreign proteins, fragments of bacteria and fungi. In this path C3 is activated to form **C3 convertase** by bacterial polysaccharides, e.g. endotoxins or cell membrane. Some serum components called factors B, D and properdin also play a role.

b. *The classic pathway (specific pathway):* This is evolutionary newer path. This path is taken for specific immunity. This is activated by immune complexes. Antibodies involved are IgG and IgM. In this path, activation is initiated by antigen-antibody complex, which activates C1. Activated C1 activates C4 + C2 forming **C3 convertase**.

c. *Mannose-binding lecting (MBL) pathway:* It is activated by microorganisms which have terminal mannose groups. MBL structure is similar to C1q. So, it activates complement by classical pathway and does not need antibody do so.

d. *Miscellaneous:* Such as:

1. By urate crystals in gout.
2. Plasmin.
3. Lysosomal proteases.
4. C3NeF—the C3 nephritic factor which is an autoantibody and activates complement by alternative pathway in type II membranoproliferative glomerulonephritis.
5. Spontaneously as seen in paroxysmal nocturnal hemoglobinuria.

Common path: Hereafter, the path is common for both the above-stated pathways as follows: **C3 convertase** breaks C3 to C3a and C3b. C3b binds to C3 convertase complex to form **C5 convertase**. C5 convertase breaks C5 to C5a and C5b. C5b together with C6, 7, 8 and 9 form the **MAC (membrane attack complex)**.

16. What are the functions of activated components of complement system?

Ans. Complement activation has 5 major biological functions:

1. Release of histamine from basophils and mast cells by **C3a, C4a** and **C5a (anaphylatoxins)**.
2. Activation of lipoxygenase pathway of arachidonic acid metabolism by **C5a**.
3. Chemotaxis of neutrophils and macrophages by **C5a**.
4. Opsonization of bacteria by coating with **C3b (opsonin)**.
5. Cytolysis of target cells by **C5b-9** the **MAC**, the membrane attack complex, which lyses the cell walls of bacteria and other cells, and also RBCs in immune hemolytic anemia.

17. Which antibodies participate in acute inflammation?

Ans. IgM and small amount of IgG. **During primary immune response (acute inflammation)**, when the foreign offending antigen is encountered by the body for the first time the B lymphocytes differentiate into plasma cells and produce IgM and a week later small amount of IgG. But, a few B lymphocytes from this clone of lymphocytes stay as **memory cells** in the blood and when the same foreign offending antigen is encountered again they respond more vigorously and rapidly with larger amount of IgG. **This response is called secondary immune response** or **acquired** or **adaptive immunity**.

18. What are the neutrophil factors, which participate in acute inflammation?

Ans. These are myeloperoxidase-containing cytoplasmic granules, **proteases**, acetyl glyceryl ether phosphoryl choline **(AGEPC)**, which was in the past called platelet-activating factor **(PAF)**.

19. What are the inhibitors of acute inflammation?

Ans.

1. *Alpha 1-antitrypsin:* It inhibits proteases.
2. *C1 esterase inhibitor:* It inhibits complement cascade.

20. What are the morphologic patterns of inflammation?

Ans. 1. *Serous:* Exudate has serum-like fluid, e.g. herpes labialis.

2. *Fibrinous:* Exudate has fibrin, e.g. fibrinous pericarditis in rheumatic heart disease.
3. *Fibrinopurulent:* Exudate has fibrin and neutrophils, e.g. streptococcal pharyngitis.
4. *Purulent:* Exudate has pus, e.g. bacterial abscess.
5. *Pseudomembranous:* Exudate has "pseudomembranous" consisting of necrotic debris, fibrin and neutrophils—no epithelial membrane is present, hence the term "pseudomembrane".
6. *Ulcerative:* Contains granulation tissue, necrotic debris and neutrophils.

21. What are the different outcomes of acute inflammation?

Ans. 1. Resolution 2. Abscess formation 3. Chronic inflammation.

22. What are the main systemic effects of inflammation?

Ans. These are under the influence of cytokines (IL-1, IL-6 and alpha-TNF). IL-1 and alpha-TNF cause leucocytosis by inducing bone marrow to release immature WBCs which have fewer nuclear lobes, called **shift to the left**. Very severe cases result in **leukemoid reaction** (described later). Fever is caused by the action of IL-1, IL-6 and alpha-TNF on hypothalamus.

23. What are the types of disorders of acute inflammation?

Ans. 1. Complement-related.

2. WBC-related.

24. What are the complement-related disorders of acute inflammation?

Ans. 1. *C1 esterase inhibitor deficiency:* Leads to: **Hereditary angioedema**. Due to: uncontrolled C1 estrase activation.

2. *C1q, C2, C4 deficiencies:* Leads to: Immune complex-mediated diseases, e.g. SLE, RA, glomerulonephritis. This happens due to impaired clearing of immune complexes from the circulation.
3. *C3 deficiency:* Leads to: Increased susceptibility to infection, mainly pyogenic infections.
4. *C5-C8 deficiency:* Increased susceptibility to recurrent Neisseria (gonococcal and meningococcal) infections.

25. What are the WBC-related disorders of acute inflammation?

Ans. 1. Defects in adhesion: LAD-1: Defective integrins. LAD-2: Defective selectin.

2. Defect in chemotaxis and phagolysosome formation **(Chediak-Higashi syndrome)**.

3. Defective microbicidal activity-**chronic granulomatous disease of childhood.** (Deficiency of NADPH oxidase causing failure of H_2O_2 formation).

26. What is the application of the knowledge of basic pathology of acute inflammation to clinical medicine?

Ans. 1. Since neutrophils from the blood are used up, the marrow produces increased number of neutrophils and pours them into the blood. This is seen as increase in white blood cell count with increased number of neutrophils in the peripheral blood. Also, since the marrow has to release these neutrophils in a hurry, less mature forms containing fewer nuclear lobes (band forms) are released into the peripheral blood **(called shift to the left)**. If the infection is very severe, the neutrophil count in the peripheral blood is more than 50,000. With many immature forms the picture may resemble leukemia. This is called **leukemoid reaction**. *This is differentiated from leukemia by:* Presence of alkaline phosphatase in these cells, which is absent in leukemia (Also, *see* Page 135).

In acute viral infections there is neutropenia and lymphocytosis.

2. Since there is an increase in immunoglobulins and fibrinogen, there is an increased erythrocyte sedimentation rate **(ESR)**.
3. *Therapeutic applications:*
   a. *Use of NSAIDs:* NSAIDs inhibit prostaglandin synthesis, thus useful in treatment of *S/S* of inflammation. COX-1 is protective for gastric mucosa. Its inhibition causes injury to gastric mucosa with gastritis and gastric ulcer formation. So, now specific COX-2 inhibitors are available which are anti-inflammatory, but do not cause injury to the gastric mucosa.
   b. Corticosteroids prevent formation of arachidonic acid from cell membrane phospholipids by inhibiting phospholipases. Useful for treatment of *S/S* of inflammations.

27. What is the application of the knowledge of basic pathology of acute inflammation to systemic pathology?

Ans. Since acute inflammation consists of 2 phases:

1. Vascular phase with dilation of vessels consequently with increased blood (hyperemia) and leakage of protein-rich fluid (exudates) from the vessels, and
2. Cellular phase, consisting of mainly infiltration of neutrophils at the site of acute inflammation.

All organs in the body have these changes present in them during acute inflammation, i.e. hyperemia, exudates formation and neutrophilic infiltrate (except in acute viral infections where there is mainly lymphocytic infiltrate). During inflammation activated phagocytes release chemicals (e.g. protease) into tissues causing injury.

28. What is chronic inflammation?

Ans. *DEF:* Features of chronic inflammation are:

1. Lasts weeks to months or years.
2. Infiltration by chronic inflammatory cells (*mononuclear cells:* lymphocytes, plasma cells, macrophages).
3. Tissue destruction.
4. Repair by new vessels proliferation (angiogenesis) and fibrosis.

29. What are some of the causes of chronic inflammation?

Ans. 1. Persisting acute inflammation.

2. Autoimmune diseases.
3. Certain infections (viral, bacterial, e.g. tuberculosis, leprosy and syphilis).

30. What are the types of chronic inflammation?

Ans. 1. Non-granulomatous 2. Granulomatous.

31. What are the non-granulomatous chronic inflammations?

Ans. Here the main cells are lymphocytes, plasma cells and monocytes-macrophages. *Application of knowledge of basic pathology of chronic non-granulomatous inflammation to systemic pathology:* Since, in chronic non-granulomatous inflammation the main participating cells are lymphocytes, plasma cells and macrophages, infiltration of these is seen in all organs and tissues suffering from chronic non-granulomatous inflammation.

32. What is a granuloma?

Ans. When the body is not able to eliminate the offending organism/substance the **activated macrophages** which look like epithelial cells (therefore, are called **epithelioid cells**) surround the area to isolate it from the rest of the body. **This collection of epithelioid cells is called a granuloma** (granuloma in Latin means a **small grain** or **granule**).

33. What are some of the granulomatous inflammations?

Ans. 1. *Bacterial:* Tuberculosis, syphilis, leprosy, cat scratch disease.

2. *Fungal:* Blastomycosis, histoplasmosis, cryptococcosis, coccidioidomycosis.
3. *Parasitic:* Schistosomiasis (bilharziosis).
4. *Foreign bodies/inorganic elements:* Suture, silica.
5. *Unknown etiology:* Sarcoidosis.
6. *Miscellaneous:* Chronic granulomatous disease of childhood, Churg-Strauss syndrome, Wegener's granulomatosis, etc.

34. What is sarcoidosis?

Ans. In early nineteenth century, Dr. Boeck thought this condition looked like a sarcoma and named it "sarcoid". It is **not** sarcoma. It is a chronic inflammatory granulomatous systemic disease of unknown etiology, which mainly affects lungs, lymph nodes, salivary glands with dry mouth **(xerostomia)**, lacrimal glands with dry eyes **(keratoconjunctivitis sicca)**, liver, skin, although it can affect any part of the body. *Common findings are:* Lymphadenopathy. *Lungs:* Enlarged hilar lymph nodes and interstitial lung disease with granulomas and restrictive changes. *Skin:* **Erythema nodosum**—Red, tender nodules on anterior legs. Parotitis + Uveitis + Fever **(uveoparotid fever or Heerfordt syndrome)**, lacrimal gland + parotid gland involvement **(Mikulikz syndrome)**; spleen, liver; (hepatosplenomegaly). *MICRO:* Small, microscopic solid, non-caseating nodules called granulomas are present which cause destruction of the tissues in these organs. Within giant cell of granuloma 2 bodies may be seen:

1. **Schaumann** = Calcium and protein in circular layers.
2. Star-shaped inclusions **(Asteroid bodies)**.

C/Fs: Hypercalcemia (Due to alpha-1 hydroxylation of vit. D in sarcoid macrophages causing increased absorption of calcium from GIT, hypercalciuria with nephrolithiasis, tiredness, loss of appetite, loss of weight, fever, night sweats, erythema nodosum, polyarthritis, dry moth, dry eyes, breathlessness, chest pain, cough.

DIAG: a. Reduced sensitivity with absent reaction **(anergy)** to skin test antigens, e.g. tuberculosis **(Mantoux test)**.

b. Polyclonal hypergammaglobulinemia.

c. Hypercalcemia and hypercalciuria.

d. Increased activity of serum angiotensin-converting enzyme.

e. Definitive diagnosis is done by biopsy showing noncaseating granulomas.

PROG: 80% get well without any treatment. 10% develop chronic illness with irreversible lung dysfunction, impaired vision, 10% develop progressive diseases with progressive pulmonary fibrosis, cor pulmonale and death.

35. What is amyloidosis?

Ans. *DEF:* Conditions in which amyloid is **extracellularly deposited** in various tissues/ organs of the body affecting their function.

Nature of amyloid: Group of insoluble proteins which form a similar structure (β-pleated sheet) with less pinkish appearance similar to carbohydrate or amylum, which are, therefore, called amyloid. It appears red when stained with congo red dye, has apple green birefringence under polarized light. It accumulates extracellularly in various tissues/organs of body in different conditions as follows:

Types of amyloidosis:

1. *Primary (immune dyscrasia) amyloidosis:* Here the amyloid is derived from immunoglobulin light chain. Therefore, it is called **AL (amyloid light chain)**

protein. It is produced by plasma cells in conditions of plasma cell disorders like **multiple myeloma** and **Waldenstrom's macroglobulinemia.** In these conditions the amyloid **deposits in tissues of mesodermal origin such as heart, muscle** and **tongue.**

2. *Secondary (reactive) amyloidosis:* Here the amyloid is derived from amyloid associated protein present in sesrum. Therefore, it is called **AA (amyloid associated)** protein. Increased AA protein is formed by the liver in conditions with chronic tissue destruction such as chronic inflammatory diseases (rheumatoid arthritis, tuberculosis, osteomyelitis, syphilis, leprosy) and non-inflammatory conditions such as renal cell carcinoma and Hodgkin's lymphoma. In these conditions amyloid is **deposited in parenchymatous organs such as kidney** (causing **nephritic syndrome, nephrotic syndrome), liver, adrenals, pancreas, lymph nodes** and **spleen**. In spleen the amyloid is deposited in perifollicular area giving it an appearance like tapioca. Therefore, in this condition spleen is called **sago spleen. Lardaceous spleen**.
3. *Alzheimer's disease:* Here the amyloid is called **A4 amyloid**.
4. *Thyroid medullary carcinoma:* Here the amyloid is derived from calcitonin.
5. *Type II diabetes mellitus:* Here the amyloid is derived from insulin or glucagons and is called islet amyloid polypeptide (IAPP).
6. *Senile amyloidosis:* Here the amyloid is derived from **transthyretin** (a serum protein which **transports thyroxine** and **retinol**).

   Dx is done by gingival or rectal biopsy.

Amyloid causes injury by causing pressure atrophy to adjacent cells when deposited in interstitial tissue, when deposited in the wall of a blood vessel, by narrowing of the lumen resulting in decreased blood supply or by causing increased permeability in glomerular vessels resulting in albuminuria.

Amyloid can be deposited almost in any organ of our body, e.g. liver, spleen, tongue, gingiva, skeletal muscles, kidneys, heart, gastrointestinal tract. However, its most harmful effects are seen in the latter three:

- In kidneys, it causes severe albuminuria leading to nephrotic syndrome.
- In heart, it causes CCF.
- In GIT, it causes diarrhea, electrolyte imbalance, malabsorption, protein loss and nutritional deficiencies.

REPAIR

36. In what ways our body repairs injuries?

Ans. In the following two ways:

1. **Regeneration:** By growth of **same type of cells.**
2. **Replacement:** By growth of **connective tissue cells.**

37. How many types of cells are in our body based on the capacity of cells to regenerate?

Ans. 1. Labile cells 2. Stable cells 3. Permanent cells.

38. What are the phases of the cell growth cycle?

Ans. Phases:

1. G1 (Presynthetic).
2. S (Synthesis of DNA).
3. G2 (Premitotic).
4. M (Mitotic).

G0 = Non-dividing resting stage.

39. What are the growth factors?

Ans. These are regulated by proto-oncogenes. If these genes get changed (mutated) they can become oncogenes and produce abnormal cells (cancer). Examples of some growth factors are:

1. *Platelet-derived growth factor (PDGF):* This factor promotes growth of fibroblast and smooth muscle.
2. *Epidermal growth factor (EGF):* This promotes growth of epithelial cells, endothelial cells and fibroblasts.
3. *Fibroblast growth factors (FGFs):* These promote production of extracellular matrix protein and promote new vessel formation (angiogenesis).
4. *Macrophage-derived growth factors (IL-1 and TNF, tumor necrosis factor):* These promote growth of fibroblasts, smooth muscle cells and endothelial cells.

40. What are the components of ECM (extracellular matrix)?

Ans. 1. *Collagen:*

a. Types I, II, III: Fibrillar: It is main part of connective tissue.

b. Type IV: Non-fibrillar: Components of BM (basement membrane).

2. *Adhesive glycoproteins:* These bind ECM to cells.
3. *Proteoglycans:* These help regulate ECM structure and permeability.

41. What are the steps in the repair process by the connective tissue?

Ans. 1. Removal of debris.

2. Formation of granulation tissue:

Granulation tissue consists of newly made fibroblasts and capillaries in loose ECM and it fills space created by liquefaction and removal of debris described above. It looks pinkish-granular on naked eye gross examination and therefore, is called **granulation tissue**. It should **not be confused with granuloma** of chronic granulomatous inflammation.

3. Scarring/remodelling of scar:

   Fibroblasts in the above granulation tissue produce collagen, which replaces the above granulation tissue and forms a scar. This also causes contraction and deformity of the original structure.

42. What are the steps of wound-healing?

Ans. 1. Acute inflammatory response.
2. Regeneration of parenchymal cells.
3. Growth of connective tissue cells.
4. Synthesis of ECM proteins.
5. Remodelling of parenchymal elements to restore tissue function.
6. Remodelling of connective tissue to achieve wound strength.

43. How do the skin wounds heal?

Ans. 1. *Healing by first intention:* This occurs in clean wounds where the two edges of the wound are in approximation. First, blood clot is formed in the wound. Then neutrophils, macrophages, and granulation tissue fill the wound and epithelium covers the wound leaving a very thin scar.
2. *Healing by second intention:* This occurs when the wound is large and the two edges of wound are not in approximation. Therefore, more granulation tissue is required and wound closes by contraction carried out by myofibroblasts. This leaves a wider scar.

44. What are the factors which delay or interfere in repair?

Ans. 1. Persistent infection.
2. Impaired circulation.
3. Retention of debris.
4. Metabolic disorders, such as diabetes mellitus, which promotes above 1 and 2.
5. Dietary deficiency of vitamin C (ascorbic acid) or protein, both of which are required for collagen synthesis.

45. What are the complications in wound-healing?

Ans. 1. *Deficient scar formation:*
   a. Wound dehiscence.
   b. Ulceration.
2. *Excessive formation of repair components:* Increased amount of granulation tissue is formed which protrudes above the surface (exuberant granulation or **proud flesh**)—can lead to hypertrophic scar—**keloid**.
3. *Contracture formation.*

46. What are the outcomes of repair process?

Ans. *These are two:*

1. Normal structure restored when
   a. The exudate is resolved,
   b. The framework of the organ/tissue is not destroyed or
   c. The cells are labile.
2. Scarring occurs when
   a. The exudate is organized,
   b. The framework of the organ/tissue is destroyed or
   c. The injured cells are permanent.

3 Disorders of the Immune System

OVERVIEW

1. Hypersensitivity reactions (types I, II, III, IV).
2. Autoimmune diseases.
3. Immune deficiency diseases.

Immunity means freedom/protection from injury. It is innate (natural) immunity or acquired immunity. This immunity is provided by the immune system of our body.

The immune system consists of:

1. Certain organs (primary: thymus, bone marrow; secondary: spleen, lymphoid tissue-encapsulated lymph nodes and non-encapsulated GALT, MALT, BALT).
2. Certain cells (neutrophils, eosinophils, basophils, mast cells, macrophages, antigen processing cells, e.g. dendritic cells, lymphocytes –T, B, NK-natural killer).
3. Certain chemicals [cytokines (interleukins, chemokines, interferons, colony stimulating factors, tumor necrotic factor, transforming growth factor)] complements, antibodies or immunoglobulins.

Our body gets injury by two mechanisms:

1. Injury by the direct action/s of the injurious agent, which could occur or be worse when due to various reasons our body's immune system is deficient; and
2. Injury by our body's reaction to injurious agent or due to various known and unknown reasons (hypersensitivity reactions of types I, II, III and IV or autoimmune diseases).

Type I (anaphylactic) hypersensitivity is mediated by IgE with release of histamine and other harmful chemical mediators from basophils and mast cells. Systemic anaphylaxis which could lead to **death** and local atopy are two types of this.

Type II (cytotoxic) hypersensitivity is mediated by IgG. It is of three types:

1. Ab-dependent, mediated by complement, e.g. Goodpasture's syndrome, pernicious anemia, some of the hemolytic anemias.
2. Ab-dependent, mediated by cells such as NK cells, macrophages, monocytes, neutrophils, eosinophils, e.g. autoimmune anemia, thrombocytopenia, leucopenia.
3. Ab-mediated cellular dysfunction, e.g. Graves' diseases, myxedema, myasthenia gravis.

Type III (immune complex) hypersensitivity is mediated by Ag-Ab complexes circulating in blood which get deposited at various tissue sites, attract and activate complement, e.g. SLE, PAN, post-streptococcal glomerulonephritis, etc.

Type IV (cell-mediated delayed) hypersensitivity is mediated by T lymphocytes, e.g. immunity and injury related to tuberculosis, leprosy, blastomycosis, histoplasmosis and conditions like contact dermatitis (poison ivy, oak), transplant rejection, etc.

Autoimmune diseases are due to certain mechanisms such as:

1. Injury, inflammation, infection, drug may modify self antigen to appear as non-self or expose an isolated antigen (thyroglobulin, lens protein, spermatozoa).
2. Foreign protein may resemble our body protein **(molecular mimicry)**.
3. Increase in T helper function or decrease in T suppressor cell function.

Some examples of autoimmune diseases are:

1. Hemolytic anemia.
2. Pernicious anemia.
3. Thrombocytopenia.
4. Myasthenia gravis.
5. Hashimoto's thyroiditis.
6. Graves' disease.
7. SLE.
8. SS.
9. PAN.
10. RA, etc.

Systemic lupus erythematosus (SLE) is due to defective helper T cells (CD4 T cells) with proliferation of B lymphocytes with antibodies production against self structures. Mechanism of injuries is by type II and III hypersensitivity. Main organs affected are heart, blood vessels, lungs, kidneys, joints, skin with a butterfly rash over the face.

Systemic sclerosis (SS) (scleroderma) consists of fibrosis with injuries to skin, GIT, heart, muscles, etc. A variant of this is **CREST** syndrome (**C** = Calcinosis, **R** = Raynaud's phenomenon, **E** = Esophageal dysfunction, **S** = Sclerodactyly, **T** = Telangiectasia).

Polyarteritis nodosa (PAN) is due to type III hypersensitivity reaction which causes arteritis of the medium- and small-sized arteries of all over the body except sparing for unknown reason the pulmonary vessels. Another peculiarity is that it is more common in young males, whereas most of the autoimmune diseases are more common in females. Common organs affected are kidneys causing hematuria, albuminuria, uremia, GIT causing abdominal pain, melena, heart, liver, spleen, skeletal muscles, nervous system, skin, etc.

Rheumatoid arthritis (RA) is a chronic systemic inflammatory disorder due to type III hypersensitivity reaction mainly involving synovial joints and may also involve skin, heart, lungs, etc.

Immune deficiency diseases are of two types:

1. Congenital.
2. Acquired.

Congenital immunodeficiency diseases are of five types due to defects in:

1. T cell.
2. B cell.
3. Both T and B cells.
4. Phagocytes.
5. Complement.

Examples of these are:

1. *T cell deficiency*—DiGeorge syndrome (thymic aplasia);
2. *B cell deficiency*—Bruton's disease;
3. *Both T and B cells*—combined B and T cell deficiency;
4. *Phagocytic disorders*—leukocyte adhesion deficiency (LAD 1 and 2), Chediak-Higashi syndrome, chronic granulomatous disease, Job's syndrome, myeloperoxidase deficiency, alkaline phosphatase deficiency;
5. *Complement disorders*—C1 esterase inhibitor deficiency, C1q, C2, C4 deficiencies, C3 deficiency, C5-C8 deficiency.

Acquired immunodeficiency diseases are:

1. HIV.
2. Acquired hypogammaglobulinemia, e.g. in lymphoma, chronic lymphocytic leukemia, multiple myeloma, nephritic syndrome, protein loosing enteropathy.
3. Acquired cell-mediated immunodeficiency, e.g. Hodgkin's disease and sarcoidosis.

Physiology of the Immune System

1. What do these terms mean: Mutualism, Commensalism, Parasitism?

Ans. Mutualism = When other organisms that live in our body are beneficial for our body. Commensalism = When other organisms that live in our body are neither beneficial nor harmful. Parasitism = When other organisms that enter our body are harmful to us. Immune system provides protection to our body from these.

2. What do you understand by immunity?

Ans. Immunity means freedom or protection from any injury.

3. What comprises the immune system of our body?

Ans. Immune system of our body is a collection of organs, cells and molecules whose main function is to free (protect) our body from exogenous (foreign bodies and organisms) and endogenous (tumors) elements and assist body in wound-healing and in removing the cells which die through natural processes. But, it can also cause problems for our body, e.g. act against endogenous autogenous tissues and cause autoimmune diseases, act against homologous elements and cause intra-uterine problems of the fetus by acting against transplacental mother's tissues, or against blood transfusion or grafts. Also, the forces which destroy harmful elements can also injure normal body tissues, e.g. various injuries during inflammation.

4. How many types of immunity our body has?

Ans. These are of 2 types:

1. Natural (innate)
2. Acquired.

5. What are the main components of natural (innate) immunity?

Ans. Its main components are:

1. *External surfaces:* Skin and mucus membranes and their secretions, e.g. mucus, tears. Skin's horny layer. Mucus membranes' cilia.
2. *Symbiotic microorganisms:* Antibiotics can interfere with this by killing these and causing diseases, e.g. thrush by *Candida albicans*.
3. *Chemicals from internal tissues:* Lysozyme, acute phase proteins (C-reactive protein produced by liver), interferon alpha and beta-protective against viruses. (Interferon beta and gamma are produced by lymphocytes during adaptive immunity and have more functions besides protecting against viruses).
4. *Phagocytic cells:* Polymorphonuclear neutrophil leukocytes (PMNs) and monocytes of blood and macrophages of tissue, natural killer (NK) lymphocytes (large granular lymphocytes).
5. *Complement system:* Alternative pathway.

6. What are the main components of acquired immunity?

Ans. Its main components are:

1. *Lymphoid system with its organs:* Primary organs (bone marrow and thymus), secondary organs [spleen, the encapsulated (lymph nodes) and non-capsulated collections of lymphoid tissue–GALT, MALT, BALT] GALT = Gut-associated lymphoid tissue, MALT = Mucosa-associated lymphoid tissue, BALT = Bronchus associated lymphoid tissue.
2. *Cells:* Lymphocytes (T, B) monocytes-macrophages, APCs (e.g. dendritic cells, macrophages, Langerhans cells which are the dendritic cells of the skin), NK cells, mast cells, basophils, eosinophils. PMNs.
3. *Cytokines:* IL 1-12, IFN-gamma, CSFs, TGF-beta, TNF, chemokines.
4. *Complement system:* Classic pathway.

7. What is the role of spleen in the immune system?

Ans. Spleen has 1/4th of all the fixed encapsulated lymphoid tissue of our body. It sits not in lymphatic drainage but in the systemic circulation. It receives 5% of total blood volume. Therefore, and because it has macrophage, dendritic cells and lymphocytes, spleen generates primary immune response to blood-borne antigens resulting in production of IgM. Also, spleen plays a role in the production of immunologic memory, suppressor T lymphocytes and immunologic mediator molecules. Hyposplenic state can be recognized by the presence of **Howell Jolly bodies** in the peripheral blood RBCs.

8. What are the main differences between natural (innate) and acquired immunity?

Ans. The main differences between the two are in:

1. Memory,
2. Specificity,
3. Cells, and
4. Molecules:

1. *Memory:* Natural immunity has no memory. Therefore, the resistance to our body from repeated infections provided by it is the same on repeated infections. Whereas, the acquired immunity has memory. Therefore, the resistance provided by it to repeated infections is improved.
2. *Specificity:* Natural immunity is generally effective against all organisms. Acquired immunity is specific for offending organisms.
3. *Main cells:* Natural immunity utilizes phagocytes and natural killer **(NK)** lymphocytes. Acquired immunity utilizes mainly lymphocytes (T and B). Also, antigen-presenting cells **(APCs)**: (dendritic cells, Langerhans cells, monocytes-macrophages), neutrophils, eosinophils, basophils.
4. *Main molecules:* Natural immunity utilizes lysozyme, complement by alternative pathway, acute phase proteins, interferons. Acquired immunity utilizes

antibodies, cytokines from lymphocytes and macrophages and other cells and complement by classic pathway.

9. How does our body recognize self from non-self tissue?

Ans. This is done by certain proteins (antigens). These are called MHC (major histocompatibility complex) so named because they were originally found to be proteins which are involved in tissue rejection from a donor. In our human body these are known as HLA (human leukocyte antigen) as they were first discovered on leukocyte, although they are present in all human body cells. In our human body there are many genes which code for these MHC. These genes are called histocompatibility genes. These are located on the short arm of chromosome 6.

HLA or MHC are mainly of 3 types: Class I, II and III.

MHC (HLA) class I proteins (antigens): These are membrane proteins of **all nucleated cells and platelets (not RBCs)**. These make complexes with proteins of virus or neoplastic cells which originate inside our body and attract cytotoxic T cells which **then destroy the virus-infected cells and the neoplastic cells**. Also, these are the **main antigens involved in the tissue graft rejection**. Main types in this class are **HLA-A, HLA-B,** and **HLA-C**.

MHC (HLA) class II proteins: These are present on **cells, which are involved in specific (acquired, adaptive) immunity** such as **B lymphocytes, some T lymphocytes** and **antigen presenting cells such as monocytes, macrophages, dendritic cells of lymphoid tissue and Langerhans cells of the skin**. These proteins present foreign proteins to T lymphocytes. The main types in this class are **HLA-D** (HLA-DP, HLA-DQ, and HLA-DR). These make complexes with outside proteins which enter our body and are engulfed (phagocytosed), e.g. exogenous products of bacteria. These complexes are then recognized by T helper cells which **stimulate B lymphocyte to produce antibodies against these complexes and thus make an immune response against them**.

MHC (HLA) class III proteins: These are complements.

10. Which are some diseases which have association with HLA (MHC) antigens?

Ans. **HLA-A3**—Hemochromatosis; **HLA-B27**—Ankylosing spondylitis, acute anterior uveitis, Postgonococcal arthritis, **HLA-DR3**—Sjogren's syndrome, chronic active hepatitis, insulin-dependent DM; **HLA-DR4**—IDDM, rheumatoid arthritis.

11. What is tolerance?

Ans. Our body's T and B lymphocytes which have the potential to react without body's tissues are killed during development. This way our body protects itself from injury by its own T and B cells and only those T and B cells remain in our body which do not react with our body, i.e. they have tolerance for our body's tissues.

Pathology of the Immune System

12. What are the pathologic disorders of the immune system?

Ans. These are of 2 types:

1. Diseases due to increased, non-protective immune reaction (hypersensitivity/autoimmune diseases).
2. Diseases due to absent/reduced immune reaction (immunodeficiency diseases).

13. What are the hypersensitivity diseases?

Ans. Normally, immune system response of our body is against foreign substances to protect and free our body from the intruding substances/organisms. Thus, it is helpful for our body. But, sometimes the response is harmful to our body. This response is called hypersensitivity.

The hypersensitivity responses are of 4 types:

1. Type I—Anaphylactic hypersensitivity.
2. Type II—Cytotoxic hypersensitivity.
3. Type III—Immune complex hypersensitivity.
4. Type IV—Cell-mediated delayed hypersensitivity.

Types I, II, and III are dependent upon antibodies produced by plasma cells, which are terminally differentiated B lymphocytes. Type IV is carried out by T lymphocytes and macrophages.

14. What is type-I (anaphylactic) hypersensitivity?

Ans. This is mediated by IgE. When some antigen enters the body it via T_H2 cells stimulates B lymphocytes to secrete IgE. These IgEs bind with the Fc receptors of tissue mast cells and basophils. When the same antigen (allergen) enters the body again it binds with the antigen-binding sites of the IgE which are bound to the tissue mast cells and basophils, causing release of histamine, and other chemical mediators of inflammation leading to harmful reactions in our body. These harmful reactions are dependent on the site of reaction taking place and also the route of entry of antigen:

Systemic anaphylaxis: When the second exposure to the same antigen is by intravenous route the reaction is systemic and can be serious causing **rapid** development of laryngeal edema, bronchospasm with asphyxia, shock and **death**.

Atopy: When the second exposure is by local route, e.g. skin, nose, etc. then the reaction is only local, e.g. urticaria (hives), eczema, hay fever (allergic rhinitis). When the reaction occurs in the airways then there is bronchoconstriction leading to difficulty in breathing and asthma attack.

15. What is type-II (cytotoxic) hypersensitivity?

Ans. This is mediated by IgG, which is bound by its two antigen-binding sites to the antigens that are part of the surface of the cells which get injured. This has three types:

1. *Antibody-dependent complement-mediated cytotoxicity (ADCom-MC):* Injury is by the activated components of the complement, which happens after IgG binds to the antigen on the cell surface, causing activation of complement and cell injury. Antigens are present on the membrane of the RBCs or basement membranes of the tissues. Examples: Hemolytic transfusion reaction, hemolytic disease of the newborn (erythroblastosis fetalis), warm antibody autoimmune hemolytic anemia, **Goodpasture's syndrome**. (Abs are against Ags of the glomerular basement membrane causing glomerulonephritis; and Abs against Ags of the alveolar wall basement membrane causing pulmonary hemorrhage), mismatched skin or organ transplant leading to rejection of the graft, **pernicious anemia** (antiparietal cell antibodies damage the parietal cells of the gastric mucosa resulting in absence of intrinsic factor necessary for the absorption of vitamin B_{12}), pemphigus vulgaris (antibodies are against keratinocyte intercellular cement).
2. *Antibody-dependent cell-mediated cytotoxicity (ADC-MC):* Mechanism of action is that after IgG is bound by its antigen-binding sites to the antigen on the cell surface and by its free Fc portion to the Fc receptors of some leukocytes, e.g. NK cells, macrophages, monocytes, neutrophils, eosinophils, which then kill the cells to which they are so attached. Complement is **not** involved in this phenomenon. ADC-MC may be important for immunity from tumors, in graft rejection and may play a role in autoimmune anemia, thrombocytopenia and leukopenia. Also, by ADC-MC parasites are destroyed where Ab is IgE.
3. *Antibody-mediated cellular dysfunction:* Mechanism of action is that antibodies react with cell-surface receptors of physiologic stimulation causing either stimulation or inhibition of functions. Examples: Antibodies react against thyroid hormone receptor causing them to either hyperact causing hyperthyroidism **(Graves' disease)** or hypoact causing hypothyroidism **(myxedema)**. In **myasthenia gravis** there are antibodies against acetylcholine receptors causing damage to the receptors, thereby acetylcholine cannot transmit impulses to the skeletal muscles resulting in muscle weakness.

16. What is type-III immune complex hypersensitivity?

Ans. Mechanism of action is that the antibodies react with antigens in the blood and the antigen-antibody complexes circulate in the blood and get deposited at various sites in our body. This attracts complement, which is activated. Activated complement components then cause inflammation, e.g. C5a is chemotactic for neutrophils, which release lysozymes causing tissue damage. Examples: **serum sickness, Arthus phenomenon, SLE, PAN, post-streptococcal glomerulonephritis, membranous nephropathy**.

17. What is serum sickness?

Ans. In the past, to induce passive immunity, preformed antibodies in some animals, e.g. horse, were injected to persons to provide passive immunity. This resulted in these foreign antibodies reacting against the antigen present in the body forming free flowing Ag-Ab complexes in the blood, which then got deposited in various tissues/organs of our body, e.g. heart, kidney, joints. Then, by activation of complement, injury to these tissues/organs occurred by the activated components of the complement and also by subsequent inflammatory reaction. Because of risk of this type of injury this practice of passive immunization is abandoned.

18. What is Arthus reaction?

Ans. **This is a localized reaction** as opposed to serum sickness which is a generalized reaction. This happens when there are already many antibodies present in the body and antigen (which is reactive against these antibodies) is introduced in the body by injection or transplantation of an organ. Ultimate injury is from Ag/Ab complexes activating complement with release of chemotactic factor, resulting in accumulation of PMNs and engulfment of host cells with release of enzymes (proteases) which destroy basement membrane, collagen, elastin and release of free oxygen radicals resulting in tissue damage. Also, by C5-C9 membrane attack complex (MAC).

19. What is type-IV cell-mediated delayed hypersensitivity?

Ans. Mechanism of action is:

1. Interaction between macrophages and CD4+ T cells of T_H1 subtype causes granuloma formation by activated macrophages and release of chemical mediators by macrophages with cell injury. Examples: **tuberculosis, leprosy, histoplasmosis, blastomycosis**.
2. CD4+, T_H1 cells activate CD8+ T cells (cytotoxic) which kill the antigen carrying cell. Examples: **contact dermatitis** (poison ivy, poison oak), **transplant rejection, tumor immunity** and response to some **viral infections**.

20. What are autoimmune diseases?

Ans. Our body's immune system is meant to attack foreign objects and organisms to keep our body free from injury and disease. It is **not** supposed to attack our own body tissue. It does **not** attack our own body tissue by recognizing it as self tissue and tolerating it. Our body achieves this by removing self-reactive lymphocytes centrally by killing the cells by apoptosis or making them inactive (anergy) in thymus and bone marrow; and, peripherally by suppression by T cells.

When due to some reason this recognition and tolerance fails our immune system attacks our own body tissue and causes disease which is known as **autoimmune disease.** This phenomenon is called **autoimmunity**, i.e. our immune system is trying to free our body from our own normal cells. The exact cause of this failure of self-recognition and failure of tolerance and development of intolerance for our own body tissue by our body's immune system is not known; but is thought to be possibly influenced by internal (genetic) and environmental (microbial) factors. Mechanisms for this are thought to be:

1. Infection, inflammation or a drug may modify the antigen for it to appear as non-self by our body's immune system.
2. Injury or inflammation may expose isolated antigens in our body to our body's immune system, e.g. thyroglobulin, lens protein, spermatozoa.
3. A foreign antigen may have common structure to our body's antigen **(molecular mimicry)**.
4. An increase in T helper cell function.
5. A decrease in T suppressor cell function.

Examples of some of the autoimmune diseases are:

1. Autoimmune hemolytic anemia.
2. Pernicious anemia.
3. Autoimmune thrombocytopenia.
4. Myasthenia gravis.
5. Hashimoto's thyroiditis.
6. Graves' disease.
7. Ulcerative colitis.
8. Primary biliary cirrhosis.
9. Chronic active hepatitis.
10. Goodpasture's syndrome.
11. Membranous glomerulonephritis.
12. Connective tissue (collagen) diseases such as:
    a. SLE (Systemic lupus erythematosus)
    b. Systemic sclerosis (scleroderma)
    c. PAN (Polyarteritis nodosa)
    d. RA (Rheumatoid arthritis).
    e. SS (Sjogren's syndrome)
    f. RS (Reiter's syndrome).
    g. Polymyositis.

21. What is SLE (systemic lupus erythematosus)?

Ans. SLE is an autoimmune disorder which affects many systems of our body, causing common clinical features of rashes and arthralgia; and serious problems of renal (with some of the manifestations being proteinuria/nephrotic syndrome, hematuria/nephritic syndrome) and cerebral (with some of the manifestations being epilepsy, psychosis) diseases.

Other manifestations can by hematologic (hemolytic anemia, leucopenia, thrombocytopenia), serositis, etc.

This is due to polyclonal B cell activation, thereby production of antibodies against structures/tissues/molecules of our own body, e.g. against our own DNA (anti-

DNA antibodies) resulting in DNA-anti DNA complexes, antinucleolar antibodies, anti mitochondrial antibodies, antierythrocyte antibodies, antithrombin antibodies, anti thyroglobulin antibodies. This information is used in clinical medicine for tests to diagnose SLE as follows: (1) *ANA (Antinuclear antibody) test:* This test is positive in certain percentage of cases with other connective tissue diseases; but, is seen with almost all cases of SLE and is almost specific for SLE when ANA react with double-stranded DNA or with Sm (Smith) antigen, which is a ribonucleoprotein. Reaction with double-stranded DNA is seen under immunofluorescence microscope by immunofluorescence technique as a **rim pattern** where the staining is present at the periphery of the nucleus. *PATHOG:* The mechanism of immune injury here is type II (cytotoxic) and type III (immune complex-mediated) injury. *MORPHO:* The general morphology of injury is fibrinoid necrosis and acute vasculitis with lymphocytic infiltration. The injury happens to many organs of our body, e.g. heart, blood vessels, lungs, kidneys, joints, skin, serosal membranes. *Heart:* Complexes of antinucleoprotein-nucleoprotein seen as **hematoxylin bodies** can be seen under atrial endocardium and at the site of closure of valve cusps causing an endocarditis known as **Libman-Sacks endocarditis**. *Blood vessels:* There is vasculitis due to immune complex deposition in the walls of the vessels. This can affect blood vessels of any organ of the body. *Lungs:* There is diffuse interstitial fibrosis seen as interstitial pneumonitis or diffuse fibrosing alveolitis. *Kidneys:* There is glomerulonephritis. The injury may vary from minimal to severe. *Joints:* This causes arthritis and arthralgia. *Skin:* This is seen as a typical **butterfly rash** over the face involving the base of the nose and adjacent malar (cheek bones) bilaterally. *Eyes:* Conjunctivitis, retinal vasculitis, optic neuritis, secondary Sjogren syndrome. *CNS:* Aseptic meningitis, vasculitis, thrombosis, CVA, cerebellar ataxia, polyneuropathy.

22. What is discoid lupus erythematosus (DLE)?

Ans. DLE is an autoimmune disease like SLE of the skin consisting of skin rash similar to malar rash seen in SLE or sharp (discoid) rash. In many years, approximately 1/10th patients develop *S/S* like SLE. ANA is present in approximately 1/3rd patients. *MICRO:* Immune complex granular deposition of immunoglobulin and C3 at the dermo-epidermal junction is seen by IM.

23. What is systemic sclerosis (scleroderma)?

Ans. The ANA in this condition is anti-Scl-70. There is fibrosis and degenerative changes affecting skin, gastrointestinal changes, heart, muscle and other organs. A variant of scleroderma is called **CREST syndrome:** (**C** = Calcinosis, **R** = Raynaud's phenomenon, **E** = Esophageal dysfunction, **S** = Sclerodactyly and **T** = Telangiectasia).

The ANA in CREST syndrome has anticentromere activity. *Calcinosis indicates* = Calcium deposition in subcutis. *Raynaud's phenomenon indicates* = Spasm of digital arteries with cyanosis. *Esophageal dysfunction indicates* = Loss of esophageal motility with dysphagia. *Sclerodactyly indicates* = Claw-like flexion deformity of fingers. *Telangiectasia indicates* = Dilatation of small vessels of the skin. Also, similar to hand, facial skin is tight giving the face a fixed appearance. Also, fibrosis of interstitial tissue of the lung can cause severe respiratory compromise.

24. What is PAN (polyarteritis nodosa)?

Ans. The mechanism of injury here is type III hypersensitivity, (Ag-Ab-immune complex-mediated). Deposition of these Ag-Ab complexes in medium and small arteries cause vasculitis with segmental fibrinoid necrosis. This can cause many features according to organs and tissues of the body affected, e.g. involvement of kidneys causes hematuria, proteinuria, uremia. Other features can be abdominal pain, hypertension, polyneuritis, splenomegaly, fever, leukocytosis. This condition for unknown reason is more common in males. All other connective tissue diseases are more common in females. Also, for unknown reason blood vessels of the lungs are not affected.

25. What is rheumatoid arthritis?

Ans. Described in Chapter 16.

26. What is Sjogren's syndrome?

Ans. It is a systemic autoimmune disease of unknown etiology commonly seen in middle-aged females as *primary form (sicca syndrome)* consisting of:

1. Xerostomia (dry mouth); and
2. Keratoconjunctivitis sicca (dry eyes).

Or as *secondary form* together with other autoimmune disease, e.g. RA, SLE, etc. ANA is anti-SS-B which is highly specific.

MORPHO:

Lymphocytic infiltration of the lacrimal and salivary glands is present causing degeneration, atrophy, necrosis, swollen and thereby decreased function. *C/Fs:* Parotid glands may be swollen and tender, some of the *D/D* of which includes suppurative sialadenitis, mumps, tuberculosis, sarcoidosis, lymphoma, etc. Also, extraglandular *C/Fs* may be present such as arthralgia, lymphadenopathy, Raynand's phenomenon, involving GIT (diarrhea, dyspepsia), renal (proteinuria, interstitial nephritis, renal tubular acidosis, glomerulonephritis), pulmonary (bronchitis, alveolitis). *COMPLI:* One of the serious complications is lymphadenopathy may develop lymphoma (Also *see* chapter 11).

27. What is polymyositis/dermatomyositis?

Ans. ANA is present in this condition also. The main body sites affected in polymyositis are proximal muscles of the limbs. Skin can also be affected with a reddish rash over the exposed areas of the face and neck. Then the condition is called **dermatomyositis**. Malignancy of some organs is also present. There is increased serum creatine kinase. Diagnosis is made by muscle biopsy. This also affects mainly females.

28. What are the immunodeficiency diseases?

Ans. These are of two types:
1. Congenital.
2. Acquired.

29. What are the congenital immunodeficiency diseases?

Ans. These are of 5 types due to defects in:
a. T cell function.
b. B cell function.
c. Combined (T and B cell).
d. Phagocytic.
e. Complement (some components).

Immunodeficiency results in increased susceptibility to infections because the immune system is responsible for protection of our body against infections. Also, it results in increased susceptibility to developing neoplasms because immune system keeps a surveillance over emergence of neoplastic cells.

30. What are the examples of the 5 types of congenital immunodeficiency diseases?

Ans. a. T cell deficiency diseases, e.g. DiGeorge syndrome (Thymic aplasia).
b. B cell deficiency diseases, e.g. Bruton's disease.
c. Combined B and T cell deficiency.
d. Phagocyte dysfunction disorders, e.g. leukocyte adhesion deficiency-1 and 2 (LAD-1 and 2), Chediak-Higashi syndrome, chronic granulomatous disease. Job's syndrome, myeloperoxidase deficiency, alkaline phosphatase deficiency.
e. Complement deficiency diseases, e.g. C1 esterase inhibitor deficiency causing hereditary angioedema; C1q, C2, C4 deficiency causing SLE, RA, glomerulonephritis; C3 deficiency resulting in susceptibility to mainly pyogenic infections, C5-C8 deficiency resulting in susceptibility to neisserial infection.

31. What is DiGeorge syndrome (thymic aplasia)?

Ans. In this condition there is failure of formation of 3rd and 4th pharyngeal pouches resulting in **absence of thymus** and **parathyroid glands**. There is depletion of T cells in the paracortical areas of the lymph nodes. There is deficient cell-mediated immune response resulting in viral and fungal infections. B-cell (immunoglobulin-antibody) response is normal. Also, there is **hypoparathyroidism** resulting in **tetany**. Child usually dies in early life.

32. What is Bruton's agammaglobulinemia?

Ans. This is a congenital condition. It is inherited as X-recessive. Therefore, males are sufferers and females are carriers. Cell-mediated immunity is normal. In this condition pre-B lymphocytes do not mature into mature B-lymphocytes which leads to inability to development of plasma cells. Thus, there is an inability to produce immunoglobulins. This makes child susceptible to bacterial infections. Lymph nodes and spleen do not have lymphoid follicles. So, after the maternal immunoglobulins (IgG, which cross the placenta) are exhausted at approximately 6 months of age, the child becomes susceptible to bacterial infections.

33. What is common variable immunodeficiency?

Ans. This has features of immunodeficiency similar to that of Bruton's agammaglobulinemia (many recurrent infections); however, these begin at later age in childhood or adolescence and affect boys and girls equally and can be congenital or acquired.

34. What is IgA deficiency?

Ans. IgA deficiency is one of the commonest immunodeficiency diseases consisting of absent serum and secretory IgA due to absent IgA positive B lymphocytes resulting in recurrent gastroenteritis, sinuses, pulmonary and urinary tract infections.

35. What is severe combined immunodeficiency disease (SCID) (swiss-type agammaglobulinemia)?

Ans. There is deficiency of both T cells and B cells with severe lymphopenia and defect in antibody-mediated and cell-mediated immunity due to autosomal recessive and X-linked. There is hypoplasia of thymus (causing defect in cell-mediated immunity) and lymph nodes MALT and other lymph tissue of the body (causing defect in antibody-mediated immunity). Patient is susceptible to severe infections, viral and fungal (due to defective cell-mediated immunity) and bacterial (due to defect in antibody-mediated immunity).

36. What is chronic granulomatous disease?

Ans. In this condition, after the phagocytes have engulfed foreign substance, due to X-linked recessive or autosomal recessive absence of NADPH oxidase, they cannot produce hydrogen peroxide, which is required to destroy the foreign substance resulting in susceptibility to recurrent infections.

37. What is Chediak-Higashi syndrome?

Ans. In this condition, the WBCs have defect in their ability to be attracted to the area where the foreign substance is (failure of chemotaxis). Also, WBCs cannot engulf the foreign substance (impairment of phagocytosis) due to defect in polymerization of microtubules. Also, there is impairment of degranulation of lysosomes into phagosomes.

38. What is Job's syndrome?

Ans. Neutrophilic chemotactic response is defective resulting in repeated staphylococcal abscesses and suppurative lymphadenitis.

39. What is angioneurotic edema?

Ans. It is intermittent acute development of local swelling of the lips, skin, respiratory and gastrointestinal mucosa. It is of two types—*sporadic* and *hereditary*. Sporadic is due to type-I hypersensitivity reaction. Hereditary is due to autosomal dominant-transmitted deficiency of C1 esterase inhibitor with increased production of C2 kinin causing increased vascular permeability resulting in edema.

40. What is acquired immunodeficiency?

Ans. This can be due to infection, malnutrition, neoplasms, iatrogenic as a result of immunosuppressive treatment.

41. What is acquired immunodeficiency syndrome (AIDS)?

Ans. This is due to infection by a virus. Virus is called human immunodeficiency virus (HIV). The resultant disease is called acquired immunodeficiency syndrome. HIV is a retrovirus. It attacks T cells. It binds to the T cell receptor which causes the stimulation of the T cell. And it inserts its genetic material into the DNA of these T cells. Thus, the stimulated T cell produces these viruses instead of T cells. Thus, virus population increases and T cell population decreases. Hence, the virus not only multiplies at the cost of our body's cells; but, at the same time, since our body's cell happens to be the T cell, which is cell of our body's immune system, our body has no means to combat this virus and therefore, it is a deadly disease. When the symptoms of HIV begin the suppressor T cells (CD_8) remain normal. The helper T cells (CD_4) decrease. So, the ratio of suppressor cells to helper cells changes from 1:2 to 1:1. Also, macrophages have receptors for HIV virus by which HIV virus enters macrophages which act as reservoirs of the virus.

Transmission: 1. Homosexual and also heterosexual intercourse.

2. IV drug abuse.

3. IV transfusions.

MORPHO: The morphological changes of HIV are those of opportunistic infections and neoplasms. Nervous system has specific changes described in the chapter of nervous system.

Course of disease: It consists of 3 phases:

1. Acute phase 2. Chronic phase 3. Crisis phase

1. *Acute phase:* Self-limited. *C/Fs*: Sore throat, myalgia.
2. *Chronic phase:* Lasts 5–10 years. *C/Fs*: Lymphadenopathy, fever, fatigue, rash towards the end. Also, slowly declining helper T cells (T_4) lymphocytes.
3. *Crisis phase:* Fast reduction in T_4 cells. *C/Fs*: Opportunistic infections (CMV, herpes simplex, mycobacteria typical and atypical, *Toxoplasma gondii*, candida, *Cryptococcus neoformans, Pneumocystis carinii*) and secondary neoplasms (Kaposi's sarcoma, non-Hodgkin's lymphoma) CNS involvement (AIDS-dementia complex, acute aseptic meningitis, vacuolar myelopathy, peripheral neuropathy).

42. What is acquired hypogammaglobulinemia?

Ans. This is seen in lymphoma, chronic lymphatic leukemia, multiple myeloma, where abnormal immunoglobulins are formed which cannot function as antibodies. Also, this is seen in conditions where there is excessive breakdown of plasma proteins, e.g. nephrotic syndrome, extensive desquamative skin diseases, protein-losing enteropathies.

43. What is acquired cell-mediated immunodeficiency?

Ans. This is seen in Hodgkin's disease and sarcoidosis.

Transplantation

44. What are the types of grafts?

Ans. 1. *Autograft:* Transplant from one region of a person to another region of the same person. Best chance of graft succeeding.
2. *Isograft:* Graft between monozygotic twins. Good chance of success.
3. *Allografts:* Graft between same members of the species. High chance of rejection.
4. *Xenografts:* Graft between members of different species. High chance of rejection.

45. What are the types of transplant rejection?

Ans. These are of three types:
1. *Hyperacute rejection:* This occurs within a few minutes of the transplantation. It is antibody-mediated **(type III)** with antibodies already present in the recipient to donor tissue. There is acute inflammation with antigen-antibody complexes deposition on the walls of small blood vessels causing fibrinoid necrosis and due to activation of Hageman clotting factor (factor XII) resulting in activation of clotting cascade, massive thrombosis of the blood vessels of the donated tissue/ organs occurs with ischemia, and necrosis.
2. *Acute rejection:* This occurs after a few days to a few months of the transplantation. It is either **type II** (antibody-mediated) or **type IV** (cell-mediated) or both. There is chronic inflammation with presence of lymphocytes and macrophages with thrombosis and necrosis of the donated organ.
3. *Chronic rejection:* This occurs after a few months to a few years of the transplantation. It is due to antibody-mediated **(type II)**. There is proliferation of the fibrous tissue with scarring of the donor organ.

46. What is graft-versus-host reaction?

Ans. Here the graft reacts against the host cells and destroys the host cells as opposed to the host cells reacting against the grafted (donor) tissue, e.g. in bone marrow transplantation because these transplanted marrow contains competent T and B cells which react against the host tissue.

4 Neoplasm/Neoplasia

OVERVIEW

1. Definitions and nomenclature.
2. Epidemiology.
3. Clinical effects.
4. Etiologic factors.
5. Molecular factors.

Neoplasm means new growth. Actually, this should be called abnormal growth because as we know new growth of several tissues occurs regularly in our body, e.g. nail, hair, blood cells, cells of the lining of the gastrointestinal tract, etc.

In nut shell, neoplasm is a **PI^{4}G** (**P**arasitic, **I**ndependent, **I**nfinite, **I**nvasive, **I**rreversible **G**rowth).

According to the type of cells all normal cells have a usual size, shape, color of cytoplasm, color of nucleus, size of nucleus in certain proportion to the cytoplasm, nucleolus in a given size, number, positioning of cells in a given order in a given tissue and dividing cells in a given number at a given location in respect to the tissue.

Atypical cell can have one or many of these features different than normal. *Dysplasia is* disorderly proliferation of cells with atypical features. It is **mild, moderate, severe dysplasia** and **carcinoma *in situ* (CIS)** when the dysplasia involves 1/4, 1/2, 3/4 and full thickness of the tissue respectively. **Dysplasia is reversible**. **Carcinoma *in situ* is not reversible**. If not timely and appropriately treated it will progress to invasive/infiltrating carcinoma, i.e. it will break through its basement/limiting membrane and spread into surrounding tissue; and, furthermore into not continuous far away tissues of the body **(metastasis, which is the most definite sign of a malignant benign neoplasm)**. *Anaplasia* is severe degree of dysplasia where the cell dedifferentiates and is seen with primitive/embryonal/fetal visual and molecular fetal features, e.g. α-fetoprotein (AFP) in embryonal carcinoma, yolk cell tumor, hepatocellular carcinoma; carcinoembryonic antigen (CEA) in colon cancer, etc. and is seen in more aggressive malignant neoplasms. *Polyp* is a benign neoplasm that projects from its surface. *Papilloma* is a benign tumor of an epithelium with finger-like architecture. *Tumor* literally means swelling and is one of the main signs of inflammation. However, traditionally it is used synonymously for neoplasm and not for inflammatory swelling.

Usually, term of a neoplasm ends with "oma". Some non-neoplastic disorders traditionally end as "oma", e.g. choristoma, hamartoma, granuloma, cholesteatoma, trachoma, glaucoma, tuberculoma, ameboma, aspergilloma, etc.

Neoplasms can be classified in various ways:

1. According to tissue of origin, e.g. parenchymal or mesenchymal.
2. Made of one cell type or mixed from one germ cell layer or more than one germ cell layer—teratoma).
3. According to the behavior (benign/malignant); malignant neoplasm according to site of origin (primary or secondary).

Also, a neoplasm with its name ending as "oma" is usually benign. However, traditionally some malignant neoplasm names end with "oma", e.g. melanoma, lymphoma, seminoma, dysgerminoma, retinoblastoma, neuroblastoma, nephroblastoma, etc.

Four main differences between benign and malignant neoplasms are:

1. Metastasis.
2. Local invasion.
3. Differentiation.
4. Rate of growth.

Malignant neoplasms **metastasize (most important difference)**, locally invade, are not differentiated and grow rapidly. Benign neoplasms do not metastasize, nor invade locally, are well differentiated and grow slowly.

Carcinoma is a name for malignant neoplasm of epithelial origin, e.g. squamous cell carcinoma, basal cell carcinoma, adenocarcinoma, bronchogenic carcinoma, hepatocellular carcinoma, renal cell carcinoma, transitional cell carcinoma, etc. **Sarcoma** is a name for malignant neoplasms of mesenchymal origin, e.g. fibrosarcoma, liposarcoma, osteogenic sarcoma, chondro sarcoma etc.

Epidemiology of neoplasms consists of certain geographic, age and sex distribution.

Clinical effects of malignant neoplasms consist of various systemic manifestations , cachexia culminating in death.

Paraneoplastic syndrome is one of the manifestations associated with different neoplasms comprising: **CONES**

1. **C** = **C**oagulopathies.
2. **O** = **O**sseous.
3. **N** = **N**eurologic.
4. **E** = **E**ndocrinopathies.
5. **S** = **S**kin.

Grading of the neoplasm is based on differentiation of neoplastic cells—least differentiated has the worst prognosis.

Staging is based on clinical spread measured by size of the neoplasm (**T**umor), spread to regional lymph **N**odes and **M**etastasis. This is known as **TNM** staging. Staging has greater predictor value than grading.

Diagnosis of neoplasms is done by:

1. Microscopic examination of cells (cytology) or tissues (histopathology).
2. Biochemical assays of the serum for the tumor markers.

Definite cause of transformation of a normal cell to a neopalstic cell is not known. It is believed that this is **due to permanent non-lethal change (mutation) in the gene/s of the cell**. This can happen in the germ cell by which it can be transmitted to the offsprings or in the somatic cell by which it can be acquired sporadically.

Development of neoplasms is affected by some:

1. Inherited; or
2. Acquired predispositions.
3. Premalignant conditions.
4. Immunosuppression.

Acquired causes of neoplasia are:

1. Physical.
2. Chemical and
3. Microbiologic.

Mechanisms of transformation of a normal cell to a neoplastic cell is a two-stage process:

1. Formation of monoclonal mass of cells.
2. Progression of the monoclonal mass of cells in multiple-steps into a heterogenous mass of subclones of cells with different aggressive properties.

Classes of genes involved in the development of neoplasms are:

1. Apoptosis regulating genes.
2. Proto-oncogenes.
3. Tumor suppressor genes.
4. DNA repair genes.

Chromosomal changes associated with neoplastic mutation of genes are:

1. Translocation.
2. Amplification.
3. Deletion.

Phenotypic properties of malignant neoplastic cells associated with abnormal growth are many, e.g.

1. Infinite.
2. Independent.
3. Invasive and metastatic.
4. Irreversible.
5. Parasitic growth.

Definitions/Terminology

1. What do you understand by the term neoplasm?

Ans. In nut shell, a neoplasm can be described as **PI^{4}G** (**P** = Parasitic, **I** = Independent, **I** = Infinite, **I** = Invasive, **I** = Irreversible, **G** = Growth). Neoplastic cell does not respond to the normal controls of growth (independent, autonomous).

2. What is the molecular basis of the origin of neoplasm?

Ans. Nonfatal irreversible injury to the genetic apparatus of the cell can convert normal cell into neoplastic cell.

3. What is the Willis definition of neoplasm?

Ans. Neoplasm is an abnormal mass of tissue, the growth of which exceeds and is uncoordinated with that of the normal tissue and persists in the same excessive manner after the cessation of stimuli which evoked the change. Fundamental to the origin of all neoplasms is: Loss of responsiveness to normal growth controls.

4. What do you understand by these terms: Neoplasia, Atypia, Dysplasia, CIS (Carcinoma *in situ*), Anaplasia, Polyp, Papilloma, Choristoma, Hamartoma?

Ans. *Neoplasia* means new growth. Actually, normal new growth occurs in our body all the time, e.g. blood cells, cells lining various surfaces of our body such as skin, GIT, etc. However, the growth in our body that is termed neoplasia is abnormal growth. Therefore, the appropriate term would be "malplasia".

Atypia: Atypia means when the cells are not typical to the normal cells. This lack of typicality could be in the following ways:

1. Loss of uniformity—cells may differ from each other in size and shape (called **pleomorphism**).
2. The nuclei become bigger and the **ratio of the nucleus to cytoplasm increases**.
3. Nuclei become darker in color (deeply stained—**hyperchromatic**).
4. The nuclear chromatin becomes clumped **focally, i.e. in some places**.
5. Nucleoli become larger and dark-colored and more than one may be present.

Dysplasia: Dysplasia is disorderly proliferation of cells. In dysplasia there is:

1. Loss in the orientation of cells, i.e. the cells are not arranged in an orderly fashion known as **loss of polarity**.
2. Loss of orderly maturation of cells, i.e. the cells do not mature in the normal order from the tall cells in the bottom basal layer of the epithelium to the flattened squamous cells in the top superficial layer of the epithelium; but, a disorderly scrambling of dark basal-appearing cells is present within the epithelium.
3. Atypia of the cells is present.
4. Mitotic figures are more in number than usual.
5. Mitotic figures appear in abnormal locations, i.e. they are not confined to the normal location of the basal layer; but, are seen in all layers of the cell.

6. In dysplasia these changes do not occupy the full thickness of the epithelium; but, **only the partial thickness of the epithelium**.
7. In dysplasia these changes are reversible, i.e. when the stimuli which evoked these changes are removed these changes revert to normal.
8. Dysplasia can progress to malignancy, as is seen in dysplasia of metaplastic squamous epithelium of cervix progresses to squamous cell carcinoma of the cervix.

CIS (Carcinoma in situ): Carcinoma *in situ* means cancer confined to the full thickness of the epithelium or epidermis, i.e. it has not broken through the basal layer and gone **(infiltrated)** the deeper tissue beneath the basal layer of the epithelium. The changes present here are those present in dysplasia with following differences:

1. The changes involve the **full thickness of the epithelium**.
2. The changes are of more severe degree than in dysplasia.
3. These changes **are not reversible** unlike in dysplasia.

Anaplasia: Anaplasia means lack of differentiation. The changes present here are those present in CIS or infiltrating carcinoma but in more severe degree as follows:

1. In anaplasia the lack of architectural and cellular differentiation (atypia) is of the most severe degree. There is a total loss of the normal architecture and the neoplastic cells are present in sheets with marked loss of polarity. Atypia is also of the most severe degree and giant cells may be present called **tumor giant cells**.
2. Mitotic figures are markedly increased in number.
3. Mitotic figures may be abnormal, i.e instead of normal bipolar, tripolar or quadripolar mitotic figures might be present.

Polyp: Tumor projecting from the surface. Sessile = without a stalk. Pedunculated = With a stalk.

Papilloma: Benign tumor of epithelium with finger-like configuration. Epithelium can be squamous skin, larynx, tongue or columnar of GIT tract or any gland or transitional of the urinary bladder, ureter, or renal pelvis.

Choristoma: It is not a neoplasm, therefore, it should not be called "oma". It is small area of normal tissue of one organ misplaced within another organ such as normal area of pancreatic tissue in the wall of the stomach.

Hamartoma: It is not a neoplasm, therefore, it should not be called "oma". It is a collection of cells normally found in an organ but not organized in a normal pattern of that organ.

5. What are the classifications of neoplasms?

Ans. A. *By behavior:*

Benign:

1. *Appearence:* Well differentiated tumor cells, resemble normal.
2. *Growth rate:* Slow, may regress; mitotic figures few and normal.
3. *Local invasion:* No local invasion; growth expansile, pushy.

4. *Distant metastasis:* Absent.

Malignant:

1. *Appearance:* Lack of differentiation (atypia, anaplasia).
2. *Growth rate:* Erratic growth rate: Slow to rapid. Mitotic figures many and abnormal.
3. *Local invasion:* Locally invasive.
4. *Distant metastasis:* Present—**This is the most definitive indication of a malignant neoplasm**.

B. *By site of origin:*

1. Primary.
2. Secondary.

C. *By tissue of origin:*

1. One parenchymal cell type.
2. Mixed from one germ cell layer.
3. Mixed from more than one germ cell layer.

"Omas" that are malignant neoplasms (not benign): Neuroblastoma, nephroblastoma, retinoblastoma, melanoma, lymphoma, seminoma, myeloma, insulinoma (approximately 10% are malignant), gastrinoma (approximately 50% are malignant).

"Omas" that are not neoplasms:

1. Choristoma.
2. Hamartoma.
3. Granuloma.
4. Pyogenic granuloma (epulis).
5. Cholesteatoma.
6. Trachoma.
7. Glaucoma.
8. Tuberculoma.
9. Ameboma.
10. Aspergilloma.

Epidemiology

Epidemiology of Neoplasia

Geographic distribution: High prevalence of cancer according to geographic regions is as follows:

1. *Esophagus:* Iran, China, India.
2. *Stomach:* Japan.
3. *Colon, breast, prostate:* USA, Europe.

4. *Liver:* SE Asia.
5. *Skin:* USA, Australia
6. *Burkitt lymphoma:* Africa.

Age Distribution

1. *Leukemia, lymphoma, nephroblastoma, neuroblastoma, retinoblastoma, rhabdomyosarcoma, yolk sac tumors of testes:* Infancy and early childhood.
2. *Medulloblastoma, osteogenic sarcoma, Ewing's tumor:* Late childhood, early adolescence.
3. *Testicular germ cell tumors:* 20–40 years.
4. *Hodgkin's lymphoma:* 2 peaks—20 years and 60 years.
5. *Colon and prostate cancers:* Increase with increasing age.
6. *Osteogenic sarcoma:* 2 peaks—20 years (primary) and 60 years (secondary).

Sex Distribution

1. *Males:* 4 commonest cancers in males are: Lungs, prostate, colorectal, urinary bladder.
2. *Females:* 4 commonest cancers in females are: Breast, uterus, lungs, colorectal.

Clinical Effects

6. What are the effects of malignant neoplasms?

Ans. In general, malignant neoplasms in our body cause weakness, weight loss, anorexia, wasting, cachexia, hypermetabolism, infection and eventual death.

7. What are paraneoplastic syndromes?

Ans. *DEF:* Various syndromes present with various neoplasms, which are not general effects of the neoplasms such as described above and are not due to direct effect of metastasis are, therefore, called paraneoplastic syndromes.

These are of the following types: **CONES**

1. **C**oagulopathies.
2. **O**sseous.
3. **N**eurologic.
4. **E**ndocrinopathies.
5. **S**kin.

1. *Coagulation abnormalities:* **Trousseau's syndrome** in carcinoma of the pancreas or some other visceral malignancies, DIC (disseminated intravascular coagulation).
2. *Osseous:* Hypertrophic osteoarthropathy and clubbing of fingers.
3. *Neurologic abnormalities:* **Lambert-Eaton myasthenic syndrome**.

4. *Endocrinopathies:*
   a. *Cushing's syndrome:* Due to production of ACTH-like substance in small cell carcinoma of the lung, renal cell carcinoma.
   b. *Hyperthyroidism:* Due to production of TSH-like substance in some lung neoplasms, hydatidiform moles and choriocarcinoma.
   c. *Hypercalcemia:* Due to production of parathormone-like substance in squamous cell carcinoma of the lung (hypercalcemia due to metastasis of a neoplasm in the bone is **not** considered as paraneoplastic syndrome).
   d. *Hypoglycemia:* Due to production of insulin-like substance in hepatocellular carcinomas, mesotheliomas and some sarcomas.
   e. *Polycythemia:* Due to production of erythropoietin in renal cell carcinoma and also with some other neoplasms.
   f. *Dilutional hyponatremia with concentrated urine:* Due to production of ADH in small cell carcinoma of the lungs and also some other neoplasms.
5. *Skin conditions:* Such as **dermatomyositis** or **acanthosis nigricans** can be present with certain visceral malignancies.

8. What is the importance of knowing about the paraneoplastic syndromes?

Ans. 1. Malignant neoplasm might initially present as paraneoplastic syndrome.
2. Paraneoplastic syndrome might cause confusion in *D/D*, staging and treatment of malignant neoplasm.
3. Paraneoplastic syndrome might cause more morbidity and even mortality than the malignant neoplasm.

Knowledge of paraneoplastic syndrome could help in dealing with these problems.

9. What are grading and staging of malignant neoplasms?

Ans. *Grading:* I to IV—based on cytological differentiation and mitoses (number and shape).
Staging: **Has greater clinical value than grading.**
1. **TNM** (Tumor size, node involvement, presence of metastasis).
2. **AJC** (American joint committee).

Staging is a clinical method based on size of the primary neoplasm, its extent of spread to the regional lymph nodes and the presence or absence of distant metastases to estimate probable aggressiveness of a given neoplasm, its apparent extent and spread in an individual patient for guidance for applying therapeutic modalities and expect prognosis.

10. What are the tests for diagnosis of neoplasms?

Ans. 1. *Microscopic examination:* Cytology, histopathology.
2. *Biochemical essays of serum tumor markers:*
   a. hCG (Human chorionic gonadotrophin)—Choriocarcinoma, hydatidiform mole.

b. PSA—Prostate cancer.

c. Alpha feto protein—Hepatocellular CA. Yolk cell tumor of ovary and testis.

d. CEA—Colon Ca.

e. 5-HT (Serotonin)—Carcinoid.

f. Calcitonin—Medullary thyroid Ca.

g. Ca-125—Ovarian cancer.

h. S-100—Melanoma, neural tumors.

Etiologic Factors

11. What are causes of neoplasia/neoplasms?

Ans. Definite cause of transformation of cells to neoplastic cells is not known. It is believed that this transformation is due to **permanent non-lethal change (mutation) in genes of the cell**. This genetic change can happen in the germ cell. Then it can be passed on to offsprings of the person as inherited disease. Or, it can happen in a somatic cell, when it affects sporadically one person only as acquired disease.

12. What are inherited predisposition to development of neoplasia?

Ans. A. *Autosomal dominant:* These are inherited by mutation of single allele of the cancer suppressor gene.

1. Retinoblastoma with incomplete penetrance.
2. Familial polyposis syndrome.
3. Neurofibromatosis-acoustic neuroma, meningioma, pheochromocytoma, gliomas of brain and optic nerve.
4. *Multiple endocrine neoplasia-I (MEN-I):* Adenoma of parathyroid, pituitary and islet cells.
5. *MEN-II:* Adenoma of parathyroid, thyroid medullary Ca, pheochromocytoma.

B. *Autosomal recessive:* These are inherited by mutation in the DNA repair gene.

1. Fanconi syndrome.
2. Ataxia telengiectasia.
3. Xeroderma pigmentosum.
4. Bloom syndrome.

C. *Familial cancers:* In these there is a familial clustering of some specific neoplasms; but, the transmission pattern is not clear. Examples of these are: cancers of colon, ovary, breast, brain.

13. What are acquired predisposition to development of neoplasia?

Ans. Some diseases increase one's risk of developing neoplasm, e.g.

1. Cirrhosis of liver—hepatocellular carcinoma.

2. Atrophic gastritis of pernicious anemia—gastric cancer.
3. Chronic ulcerative colitis—carcinoma of colon.
4. Leukoplakia of the oral and genital mucosa—squamous cell carcinoma.

14. What are some of the premalignant conditions?

Ans. *GIT:* Leukoplakia, erythroplasia, Barrett's esophagus, atrophic gastritis in pernicious anemia, ulcerative colitis, Peutzs-Jeghers syndrome, familial polyposis syndromes, *Respiratory system:* Bowen's disease, bowenoid papulosis, erythroplasia of Queyrat, *Skin:* Dysplastic nevus.

15. What is the relationship of immune suppression to causation of cancer?

Ans. Both antibody- and cell-mediated immune responses to cancer cells have been identified. Primary immune deficiency diseases-likelihood of cancer is 10,000 times than normal. Secondary immune suppression due to drugs-prone to cancer.

16. What are the acquired causes of neoplasia?

Ans. 1. Physical agents 2. Chemical agents 3. Microbiologic agents.

17. What are the physical causative agents of neoplasia?

Ans. 1. *Ionizing radiation:*
   a. Skin cancer in radiologist.
   b. Lung cancer in uranium miners.
   c. Thyroid cancer in people treated with radiation therapy to head/neck area for other diseases.
   d. Acute and chronic myeloid leukemia in people of Hiroshima and Nagasaki, who survived atomic blasts.
   e. Osteogenic sarcoma in radium watch dial workers.
2. *Ultraviolet radiation:* Ultraviolet radiation in sunlight causes increased incidence of skin cancer such as melanoma, basal carcinoma and squamous cell carcinoma.
3. *Heat:* Kangri cancer (squamous cell carcinoma of the abdominal skin) in Kashmiri people who used kangri (fire basket) to stay warm.
4. *Soot:* **Chimney-sweep's cancer** (squamous cell carcinoma of the scrotal skin) in chimney sweepers due to chronic irritation from the soot. **First environmental cancer recognized by Sir Pott (English surgeon 1744-1788).**
5. *Chronic irritation:* Squamous cell carcinoma of sinus tract in chronic osteomyelitis.

18. What are the chemical causative agents of neoplasia?

Ans. Several chemical agents are linked to carcinogenesis such as: Naphthylamines—carcinoma of urinary bladder, aniline dyes—bladder cancer, aromatic amines and azo dyes—hepatocellular carcinoma, vinyl chloride—angiosarcoma of liver, arsenic—skin cancer, asbestos—cancer of lung/mesothelioma of pleura and peritoneum, agent orange which has dioxins—lymphoma, Hodgkin's disease. Smoking—cancer of lungs, urinary bladder, kidneys. Chemotherapeutic drugs (alkylating agents)—leukemia.

Diet:

1. High fat low calorie diet—breast/prostate/colon cancer.
2. Low fiber diet—colon cancer.

19. What are the microbiologic causative agents of neoplasia?

Ans. 1. *Bacteria: H. pylori*—gastric carcinoma, gastric B-cell lymphoma (MALTomas).

2. *Parasites:*
   a. *Schistosoma hematobium*—bladder cancer.
   b. *S. mansoni*—colon cancer.
3. *Fungi: Aspergillus flavus* aflatoxin—liver cell cancer (in grains and nuts).
4. *Viruses*:
   1. HPV (Human papilloma virus):
      a. Warts
      b. Squamous cell carcinoma of cervix, vulva, vagina, anus, larynx.
   2. *E-B virus:*
      a. Burkitt's lymphoma
      b. B-cell lymphoma
      c. Hodgkin's disease
      d. Nasopharyngeal carcinoma.
   3. *Hepatitis B and C viruses:* Hepatocellular carcinoma.
   4. *HTLV-1:* Human T-cell leukemia.

Molecular Factors

20. What are the mechanisms of transformation of a normal cell to a neoplastic cell?

Ans. Our body's cells are exposed to injurious carcinogenic agents/stimuli on a regular basis. Our body's various defense mechanisms protect our cells from becoming neoplastic. Mechanism of development of cancer cell is a 2-stage process consisting of:

1. First stage of multi-step transformation of a normal cell into a **monoclonal** mass of malignant neoplastic cells, and
2. Second stage of progression of the cells of this neoplastic mass in multiple steps into a **heterogenous mass of sub clones** of cells with different aggressive properties thereby making the tumor mass more aggressive as a whole as follows:

1. *Stage-1:* Initial monoclonal neoplastic transformation of the normal cell:

   One single cell escapes protective mechanism by non-lethal irreversible injury to one of its pertinent growth-related gene with a permanent **change (mutation)** in it. From this single cell several new cells arise (thus they are monoclonal), which during successive generations go through several steps in which there is genetic/molecular and phenotypic/morphologic changes during which the daughter cells of this single cell become transformed from a normal cell to hyperplastic cells to dyplastic cells/benign neoplastic cells to malignant neoplastic cell (cancer cells).

   These steps are mutations in **4 different pertinent genes.** These can sometimes involve **chromosomal changes**. These changes in the genes give the cells various **phenotypic properties of neoplasia** thus making it a neoplasm.

2. *Stage-2:* Tumor progression with acquisition by different daughter cell different aggressive properties with development of heterogeneity of the monoclonal cancer cells. Thereafter, the daughter cells of these neoplastic cells during subsequent division develop independent genetic mutations thereby they acquire different properties and become a heterogenous mass of cells by virtue of which the malignant neoplasm becomes more aggressive. This phenomenon is called **tumor progression**.

21. What are the 4 classes of genes involved in the development of neoplasms?

Ans. Four types:

a. **A**poptosis-regulating genes.

b. Growth-promoting proto-oncogenes, i.e. genes which **b**ring about growth.

c. Growth-inhibiting tumor-suppressor genes, i.e. genes which **c**ut down growth.

d. **D**NA repair-regulating genes.

a. *Apoptosis-regulating genes:*

   Example of these genes is **bcl-2. It prevents apoptosis**. Over expression of bcl-2 extends cell survival. So, if there are cells present with damage to proto-oncogene or tumor suppressor gene these will **not** undergo apoptosis resulting in tumor formation. Example of this is **B-cell lymphomas of follicular type** and **Burkitt lymphoma**. Here there is a t(14:18) translocation. This places bcl-2 on chromosome 18 near active heavy chain locus on chromosome 14 resulting in over expression of bcl-2. Other examples of this are: **MALTomas**, due to t(11:18).

b. *Proto-oncogenes:*

   These genes are normally present in our cells. These affect normal growth and differentiation of the cells. These can be converted into oncogenes. This conversion can happen inside a retrovirus. These genes are then called **v**irus-associated **onc**ogenes **(v-onc)**. This happens rarely. This conversion can also commonly occur inside our cells. These genes are then called **c**ell-associated **onc**ogenes **(c-onc)**. **This happens more commonly**.

Oncogenes: Oncogenes are associated with development of neoplasms. These genes are **not** normally present in our cells. These are converted from proto-oncogenes mainly in 4 ways:

TAPE

1. Translocation.
2. Amplification.
3. Point mutation.
4. (Extra) Over expression.

Following are some examples of oncogenes, their mode of activation and resultant tumors:

1. Translocation: **abl:** translocation of gene leads to **CML**.
2. Amplification: N-*myc*: amplification implicated in **neuroblastoma**.
3. Point mutation: **ras** oncogene implicated in many cancers.
4. (Extra) Over expression: **erb-b1** implicated in **squamous cell carcinoma of lung, erb-b2** implicated in breast cancer, **hist-1** implicated in **stomach** and **bladder cancers, sis** implicated in **astrocytoma, osteosarcoma**.

c. *Tumor-suppressor genes:*

These genes suppress cell proliferation, thereby suppress formation of cancer. Therefore, these genes are called cancer-suppressor or anti-oncogenes. Mutations with **inactivation** of these genes leads to unregulated cell growth and tumor formation. **Both alleles of these genes have to be muted (inactivated) for the development of the disease**. Therefore, these are known as **recessive genes. Rb gene** located on chromosome 14 is one example of it. Mutation in **Rb** gene leads to retinoblastoma. Approximately 1/2 patients inherit this (familial) and ½ acquire (sporadic) it. In sporadic type, both the alleles are inactivated by somatic mutation. In familial type, one allele is inactivated in the germ line **(one-hit)** and, only one (the second allele) has to be inactivated by somatic mutation **(second-hit). Therefore, familial retinoblastoma is considered to be inherited as autosomal dominant**. (**The "two-hit" hypothesis of Knudson**, which states that two mutagenic alterations are required to cause alterations on both chromosomes, which is necessary for the formation of retinoblastoma). Inactivation of Rb gene is also seen in formation of **osteogenic sarcoma**. Most common method of inactivation of anti-oncogene is by deletion of short arm of chromosome 11, where WT-1 gene is located resulting in **Wilms' tumor**. Some other examples of inactivation of tumor suppressor genes and associated neoplasms are:

1. **TP53: Most cancers**.
2. **NF1: Neuroblastoma**.
3. **NF2: Meningioma, schwannoma**.
4. **APC: Colon, stomach, pancreas**.
5. **BRCA1 and 2: Breast cancer**.

d. *DNA repair genes:*

With few exceptions of CNS, cardiac and skeletal muscle cells, most of our body cells die and are regularly replaced by new dividing cells. During this division of so many cells, mutations in the proto-oncogenes, tumor suppressor genes and apoptotic genes occur regularly. However, only rarely do these new cells acquire malignant properties because the DNA repair genes repair defects in these 3 genes on regular basis as and when they occur thereby preventing development of malignant neoplasms. But, when there is defect in the DNA repair gene, mutations in the proto-oncogenes, tumor suppressor genes and apoptotic genes cannot be corrected resulting in development of malignant neoplasms. Some of the DNA repair genes are: **hMSH2, hMLH1**. Some examples of diseases due to defect of these DNA repair genes are as follows:

1. In **HNPCC (hereditary non-polyposis colon cancer)** patients are born with one of the defective repair genes.
2. **In xeroderma pigmentosum** patients are susceptible to develop skin cancer from damage by UV light preventing normal DNA replication, which cannot be repaired due to loss of repair genes.
3. **In hereditary breast and ovarian cancers** there is defect in tumor suppressor genes BRCA1 and BRCA2, which cannot be repaired due to defect in DNA repair genes.
4. Similar problem also exists in the development of **ataxia-telangiectasia, Bloom syndrome** and **fanconi anemia**.

22. What are the changes in the chromosomes associated with neoplastic mutation of genes?

Ans. These are of three types:

1. Translocation.
2. Deletion.

1. *Translocation:* An important mechanism by which c-oncs become tumorigenic is by chromosomal translocation as seen in following examples:
   a. *Fusion of 2 genes with formation of a hybrid gene with expression of tumor-promoting protein (9:22 translocation and chronic myeloid leukemia development):* c-abl proto-oncogene on chromosome 9 is transposed to chromosome 22 near bcr (breakpoint cluster region) which is an oncogene. This results in union of abl and bcr genes with formation of **hybrid** or **chimeric gene: c-abl-bcr** gene, the protein product of which facilitates chronic myeloid leukemia (CML) formation. The so changed **chromosome 22** is known as **Philadelphia chromosome** as it was first discovered in Philadelphia.
   b. *14:18 translocation and follicular lymphoma:* Immunoglobulin heavy chain on chromosome 14 is transposed to chromosome 18 near bcl-2 oncogene with increase in expression of bcl-2 with formation of **follicular lymphoma**.
   c. *8:14 translocation and Burkitt's lymphoma:* c-myc proto-oncogene on chromosome 8 is transposed to chromosome 14 to a site near to the immunoglobin heavy chain gene with increase in the expression of c-myc

with formation of **Burkitt's lymphoma**. Other chromosomal defects implicated in oncogenesis is trisomy 21 **(Down's syndrome) resulting in acute leukemias**.

2. *Deletion:* Wilms' tumor–*see* above.

23. What are the phenotypic properties of malignant neoplastic cells?

Ans. There are 4 main properties of malignant neoplastic cells. These are "**4 Is**" s as follows:

1. Infinite growth.
2. Independent growth.
3. Invasive and metastatic.
4. Irreversible.

1. *Infinite growth:* This is achieved as follows:
   a. Telomere length maintained same by activation of telomerase with limitless multiplication.
   b. *Evading death (apoptosis):* Over expression of antiapoptotic genes, BCL-2, BCL-XL, e.g. over expression of BCL-2 gene in follicular B cell lymphomas.
   c. Not responding to growth-suppressor signals (by mutation in Rb, TGF-beta, APC and TP53 genes).
2. *Independent growth:* This is achieved by making own growth signals.
3. *Invasion and metastasis:* This is achieved as follows:
   a. Growth of the neoplasm and formation of new vessels.
   b. Detachment of tumor cells from each other.
   c. Attachment of tumor cells to matrix components of blood vessels.
   d. Invasion of the tumor cells into lymphatics and blood vessels by their ability to penetrate the basement membranes of the vessels.
   e. Survival and transport of neoplastic cells inside the vessels as emboli.
   f. Passage out of the vessels by penetrating again through the basement membrane at the implantation site.
   g. Overcoming the defense mechanisms of the tissue at the site of implantation and grow at the implantation site.

Other special features are as follows:

Some of these features help us understand how and why these cells behave in such a different manner than our normal body cells. Some features help us identify them and assess them. These are:

1. *Loss of contact inhibition:* In vitro tissue culture the normal cells stop growing when they touch each other. But, the neoplastic cells continue to grow even after they touch each other.

2. *Loss of adhesion:* Normal cells grow in clusters. Neoplastic cells grow separately.
3. *Loss of anchorage dependence:* Normal cells need to be anchored to a solid surface for their growth. But, neoplastic cells do not need to be so anchored.
4. *Presence of proteases over the cell surface:* Normal cells do not have protease over their surface but, neoplastic cells have protease over their surface.
5. *Increased laminin receptors over the cell surface:* Neoplastic cells have increased laminin receptors over their surface. This may help them to attach to basement membranes.
6. *Production of oncofetal proteins or antigens:* Some of our normal cells produce certain proteins only when they are in embryonic or fetal stage of development, when they are undifferentiated. These proteins are called **oncofetal proteins** or **antigens**. These oncofetal proteins or antigens are produced by certain neoplastic cells. This indicates that these neoplastic cells lack differentiation, e.g. alpha fetoprotein in liver cancer, yolk sac tumor of the ovary, and testis; carcinoembryonic antigen (CEA) in colon.
7. *Monoclonal origin:* Most of the neoplastic cells are monoclonal, i.e. originate from a single precursor cell, which has developed neoplastic characteristics.
8. *Invasiveness:* Normal cells cannot infiltrate into neighboring tissues. Neoplastic cells can infiltrate into neighboring tissues.
9. *Metastatic features:* Metastasis means implantation of neoplastic cell at the site non-contiguous and distant from the site of the origin of the neoplasm. Normal cells stay where they develop. Malignant neoplastic cells have properties by which they can spread to sites away from the site of their development, such common sites are lymph nodes, lungs, liver, bone marrow, brain. They spread via either **lymphatics (most carcinomas)** or **blood vessels (most sarcomas)**, or by seeding of pericardial, pleural or peritoneal (ovarian cancer to liver) surfaces or by CSF (brain tumors).

5

Hemodynamic Disorders

OVERVIEW

1. Hemostasis.
2. Edema.
3. Hyperemia and congestion.
4. Hemorrhage.
5. Thrombosis.
6. Embolism.
7. Infarction.
8. Shock.
9. Disseminated intravascular coagulation (DIC).

Blood in our body carries all the necessary elements (oxygen, nutrients, hormones, defensive cells and chemicals, etc.) to all the organs, tissues and cells of our body and removes from there all the products of metabolism (carbon-dioxide, urea, creatinine, ammonia, bilirubin, etc.).

To achieve this, the blood must be maintained in a free-flowing, clot-free-fluid state in normal blood vessels; and a plug should form at the site of break in the blood vessel wall to prevent blood from flowing out of the blood vessels. This maintenance is called **hemostasis**, which is dependent upon:

1. Normal vessel wall (structure and function).
2. Platelets (number, structure and function).
3. Coagulation cascade (components and function).

Disorders of this orderly system consist of:

1. Edema.
2. Hyperemia and congestion.
3. Hemorrhage.
4. Thrombosis.
5. Embolism.
6. Ischemia.
7. Infarction.
8. Shock.
9. Disseminated intravascular coagulation (DIC).

Edema is increased fluid within the tissues. *It is mainly due to:*

1. Increased hydrostatic pressure, which pushes excessive fluid out of the blood vessels or
2. Decreased plasma osmotic pressure, which precludes pulling back of the pushed out fluid back into the blood vessels.
3. Increased sodium along with water causing increased blood volume which contributes to both (1) and (2).
4. Lymphatic obstruction.
5. Inflammation as described in Chapter 2.

Edema fluid is of two types:

1. **Transudate** which is non-inflammatory, having specific gravity of < 1.012, no proteins or cells.
2. **Exudate** which is inflammatory, having specific gravity of >1.020, and containing protein and cells.

Hyperemia and *congestion* mean increased blood volume in a particular tissue. Hyperemia is an active process, e.g. as in inflammation and congestion is a passive process, e.g. as seen in CCF.

Hemorrhage is extravasation of blood from the circulatory system, e.g. through GIT, upper and lower respiratory tract, urinary tract, genital tract, skin, etc.

Thrombosis is pathologic blood clotting within the cardiovascular system. *Its predisposing conditions are*: (described by **Virchow's triad**) **ABC**

1. **A** = **A**bnormal (injured) surfaces, endothelial or endocardial.
2. **B** = **B**lood flow abnormal (stasis or turbulence).
3. **C** = **C**oagulation abnormal.

Fate of thrombus is: **DOPE**

1. **D** = **D**issolution.
2. **O** = **O**rganization and recanalization.
3. **P** = **P**ropagation.
4. **E** = **E**mbolization.

Embolus is a detached intravascular solid, liquid, gaseous mass that is carried by the blood to a site distant from its site of origin and getting stuck at the narrowest portion, mostly resulting in cut off blood supply to the organ distal to it resulting in ischemia or infarction or **shock** and **death** when together in both the large pulmonary arteries. *Some of the types of emboli are:*

1. Dislodged thrombi (~ 99% of emboli–thromboemboli).
2. Fat from major fracture.
3. Air from chest wall injury, obstetric injury, decompression sickness.
4. Amniotic fluid.

Paradoxical embolus is an embolus in systemic circulation instead of pulmonary circulation due to ASD/VSD. **Saddle embolus** is an embolus across the bifurcation of pulmonary artery.

Ischemia is reduced blood supply to an organ or part of the body.

Infarction is ischemic necrosis of a tissue due to occlusion of either arterial blood supply or venous drainage.

Shock is systemic hypoperfusion due to reduction in cardiac output or in the effective circulating blood volume resulting in impaired tissue circulation and hypoxia. Reduction in cardiac output could be due to cardiac failure or obstruction within the circulation. Reduction in effective circulatory volume could be due to loss of blood or pooling of blood within the circulation which could be septic, neurogenic, anaphylactic or heat stroke. **Earliest sign of shock is tachycardia**.

Disseminated intravascular coagulation (DIC) is not a disease but a potential complication of any condition causing generalized activation of thrombin leading to exhaustion of all coagulation protein resulting in generalized bleeding. *Its causes are:* **DIC** and **M**

1. **D** = **D**elivery-related, e.g. amniotic fluid embolism, septic abortion, retained dead fetus, toxemia, abruptio placenta.
2. **I** = **I**nfections, e.g. septicemia, meningococcemia.
3. **C** = **C**ancer, e.g. carcinoma of lung, pancreas, prostate, stomach, acute promyelocytic leukemia.
4. **M** – **M**iscellaneous, e.g. severe trauma, shock, etc.

Hemostasis

1. What is the importance of normal circulation in our body? What does it depend on? What is circulation homeostasis?

Ans. Health of cells, tissues, organs and organ systems of our body depends on the normal circulation, to deliver oxygen, nutrients and hormones and remove waste products. Normal circulation depends on circulation homeostasis, which depends on normal:

1. Vessel structure (macroscopic and microscopic).
2. Intravascular pressure.
3. Intravascular osmolarity, and
4. Hemostasis.

2. What is hemostasis? What does it depend on?

Ans. Hemostasis means maintaining blood in a free-flowing, clot-free fluid state in normal vessels and rapid formation of a hemostatic plug at the site of breach in the continuity of the vessel to prevent bleeding. This depends on normal:

a. Vessel wall (structure and function).

b. Platelets (number, structure and function), and

c. Coagulation cascade (components and function).

3. What are the hemodynamic disorders?

Ans. Hemodyanamic disorders are as follows:

1. Edema.
2. Hyperemia and congestion.
3. Hemorrhage.
4. Thrombosis.
5. Embolism.
6. Ischemia.
7. Infarction.
8. Shock.
9. Disseminated intravascular coagulation (DIC).

Edema

4. What is edema?

Ans. *DEF:* A local or generalized condition in which there is excessive amount of fluid in the tissues of our body.

5. What do the terms anasarca, hydrothorax, hydropericardium, hydroperitoneum mean?

Ans. Anasarca = severe, generalized edema of the whole body. Hydrothorax = excessive fluid in the pleural cavity. Hydropericardium = excessive fluid in the pericardial cavity. Hydroperitoneum = excessive fluid in the peritoneal cavity. Also called ascites.

6. How many types of edema fluids there are?

Ans. These are of two types:

1. Transudate.
2. Exudate.

7. What is exudate? What is transudate?

Ans. *Exudate:* Inflammatory, caused by increased permeability of blood vessels. Specific gravity more than 1.020. Has high protein and cell contents.

Transudate: Non-inflammatory, caused by increased hydrostatic pressure and/or decreased plasma oncotic pressure. Specific gravity less than 1.012. No protein or cells content.

8. What are the causes of edema?

Ans. Two main causes of edema:

a. Inflammatory: Acute or chronic.
b. Non-inflammatory.

9. What are the causes of noninflammatory edema?

Ans. 1. Increased hydrostatic pressure.

2. Reduced plasma proteins with reduced plasma osmotic pressure.
3. Lymphatic obstruction.
4. Increased intravascular sodium with water retention.

1. *Causes of increased hydrostatic pressure:*
   a. Congestive cardiac failure.
   b. Constrictive pericarditis.
   c. Cirrhosis of the liver (ascites).
   d. Thrombosis of a vein.
   e. External pressure on a vein.
   f. Prolonged lower limb dependency due to inactivity.
2. *Causes of reduced plasma proteins and osmotic pressure:*
   a. *Reduced intake:* Malnutrition.
   b. *Reduced synthesis:* Liver failure–cirrhosis.
   c. *Increased loss:* Protein loosing gastroenteropathy or glomerulopathy (nephrotic syndrome).

3. *Causes of lymphatic obstruction:*
   a. Inflammatory.
   b. Neoplastic.
   c. *Iatrogenic:* Surgery, radiation.
4. *Causes of increased sodium:*
   a. Increased intake.
   b. Increased renal reabsorption: Reduced renal perfusion–Increased renin-angiotensin-aldosterone mechanism.

Pathogenesis of edema formation: Normally, the fluid from our circulation circulates through our tissues by exiting at the arteriolar end under the influence of hydrostatic pressure and reenters at the venular end under the influence of plasma osmotic pressure–a little residual amount is drained by the lymphatic vessels. When this normal system fails due to above causes, edema develops. Also in congestive cardiac failure there is decreased blood supply to the kidneys causing increased renin release from the juxtaglomerular cells. Renin converts blood angiotensinogen to angiotensin I, which is converted to angiotensin II by angiotensin-converting enzyme (ACE), which stimulates aldosterone secretion from the adrenal cortex. Aldosterone causes increased sodium and water reabsorption from the renal tubules thereby increasing plasma volume leading to further increase in plasma hydrostatic pressure and more edema. **This is the rationale of treatment with aldosterone antagonists for treatment of edema, besides the obvious measures consisting of sodium restriction and other diuretics**.

MORPHO: Edema can be present in any part of the body. Commonly it is seen in the subcutaneous tissue of the dependent parts due to gravity, also, in the lungs, brain, and in potential spaces (pleura, pericardium, peritoneum).

Subcutaneous edema: Usually seen in dependent areas of the body due to gravity. When pressure is applied by finger the fluid is displaced leaving a finger-shaped depression, called **pitting edema**. Subcutaneous edema in early stage is seen in areas with loose connective tissue such as periorbital area.

Pulmonary edema: Weight of the lungs is 2–3 times the normal weight. Edema fluid can be removed from the lungs by suction and can be blood-tinged with extravasated RBCs.

Brain edema: Gyri are distended, flattened and sulci narrow. Brain herniation can occur and when in the foramen magnum area can cause compromise of the cardiopulmonary center with **death**.

C/Fs: Pulmonary edema can give rise to dyspnea—initially upon exertion, then at rest and later orthopnea (inability to lie flat)—can lead to respiratory failure and **death**.

Hyperemia and Congestion

10. What are hyperemia and congestion?

Ans. *DEF:* Both terms mean local increased volume of blood in a particular tissue.

Hyperemia: It is an active process. It results from increased tissue inflow of blood due to arteriolar dilation, e.g. sites of inflammation. The affected tissue is redder due to engorgement with oxygenated blood.
Congestion: It is a passive process. It results from impaired venous outflow from a tissue, e.g. systemic, such as cardiac failure or local, such as isolated venous obstruction. The affected tissue is of bluish-red color (cyanosis) due to deoxygenated blood.

Hemorrhage

11. What is hemorrhage?

Ans. DEF: Extravasation of blood due to rupture of a blood vessel.
Epistaxis = hemorrhage from nose. Hematemesis = blood in vomitus. Common cause: stomach ulcer, ruptured esophageal varices secondary to portal hypertension. Hemoptysis = presence of blood in sputum. Common causes: bronchitis, bronchiectasis, pulmonary TB, pulmonary neoplasms, mitral stenosis. Melena = presence of dark-digested (blackish in color) blood in feces. Common cause: duodenal ulcer. Petechia = minute hemorrhages into skin, mucus membranes or serosal surfaces. Purpura = slightly larger hemorrhages than petechia. Hematoma= accumulation of blood into a tissue. Ecchymoses = accumulation of blood in subcutaneous tissue.

Thrombosis

12. What is thrombosis?

Ans. It is **pathologic blood clotting** with formation of blood clot **in an unbroken blood vessel** with several pathologic consequences as opposed to **hemostasis** which is **physiologic blood clotting** with formation of blood clot **in a broken blood vessel** to prevent bleeding.

13. How does our body achieve physiologic clotting?

Ans. *Physiologic clotting is achieved by a well-balanced system between 2 sets of factors:*

A. Facilitate clotting.

B. Inhibit clotting.

14. What are the phases of physiologic clotting?

Ans. It has four phases:

1. Vasoconstriction.
2. Primary hemostasis.
3. Secondary hemostasis.
4. Thrombolysis.

1. *Vasoconstriction:* Neurogenic and by endothelin from endothelial cells.
2. *Primary hemostasis (plug formation):* Exposed subendothelial extracellular matrix (ECM) of the broken blood vessel (BV) attracts platelets which **adhere** to ECM with the help of **von Willebrand factor**, change shape and secrete thromboxane A2 (TXA_2) which attract more platelets resulting in their **aggregation** with formation of a plug at the broken site of BV.
3. *Secondary hemostasis (fibrin clot formation):* Its components are coagulation factors which are plasma proteins which circulate in blood in inactive form and get serially activated when needed as described below. These are: Factor I (fibrinogen, made in liver), Factor II (prothrombin, made in liver) (IIa is called thrombin), Factor III (tissue thromboplastin derived from injured tissue), Factor IV (calcium), Factor V (proaccelerin, made in liver), Factor VI (activated factor V), Factor VII (proconvertin made in liver), Factor VIII (antihemophilic factor made by endothelial cells), Factor IX (Christmas factor made by liver), Factor X (Stuart-Prower factor made by liver), Factor XI (plasma thromboplastin antecedent made by liver). Factor XII (Hageman factor made by liver), Factor XIII (fibrin-stabilizing factor made by platelets). **Factors II, VII, IX and X synthesis requires vit K by the liver**. Coagulation pathway is activated. Two pathways are involved:
   A. Intrinsic pathway activated by platelet factor 3.
   B. Extrinsic pathway activated by tissue factor from injured tissue.
   Both pathways meet at Factor X. Intrinsic arrives here through serial activation of Factor XII, XI, IX, VIII; and, extrinsic through activation of Factor VII. Thereafter the pathway is common with activation of factor X, V, II and I with formation of fibrin which forms a meshwork at the site of the plug.
4. *Thrombolysis:* This formed clot has to be confined to the site of injury and later dissolves to maintain free circulation.
   This is achieved by: **TAP**
   A. **T**issue plasminogen activator (tPA) from endothelial cells breaks fibrin causing dissolution of clot. **(It is therapeutically used for this purpose in acute myocardial infarction)**.
   B. **A**ntithrombin III binds with heparin-like molecule on endothelial surface and inactivates IIa, XIIa, IXa, XIa, Xa.
   C. **P**roteins C and S inhibit clotting by inactivating factors Va and VIIa.
   All these coagulation factors (plasminogen, antithrombin III, proteins C and S) are made by the liver.

15. What are the predisposing factors of pathologic clotting (thrombosis)? What is Virchow's triad?

Ans. Predisposing conditions to thrombus formation: **Virchow's triad:** **ABC**

A. **A**ttacked (injured) surfaces (endothelial or endocardial).
B. **B**lood flow disturbances (stasis or turbulence).
C. **C**oagulation defects.

A. *Endothelial injury:* This is the main predisposing condition. Particularly important in thrombus formation in heart and arterial circulation:

1. Myocardial infarction.
2. Valvulitis.
3. Ulcerated plaques in severe atherosclerosis.
4. Hypertension.
5. Scarred valves.
6. Bacterial endocarditis.
7. Cigarette smoke.

   Endothelial/endocardial injury causes exposure of the underlying collagen with adherence of platelets and release of tissue factor leading to clotting.

B. *Alteration in normal blood flow:* Turbulence: contributes by:

1. Causing endothelial injury.
2. Forming counter currents.
3. Forming stasis. Stasis is the dominant factor in development of venous thrombi. Seen in prolonged bed rest, immobilization, MI, AF, sickle cell anemia, polycythemia.

C. *Abnormal coagulation:*

a. *Genetic:* Factor V mutation, deficiency of antithrombin III, protein C or S.
   Factor V mutation makes it resistant to inactivation by protein C.

b. *Acquired:*

1. Cancer, e.g. acute promyelocytic leukemia, pancreas cancer.
2. Tissue injuries.
3. DIC.
4. Lupus anticoagulant.
5. Increased estrogen, oral contraceptives.
6. Nephrotic syndrome.
7. Smoking.

16. How is the knowledge about clotting system in our body applied for therapeutic purpose?

Ans. 1. Tissue plasminogen activator (tPA) from endothelial cells breaks fibrin causing dissolution of clot. Therefore, it is used for this purpose in acute myocardial infarction.

2. Heparin-like molecule on the endothelial surface binds with antithrombin III and inactivates clotting factors IIa, XIIa, XIa, IXa, Xa. Therefore, heparin is used as an anticoagulant.
3. Vit. K is necessary for the liver to make clotting factors II, VII, IX and X. Therefore, drugs which interfere with vitamin K metabolism are used as oral anticoagulants.
4. Aspirin inhibits platelet production of TXA_2 thereby interferes in platelet aggregation. Therefore, aspirin is used in treatment and prevention of ischemic diseases of the cardiovascular system.

17. What is the morphology of thrombus?

Ans. Head of thrombus is made of platelets and fibrin. Tail is made of RBCs and fibrin. **Lines of Zahn** are alternating layers of fibrin, platelets and RBCs within the tail of thrombus. Thrombi can be small and partially block the flow of blood (mural thrombi) or large and completely block the flow of blood (occlusive thrombi), which are commonly seen in coronary arteries with myocardial infarction, cerebral with stroke, mesenteric with intestinal infarction.

18. What is the fate of thrombus?

Ans. **DOPE**

1. *Dissolution:* Fibrinolysis.
2. *Organization and recanalization:* Inflammation and fibrosis may occur (organization). Eventually a vascular channel may be re-established (recanalization).
3. *Propagation:* Collect more platelets and fibrin (propagate)-eventually obstructing some critical vessel.
4. *Embolization:* Detach from the site of origin-Dislodge-get transported in BV-get stuck at some other site.

19. What is mycotic aneurysm?

Ans. In large thrombi within aneurysmal dilations or cardiac chambers, instead of organization, center of thrombus undergoes enzymatic digestion (due to release of lysosomal enzymes from the WBCs and platelets) and if bacterial seeding occurs at the site, this degraded thrombus becomes an ideal culture medium and becomes infected and is called mycotic aneurysm.

20. What is migratory thrombophlebitis (Trousseau's syndrome)?

Ans. In cancers tumor-associated procoagulant release causes thrombosis at different sites in body which is known as migratory thrombophlebitis or Trousseau's syndrome.

Embolism

21. What is an embolus?

Ans. Embolus is a detached intravascular solid, liquid, or gaseous mass that is carried by the blood to a site distant from its point of origin. 99% of the emboli are dislodged thrombi. Hence, the term thromboembolism. Simply put, it is like a bullet. A bullet moves out of a place and lodges at a different place. Embolus does the same. A bullet can be made of metal, rubber or other substance. Similarly, an embolus can be made of blood, air, fluid, fat, etc. A bullet can be one large piece and make a big injury, even death, or several small pellets and make several small injuries. Similarly, an embolus can be large causing a big injury, even death, or several small pieces causing small areas of injuries (infractions).

22. What are the types of emboli?

Ans. Thrombus, fat, amniotic fluid, air, nitrogen, tumor, septic, etc.

23. What are the disorders due to an embolus?

Ans. Potential consequence of embolism is infarction of the tissue distal to it. Clinical outcome of thromboembolism depends on whether it lodges in pulmonary or systemic circulation. 95% arise from deep lower limb veins above knee. These occlude the pulmonary artery or lodge across the bifurcation of the pulmonary artery **(saddle embolus)** or pass into smaller branching arterioles. Often, they are multiple, recurrent emboli. In general, one pulmonary embolus is risk factor for future pulmonary emboli.

24. What is paradoxical embolism?

Ans. With ASD or VSD the venous embolus instead of following the normal path of circulation and going into lungs might go into systemic circulation.

25. What are some important points about pulmonary thromboembolism?

Ans.
1. Approximately 2/3rd of the pulmonary circulation obstruction results in **sudden death**, right heart failure, or cardiovascular shock.
2. Recurrent emboli in several months to years cause pulmonary hypertension and right heart failure.
3. Majority of pulmonary emboli are clinically silent.

26. What is systemic thromboembolism?

Ans. Embolism in arterial circulation.

Origin: 1. Majority are intracardiac mural thrombi.

2. Some are from atherosclerotic plaque or cardiac valve vegetations. Most of these get stuck in lower limbs. Other in brain, intestine, kidneys, spleen.

27. What is FAT embolism?

Ans. From fracture of a large bone. Only very few of these have clinical findings consisting of pulmonary insufficiency, neurologic symptoms which appear 1–3 days after injury with sudden onset of dyspnea, and tachycardia, irritability, restlessness.

PATHOG: Due to both mechanical obstruction and toxic injury.

PROG: Causes death in approximately 1 in 10 patients.

28. What is air embolism?

Ans.
1. *Chest wall injury:* More than 100 ml air is required to produce clinical effect.
2. Obstetric procedure.
3. *Decompression sickness:* Sudden changes in atmospheric pressure seen in cases such as deep sea divers, under water construction workers.

29. What is amniotic fluid embolism?

Ans. *Cause:* Tear in placental membrane and rupture of uterine veins. *S/S*: Sudden onset of SOB (shortness of breath), cyanosis, shock. Findings: In lungs: squamous cells, from fetal skin, lanugo hair, fat from vernix caseosa, pulmonary edema, DIC.

30. What is ischemia? What are some of the common causes of ischemia?

Ans. Reduced blood supply to an organ or part of the body. (Greek-Isch = restriction, hemia = blood, restricted blood supply).

Some of the common causes of ischemia are:

Low blood volume (due to hemorrhage, dehydration), decreased circulation, e.g. congestive cardiac failure (CCF), or thickening of the blood vessels (atherosclerosis), blockage of the blood vessels either internal, e.g. thrombosis, embolism or external from compression from various causes such as mass of a neoplasm or inflammatory mass or torsion of an organ, etc.

Infarction

31. What is infarction?

Ans. *DEF:* Area of ischemic necrosis caused by occlusion of either arterial supply or the venous drainage in a particular tissue, e.g. MI, CVA, pulmonary, bowel, limbs. 99% infarcts are from thrombotic/embolic events and almost all are from arterial occlusion.

Types: 1. Red-hemorrhagic.

2. White-anemic.

1. *Red:* Seen in tissues with dual circulation, e.g. lungs, small intestine, or with venous occlusion, e.g. ovarian or testicular torsion.
2. *White:* Occurs with arterial occlusion and in solid organs, e.g. heart, kidneys, spleen.

   MORPHO: GROSS: Infarcted area is wedge-shaped.

   MICRO: 1. *Coagulative:* Faint outline of the tissue visible.

   2. *Liquefactive:* Outline of the tissue is not visible.

Shock

32. What is shock?

Ans. *DEF:* Systemic hypoperfusion, due to reduction in cardiac output or **in effective** circulating blood volume resulting in hypotension, decreased tissue perfusion, and cellular hypoxia. Initially hypoxic and metabolic effects of hypoperfusion cause reversible cellular injury, persistence of shock eventually causes irreversible cellular injury and can result in **death** of patient. Therefore, early recognition and treatment is crucial.

33. What are the types of shock?

Ans. 1. Hypovolemic.
2. Circulatory.
3. Distributive.
   a. Septic.
   b. Neurogenic.
   c. Anaphylactic.
   d. Heat stroke (shock).

1. *Hypovolemic:* E.g. from hemorrhage due to various causes, dehydration from excessive sweating, vomiting, diarrhea, severe burns.
2. *Circulatory:* Due to myocardial pump failure. Causes: Myocardial infarction (MI), arrhythmia, pericarditis. Or obstruction by a thrombus or embolus in the circulation, e.g. large pulmonary embolus.
3. *Distributive:* Widespread vasodilation causes a sudden increase in capacity of vascular bed, which cannot be filled adequately by the normal circulating blood volume. Thus, tissue hypoperfusion and cellular anoxia result.
   a. *Septic:* Mostly due to gram –ve sepsis (endotoxic shock). But, can occur with gram +ve and fungal infections. Endotoxins are bacterial wall lipopolysaccharides (LPS), which induce inflammatory events with release of cytokines which cause systemic vasodilation (hypotension), diminished myocardial contractility, generalised endothelial injury with activation of coagulation system leading DIC.
   b. *Neurogenic:* Due to spinal cord injury—causing loss of vascular tone and peripheral pooling of blood.
   c. *Anaphylactic:* IgE-mediated hypersensitivity response—associated with systemic vasodilation and increased vascular permeability.
   d. *Heat stroke (shock):* Due to peripheral vasodilation with peripheral pooling of blood and decreased effective circulating blood volume.

34. What are the stages of shock?

Ans. 1. Compensatory stage.
2. Progressive stage.
3. Irreversible stage.

1. *Compensatory stage:* Neurohumoral mechanisms help maintain cardiac output (CO) and blood pressure (BP) as normal. This results in **tachycardia**, peripheral vasoconstriction, renal conservation of fluid. Skin vasoconstriction causes **coolness and pallor of skin. (In septic shock due to vasodilation skin may feel warm and flushed)**. Coronary and cerebral vessels are less responsive to above mechanisms and hence maintain their blood flow.
2. *Progressive stage:* In this there is severe generalized hypoxia causing anaerobic glycolysis thereby lactic acidosis, arteriolar dilation with pooling of blood in

them and reduction in cardiac output, fall in blood pressure and reduction in urine output. Hypoxia to brain causes confusion. Also, endothelial cells become exposed to injury with risk of developing DIC.

3. *Irreversible stage:* Lysosomal enzyme leakage from generalized cell injury leads to irreversible shock with acute tubular necrosis and complete renal function failure **with almost inevitable death**.

   MORPHO: Brain, heart, kidneys, lungs, GIT, liver show focal ischemic necrosis.

DIC

35. What is disseminated intravascular coagulation (DIC) (consumption coagulopathy)?

Ans. DIC is not a disease; but, a potential complication of any condition associated with widespread activation of thrombin. This causes generalized formation of microscopic fibrin thrombi in the microcirculation and generalized circulatory insufficiency. Due to the development of multiple thrombi there is rapid consumption of platelets and coagulation proteins. Hence, the term consumption coagulopathy. Simultaneously, fibrinolytic mechanisms are activated. So, the initial thrombotic disorder ends as a serious bleeding disorder.

Causes:

1. ***D:*** Delivery-related: Amniotic fluid embolism, septic abortion, retained dead fetus, toxemia, abruptio placenta.
2. ***I:*** Infections: Septicemia, meningococcemia.
3. ***C:*** Cancer: Acute promyelocytic leukemia, carcinoma of lung, pancreas, prostate, stomach.
4. Miscellaneous: Severe trauma, shock.

C/Fs: Presentation is usually bleeding-related in acute DIC, which is commonly due to above delivery-related problems. Whereas, usually it is thrombosis-related in chronic DIC, which is commonly due to cancers.

The usual *C/Fs* are: Renal failure with shock; nervous system failure with coma; cardiopulmonary failure with dyspnea, cyanosis, shock; mechanical hemolytic anemia due to many thrombi in small blood vessels.

6 Genetic and Congenital Diseases

OVERVIEW

1. Definitions and nomenclature.
2. Genetic diseases.
3. Congenital diseases.

Genetic diseases are diseases due to abnormalities of the chromosome or the gene.

Congenital diseases are diseases which are present at birth.

Unit of a gene is a **nitrogenous base:** Purine (adenine and guanine) and pyrimidine (cytosine and thymine–uracil in RNA). One purine nitrogenous base paired with one pyrimidine nitrogenous base makes a **base pair**. Many base pairs together make a **gene** (approximately 50,000 in one person). Many genes together make a **DNA**. One DNA wrapped in some protein makes one **chromosome**. Humans have 46 chromosomes (23 pairs, one of each pair from each parent). 22 pairs are **autosomes** and one pair is **sex chromosome** (XX for female and XY for male). So, each gene is in a pair (one from each parent), (except XY in male).

Genetic diseases can be due to various abnormalities of the chromosomes or due to mutation (permanent change) of the gene. When mutation is of one of the pair of the gene (genotype) and it results in a structural or functional body defect (phenotype) it is known as **dominant gene**. Whereas, when mutation is necessary in both the pairs of the gene for phenotypic effect, then the gene is known as **recessive gene**.

Chromosomal abnormalities can be of the 22 autosomes or of the X or Y sex chromosomes. These abnormalities can be either of **number** (increased or decreased) or **structure** (addition, deletion or configuration change) of the chromosomes.

Congenital diseases can be due to various known causes such as genetic, teratogenic agents or due to unknown causes.

Genetic diseases can be classified as:

1. *Chromosomal disorders:*
   - I. *Hereditary disorders:* E.g. Down syndrome with Robertsonian translocation.
   - II. *Non-hereditary disorders* (due to abnormalities during gametogenesis).
     - A. Autosomal numerical.
     - B. Sex (X or Y) chromosomal numerical.
     - C. Autosomal structural.

2. *Genic disorders:*
   I. *Mendelian:*
      a. Autosomal dominant.
      b. Autosomal recessive.
      c. X dominant.
      d. X recessive.
   II. *Non-mendelian:*
      a. Genomic imprinting (not inherited, due to abnormalities during gametogenesis).
      b. Mitochondrial gene.
      c. Triplet nucleotide repeat mutations.
   III. Gene + environment (multifactorial, polygenic, familial).
   IV. Somatic cells genes (after birth–mostly neoplastic effects).

Congenital diseases can be classified as:

1. Genetic (as above, except some genetic diseases are not congenital, e.g. Huntington's disease).
2. Environmental (in utero)
3. Unknown.

1. What do you understand by the term congenital diseases?

Ans. Diseases present at the time of birth.

2. What do you understand by the term genetic diseases?

Ans. Diseases due to the disorders of the chromosomes or genes. Congenital disease can be genetic or **not (e.g. develop during embryogenesis)**. Genetic diseases can be congenital or **not (e.g. Huntington's disease, adult cystic kidney disease)**.

3. What do you understand by these terms related to the gene: Nitrogenous bases, nucleoside, nucleotide, base pair, codon, anticodon, gene, genome, DNA, gene mutation?

Ans. *Nitrogenous bases:* Purine (adenine, guanine); pyrimidine (cytosine, thymine—uracil in RNA).

Nucleoside: Nitrogen base with sugar (deoxyribose in DNA, ribose in RNA).

Nucleotide: Nucleoside + phosphate.

Base pair: 1 purine base paired (bounded by H) with 1 pyrimidine base (approximately 3 billion in a person).

Codon: 3 nucleotide base pairs together made from DNA as template.

Anticodon: 3 nucleotide base pairs brought together by tRNA for transcription–reciprocal to codon.

Gene: Many base pairs make 1 gene (approx. 50,000 in 1 person).

Genome: All genes in 1 person.

DNA: Many genes together.

Gene mutation: Permanent change in a gene.

4. What do you understand by these terms related to the chromosome: chromosome, karyotype, centromere, isochromosome, deletion, inversion, translocation, robertsonian translocation, ring chromosome, band of a chromosome, region of a chromosome, haploid (n), diploid (2n), polyploidy, euploid, aneuploid, trisomy, monosomy, mosaicism, chimera, nondisjunction?

Ans. *Chromosome:* 1 DNA wrapped in some protein.

Karyotype: In humans, 46 chromosomes (22 pairs + XX in females, 22 pairs + XY in males).

Centromere: A constricted part of the chromosome. The part of the chromosome on each side of the centromere is called an arm. During division, the chromosome normally divides vertically into two chromatids. These chromatids are held together at the centromere. Depending on the site of location of the centromere chromosomes have different terms:

Metacentric chromosome: Chromosome whose centromere is located in the middle of a chromosome with arms on each side of the centromere being equal.

Submetacentric centromere: It is located off-centre with one arm being short than the other.

Acrocentric centromere: It is located near one end of chromosome with one arm being very short than the other.

Isochromosome: When centromere divides horizontally instead of vertically leaving 2 short arms only or 2 long arms only, e.g. i(Xq).
Deletion: Loss of a portion of a chromosome, e.g. Cry-du-chat (deletion of short arm of 5 chromosome).
Inversion: When there are 2 interstitial breaks in a chromosome and the broken segment reunites after a complete turnaround.
Translocation: When chromosomal segments are exchanged between nonhomologous chromosomes, e.g. in translocation type of Down's syndrome a segment from long arm of chromosome 14 is translocated to long arm of chromosome 21 and vice versa. It is written as: "t" followed by the involved chromosomes in numerical order within parenthesis (bracket), e.g. for translocation type of Down's syndrome: t(14q;21q).
Robertsonian translocation: When the exchange is equal between the two chromosomes.
Ring chromosome: A variant of deletion: After loss of segments from each end of the chromosome, the arms unite to from a ring.
Band of a chromosome: Part of chromosome distinguishable from adjacent parts by lighter or darker staining.
Region of a chromosome: An area of chromosome lying between 2 adjacent landmarks. Chromosome landmark is a constant and distinct morphologic feature that helps to identify a specific chromosome.
Haploid (n): Number of chromosomes in a gamete (sex cell) is 23 and this is the haploid no.(n).
Diploid (2n): 46 is called diploid number (as it is double of 23).
Polyploidy: Euploid condition beyond diploid, e.g. 69 ($3n$-triploid), 92 ($4n$-tetraploid), etc.
Euploid: An exact multiple of haploid is euploid number, e.g. 46, 69, 92, etc.
Aneuploid: A chromosome number that is not exact multiple of 23 is called aneuploid, e.g. Down syndrome with 47 chromosomes, Turner's syndrome with 45 chromosomes.
Trisomy: An aneuploid state in which a third chromosome is present in addition to the normal autosomal pair (as in Down syndrome) is called trisomy.
Monosomy: Absence of one chromosome of a pair is called monosomy, e.g. monosomy for X chromosome in Turner's syndrome. Trisomy and monosomy occur due to non-disjunction of chromosomes during gametogenesis.
Mosaicism: More than one populations of cells are present, where some have normal number of chromosomes and others have increased or decreased number of chromosomes. This happens due to nondisjunction of chromosomes during mitosis in the zygote.
Chimera: More than one cell population derived from different zygotes. (This term is derived from a mythological animal whose head was of a lion, body of a goat and tail of a snake).
Nondisjunction: Failure of disjoining of a homologous pair of chromosomes during meiosis.

5. What do these genetic "shorthand" terms mean: p, q, –, +, t, q31, p14, 46, XX, t(2;5)(q31, p14)?

Ans. "p" = Short arm of chromosome (p for petit). "q" = Long arm of chromosome. – / + = Absence or addition of a whole chromosome is indicated by a [–] or a [+] sign respectively before the number of that chromosome, e.g. 47 + 21. Decrease or increase in length of a chromosome is indicated by a [–] or a [+] sign respectively after the number of that chromosome, e.g. a short arm deletion of chromosome number 5 is: 5p–. "t" = Translocation. q31 = Long arm/region 3/b and 1. p14 = short arm/region 1/band 4. 46, XX, t(2;5)(q31,p14) = Reciprocal translocation involving the: long arm (q) of chromosome 2, region 3, band 1 and short arm (p) of chromosome 5, region 1, band 4.

6. What do these terms mean: mutation, missense, nonsense, frameshift, point mutation penetrance, expressivity, polymorphism, pleiotropy, genetic heterogeneity, Mendel's laws, autosomal dominant, autosomal recessive, X-dominant, X-recessive, codominance?

Ans. ***Mutation:*** Permanent change in a gene.

Missense: Muted gene codes for a different protein than normal.

Nonsense: Muted gene codes which results in early termination.

Frameshift: Muted gene codes for an abnormal short protein.

Point mutation: One single nucleotide is substituted for another, e.g. substitution of GUA or GUG of valine for GAA or GAG of glutamic acid at the 6th position of beta globulin chains of hemoglobin in sickle cell anemia.

Penetrance: Percentage of persons with an autosomal dominant gene showing the trait.

Expressivity: Different expressions of autosomal dominant trait in affected persons.

Polymorphism: Many allelic forms of a single gene.

Pleiotropy: Many phenotypic end-effects of a single mutant gene.

Genetic heterogeneity: Different mutant genes showing one end-effect (trait).

Mendel's laws: Single gene mutations inherited as autosomal dominant or recessive, sex dominant or recessive.

Autosomal dominant: Gene located on one of the 22 pairs of autosome chromosomes manifests in heterozygous state.

Autosomal recessive: Gene located on one of the 22 pairs of autosome chromosomes manifests in homozygous state.

X-dominant: Gene located on one of the 2X chromosomes manifests in heterozygous state.

X-recessive: Gene located on the 2X chromosomes manifests in homozygous state.

Codominance: Both alleles of a gene pair are expressed fully, e.g. blood groups such as blood group AB.

7. What is a Punnett square?

Ans. Punnett square is used to visualize the chances of inheriting a particular gene. Using G for a healthy gene and g for an affected recessive gene, the Punnett square shows which offspring are likely to inherit two healthy genes, which offspring are likely to be carriers of the gene, and which are likely to have the disorder caused by the defective gene.

8. Classify genetic diseases.

Ans. 1. *Chromosomal disorders:*

I. *Hereditary:* Down syndrome with 21 to 14 or 22 Robertsonian translocation.

II. *Non-hereditary (due to abnormalities during gametogenesis):*

A. Autosomal numerical
- a. Trisomy 21 (Down syndrome).
- b. Trisomy 18 (Edward syndrome).
- c. Trisomy 13 (Patau syndrome).

B. Sex (X or Y) chromosomal numerical
- a. 47, XXY (Klinefelter syndrome).
- b. 47, XYY Males.
- c. 45, XO (Turner's syndrome).

C. Autosomal structural
- a. Cri-du-chat syndrome (deletion of part of the short arm of chromosome 5).

2. *Genic disorders:*

I. *Mendelian (due to disorders of one gene, monogenic, nuclear gene):*
- a. Autosomal dominant disorders.
- b. Autosomal recessive disorders.
- c. X Dominant disorders.
- d. X Recessive disorders.

II. *Non-mendelian monogenic:*
- a. Genomic imprinting (not inherited, due to abnormalities during gametogenesis).
- b. Triplet nucleotide repeat mutations.
- c. Mitochondrial gene.

III. Genes + environment (multifactorial, polygenic, familial).

IV. Somatic cells genes *(after birth, mostly neoplastic cells).*

9. Classify congenital diseases.

Ans. 1. Genetic (as above, *except* some genetic diseases are not congenital, e.g. Huntington's diseases and somatic cell gene mutations).

2. Non-genetic (due to physical, chemical, microbiological environmental factors during development in the uterus).
3. Unknown causes.

10. What are the hereditary diseases due to disorders of the chromosomes?

Ans. Most chromosomal disorders are due to de novo (new) changes, i.e. during *gametogenesis* in normal parents. Therefore, risk of recurrence in siblings is low. One example of inherited chromosomal disorder is the *Down syndrome due to robertsonian translocation.* This is seen in approximately 4% of Down syndrome. Extra 21 chromosomal material is not present as an extra chromosome numerically; but, as a translocation of long arm of 21 chromosome on chromosome 14 or 22. This is transmitted either from father or mother, who would have chromosome count of 45; but, chromosomal material of 46 due to long arm of chromosome 21 attached to chromosome 14 or 22. Therefore, he/she would be phenotypically normal. During gametogenesis his/her one of the gametes will get numerically 23 chromosomes (with chromosomal material of 24), which will unite with opposite gamete consisting of chromosome 23 resulting in total chromosomal material of 47 leading to Down syndrome.

11. What is trisomy 21 (Down syndrome)?

Ans. Three 21 chromosomes or material of three 21 chromosomes instead of two. *C/Fs*: Upward slanting eyes, prominent epicanthal folds, simian crease, mental retardation, congenital heart disease, most common is VSD; increased susceptibility to acute leukemias, alzheimer's disease.

Types: 3 Types: 1. *Nondisjunction:* 95% of cases. An extra chromosome is present (47+21). **Parents are of normal karyotype**. Associated with increasing maternal age.

2. *Translocation:* 4% of cases. One of the two parents has an abnormal chromosome where one of the 21 chromosomes is attached to either chromosome 14 or 22. **The affected child has normal number of 46 chromosomes; but, either his chromosome 14 or 22 has an extra chromosome 21 attached to it. So, in effect he has a complement of three chromosomes 21**. This is not associated with increased maternal age; but, the **carrier parent can produce further children with same abnormality**.
3. *Mosaic:* 1% of cases.

12. What is trisomy 18 (Edward syndrome)?

Ans. Three 18 chromosomes instead of two. *C/Fs:* Mental retardation, prominent occiput, micrognathia, low set ears, short neck, overlapping fingers, congenital heart disease (VSD, ASD, PDA), rocker bottom feet. Life span is 2–3 months.

13. What is trisomy 13 (Patau syndrome)?

Ans. Three 13 chromosomes instead of two. *C/Fs:* Mental retardation, microcephaly, microphthalmia, cleft. Lip and palate, congenital heart disease (VSD, ASD, PDA, dextrocardia), renal malformations. Death is usually in neonatal period.

14. What is 47, XXY (Klinefelter syndrome)?

Ans. Defect consists of nondisjunction during meiosis either in the sperm or ovum resulting in either an ovum having 2 X chromosomes being fertilized by a normal sperm with one Y chromosome or a normal ovum having one X chromosome being fertilized by a sperm having both X and Y chromosomes.

C/Fs: Phenotype is male. Male hypogonadism (eunuchoid). Testis atrophied with sterility. Low serum testosterone because testes atrophied. Increased pituitary gonadotrophins in the absence of loss of feedback inhibition because testosterone low. Gynecomastia because testosterone low. Reduced facial and body hair because testosterone low. Patient also has mental retardation.

15. What is 47, XYY males?

Ans. Defect is in the sperm. This defect happens during spermatogenesis during second meiotic division. Defect is nondisjunction resulting in both Y chromosomes going into one spermatozoon. When this sperm fertilizes the ovum there are 3 sex chromosomes: XYY.

C/Fs: Phenotype is male. These people are physically normal (but, may be tall). But, approximately 1% have behavioral problems, e.g. antisocial behavior.

16. What is 45, XO (Turner's syndrome)?

Ans. Defect is in the ovum. Defect is of the X chromosome. Defect is of more than one type:

1. One X chromosome is absent in all the cells of the affected person's body (45 XO karyotype). This is seen in approximately 1/2 of the cases.
2. One X chromosome is absent in only some of the cells of the affected person's body *(mosaics) (45 XO/46 XX). This is seen approximately in other 1/2 of the cases.*

C/Fs: Phenotype is female. Hypogonadism (ovaries are atrophied). External genitalia atrophied, short stature, primary amenorrhea, ovaries only as fibrous streaks without any follicles, low ovarian estrogen with elevated pituitary gonadotrophin, no breast, webbing of neck, cubitus vulgus (increased carrying angle of the elbow), widespread nipples, horseshoe-shaped kidney, coarctation of the aorta, CHF.

In mosaics variants (45 XO/XX): Body appearance may be normal and person might have only primary amenorrhea.

17. What is hermaphroditism?

Ans. One ovary and one testis. Karyotype: 50%XX, 25%XY, 25% 45 XO/46 XY.

18. What is pseudohermaphroditism?

Ans. *Female:* 46,XX ovaries and internal genitalia normal. External genitalia virilized due to increased androgens.

Male: 46,XY. Testis present. External genitalia like female due to decreased androgens.

19. What is deletion of short arm of chromosome 5 (cri du chat syndrome)?

Ans. Portion of short arm of chromosome 5 is lost. *C/Fs:* Affected children have high-pitched, cat-like cry, mental retardation, microcephaly and congenital heart defects.

20. What are general features of autosomal dominant disorders?

Ans. 1. Manifested in heterozygous state.
2. At least one of the parents is affected.
3. Both males and females are equally affected.
4. Both males and females can transmit it.
5. When an affected person marries an unaffected person, 1 in 2 children (50%) has the chance of getting the disease.
6. There may be low penetrance or variable expressivity.

21. What are general features of autosomal recessive disorders?

Ans. 1. Largest group of mendelian disorders.
2. Occur when *both* alleles at a given locus are mutants (one from each parent).
3. Both parents are heterozygote careers.
4. Siblings have 1 in 4 chance of having the disease, i.e. recurrence risk is 25% for each birth.
5. Males and females are affected equally.

22. What are the general features of X-linked dominant disorders?

Ans. Very few cases. Affected heterozygous female transmits to 50% of sons and daughters. *All males* transmit to *all* daughters and cannot transmit to sons. *Example:* Vitamin D-resistant rickets.

23. What are general features of X-linked recessive disorders?

Ans. 1. Gene is transmitted by mother.
2. Her 50% daughters are asymptomatic careers.
3. All her sons are affected. All his daughters are asymptomatic careers. All his sons are neither affected nor careers.

24. Give some examples of:
A. autosomal dominant disorders,
B. autosomal recessive disorders,
C. X-linked dominant disorders,
D. X-linked recessive disorders.

Ans. A. *Some of the autosomal dominant disorders:*
a. Marfan syndrome.
b. Hypercholesterolemia, familial.

c. Acute intermittent porphyria.
d. Hereditary spherocytosis.
e. von Willebrand disease.
f. Huntington disease (triplet repeat-CAG).
g. Neurofibromatosis types 1 and 2.
h. Tuberous sclerosis.
i. Hereditary nonpolyposis colorectal cancer.
j. Familial polyposis syndrome (Gardner's and Turcot's syndromes).
k. Peutz-Jegher's syndrome.
l. Adult polycystic kidney disease.
m. Nephroblastoma (Wilms' tumor).
n. Achondroplasia.
o. Osteogenesis imperfect.
p. Myotonic dystrophy (triplet repeat-CTG).
q. Hereditary hemorrhagic telangiectasia (Osler-Weber-Rendu syndrome).
r. von Hippel-Lindau disease.
s. Familial retinoblastoma.
t. Multiple endocrine neoplasia.

B. *Some of the autosomal recessive disorders:*

a. Mucopolysaccharidosis.
b. Phenylketonuria.
c. Glycogen storage diseases.
d. Cystic fibrosis.
e. Hereditary hemochromatosis.
f. Wilson disease.
g. Alpha 1-antitrypsin deficiency.
h. Homocystinuria.
i. Lysosome storage diseases (type II glycogen storage disease-Pompe disease, Tay-Sachs disease, Gaucher disease, Niemann-Pick disease, Hurler disease).
j. Sickle cell anemia.
k. Thalassemias.
l. Friedrich ataxia (spinocerebellar degeneration-triplet repeat-GAA).
m. Childhood polycystic kidney disease.
n. Neurogenic muscular atrophies.
o. Spinal muscular atrophy.
p. Galactosemia.
q. Alkaptonuria.
r. Chronic granulomatous disease (cytoplasmic NADPH oxidase deficiency).
s. Cockayne syndrome.

t. Xeroderma pigmentosum.
u. Ataxia telangiectasia.
v. Bloom syndrome
w. Fanconi syndrome.
x. Albinism.
y. Abetalipoproteinemia.

C. *Some of the X-linked dominant disorders:*
a. Vitamin D-resistant rickets.

D. *Some of the X-linked recessive disorders:*
a. Type II mucopolysaccharidosis (Hunter's syndrome).
b. Lesch-Nyhan syndrome.
c. Wiskott-Aldrich syndrome.
d. Agammaglobulinemia.
e. Chronic granulomatous disease (membrane NADPH oxidase deficiency).
f. G-6-P D deficiency.
g. Hemophilia A and B.
h. Duchenne muscular dystrophy.
i. Becker muscular dystrophy.
j. Fragile X syndrome, triplet repeat-CGG.
k. Diabetes insipidus.
l. X-linked spinal muscular atrophy.

25. What is Marfan syndrome?

Ans. *DEF/DES:* Autosomal dominant disease. Defect of fibrillin. Leads to qualitative and quantitative disorder of the connective tissue of the whole body mainly affecting eyes (dislocation of lens, long eyeballs with susceptibility to retinal detachment); CVS (aortic aneurysm, aortic dissection, loose mitral and tricuspid valves, CCF). Skeletal system (long legs, arms, fingers).

26. What is Ehlers-Danlos syndrome?

Ans. Autosomal dominant disease. Defect in collagen. *C/Fs:* Skin is hyperextensible and fragile. Joints are hypermobile. Susceptibility to rupture of colon and large arteries, eyes are fragile with susceptibility to corneal rupture and retinal detachment, susceptibility to diaphragmatic hernia.

27. What is myotonic dystrophy (MD)?

Ans. Autosomal dominant. There is a triplet repeat mutation. Defect is in muscle spindles with fiber splitting, necrosis and degeneration. *C/Fs:* Abnormalities of gait due to weakness in foot dorsiflexor. Myotonia (Sustained involuntary contraction of a group of muscles is the main symptom). Other features are: cataract, frontal balding, gonadal atrophy, cardiomyopathy.

28. What is neurofibromatosis type I?

Ans. Autosomal dominant. *C/Fs:* Neurofibromas, optic nerve gliomas, meningiomas, pigmented nodules of iris *(Lisch nodules)*, cutaneous hyperpigmented macules *(cafe-au-lait spots)*.

29. What is neurofibromatosis type II?

Ans. Autosomal dominant. VIII cranial nerve schwannomas bilaterally, multiple meningiomas.

30. What is tuberous sclerosis?

Ans. Autosomal dominant. Cerebral cortical tubers (hamartomas made of neural and glial cells), angiofibromas, seizures, mental retardation, renal angiomyolipomas, cardiac rhabdomyomas.

31. What is hypercholestrolemia, familial?

Ans. Autosomal dominant. Gene responsible for production of receptors on cells for the LDL (low-density lipoprotein) is affected with increase in LDL cholesterol in blood with increased incidence of atherosclerosis and its complications, e.g. myocardial ischemia and infarction.

32. What is acute intermittent porphyria?

Ans. Autosomal dominant. Enzyme involving biosynthesis of heme is affected with overproduction of intermediate compounds (porphyrins), which are toxic leading to mainly 3 patterns of symptoms:

a. Neurovisceral b. Photosensitive c. Hemolytic anemia.

33. What is phenylketonuria?

Ans. Autosomal recessive. One of the errors of amino acid metabolism. Defective enzyme is phenylalanine hydroxylase with accumulation of phenylalanine leading to mental retardation of the newborns; avoiding phenylalanine in diet prevents this.

34. What is alkaptonuria?

Ans. Autosomal recessive. One of the errors of amino acid metabolism. Defective enzyme is homogentisic oxidase with accumulation of homogentisic acid, which binds to connective tissue and cartilage (nose, ears, cheek) making them blue-black in color *(ochronosis)* and less resilient causing arthropathy; usually affecting vertebral, shoulder, hip and knee joints.

35. What is albinism?

Ans. Autosomal recessive. One of the errors of amino acid metabolism. Tyrosinase is defective with deficiency of melanin in skin, eyes leading to photophobia, strabismus, nystagmus, decreased visual acuity, increased incidence of squamous cell carcinoma.

36. What is maple syrup urine disease?

Ans. Autosomal recessive. One of the errors of amino acid metabolism. Ketoacid oxidase is deficient affecting leucine, valine, isoleucine leading to mental retardation and urine smells like maple syrup.

37. What is homocystinuria type I?

Ans. Autosomal recessive. One of the errors of amino acid metabolism. Cystathionine is the defective enzyme. Homocystine is excreted in urine. Patients have learning difficulties, Marfan-like syndrome, thrombotic episodes.

38. What are glycogen storage diseases?

Ans. a. *Type I (von Gierke's disease):* Defective enzyme is glucose-6-phosphatase: Hepatomegaly, hypoglycemia with seizure episodes, hyperlipidemia, failure to thrive, 50% mortality in early childhood.

b. *Type II (Pompe's disease) (lysosomal storage disease):* Defective enzyme is lysosomal alpha glucosidase. *C/Fs*: Affects all organs of our body, mainly heart, brain and skeletal muscles with cardiomegaly, neurologic impairment and muscle weakness. Death occurs by 2 years of age, mainly due to heart failure.

c. *Type III:* Defective enzymes are glycogen debranching enzymes. *C/Fs:* Mild hepatomegaly, hypoglycemia, growth retardation.

d. *Type IV:* Defective enzymes are branching enzymes. *C/Fs:* Affects all organs, mainly liver with cirrhosis. Death occurs by 3 years of age.

e. *Type V (Mc Ardle's disease):* Defective enzyme is striated muscle phosphorylase. *C/Fs:* Mild muscle weakness.

39. What are lysosomal storage diseases?

Ans. a. *Gaucher's disease (sphingolipidoses):* Beta glucosidase is deficient resulting in storage of glucosylceramide in lysosomes of macrophages of liver, spleen, bone marrow, lymph nodes. **Gaucher cells** (macrophages with stored glucosylceramide) are seen in liver, spleen, marrow and lymph nodes. These show by *LM:* Fibrillary cytoplasm **(wrinkled tissue paper-like appearance)**, by *EM:* Linear stacks. There are 2 forms: Infantile and adult. There is hepatosplenomegaly, pancytopenia, fractures.

b. *Niemann-pick disease (Sphingolipidoses):* Deficient enzyme is sphingomyelinase with storage of sphingomyelin in cells which show by *LM:* **Foamy cytoplasm**, by *EM:* **Zebra bodies** (parallel lamellas). Tissues affected are brain, liver, spleen.

c. *Tay-Sachs disease (sphingolipidoses):* Hexosaminidases is deficient resulting in storage of ganglioside GM2 in lysosomes of neurons and macrophages. These show by *LM:* **Foamy cytoplasm**, by *EM*: **Whorled distended lysosomes**. Clinically, patient has **cherry red spots on retina**, blindness, mental retardation, seizures.

d. *Hurler's syndrome (MPS 1-mucopolysaccharidoses I):* Inheritance is autosomal recessive. Defective enzyme is L-iduronidase with storage of mucopolysaccharides heparan and dermatan sulfate. Tissues affected are: skin, cornea, bone, heart, brain, liver, spleen. *Results in* mental retardation, heart failure.

e. *Hunter's syndrome (MPS II):* X-linked recessive. (*see* below).

40. What is type II mucopolysaccharidosis-Hunter syndrome?

Ans. X-linked recessive. Defective enzyme is L-iduronate sulfatase.

41. What is fragile X syndrome?

Ans. X-linked recessive. Mutation of a gene on the long arm of X chromosome. Mutation involves repetition of 3 nucleotides in a long sequence. This disrupts their function causing mental retardation of moderate to severe degree. **It is the second most common causes of familial mental retardation after Down syndrome**. The X chromosome breaks easily in vitro. Hence, it is called fragile X syndrome.

42. What is genomic imprinting?

Ans. *General features:* Not inherited like mendelian. Generally, inheriting an allele from the father or mother has the same effect because there is no structural differences between normal homologous paternal and maternal genes. However, expression of some genes depends on whether they are inherited from the father or the mother because there is functional difference between several paternal and maternal genes. These are due to epigenetic process called genomic imprinting. Epigenetic means: Phenotypic effect independent of genotype. This is due to DNA methylation that occurs during gametogenesis which can affect gene expression in zygotic cells. Paternal imprinting means paternal gene is inactivated. Maternal imprinting means maternal gene is inactivated. This can cause disorders. One example of this from each parent is:

1. *Prader-Willi syndrome:* (Maternal imprinting) **Gene on maternal chromosome 15 is imprinted (inactivated)**. Corresponding **paternal gene (allele) is deleted**. *C/Fs*: Mental retardation, hypogonadism, hypotonia.
2. *Angelman (happy puppet) syndrome:* (Paternal imprinting) **Gene on paternal chromosome 15 is imprinted (inactivated)**. Corresponding **maternal gene (allele) is deleted**. *C/Fs:* Mental retardation, seizures. Ataxic gait and inappropriate laughter (happy puppet).

43. What is triplet nucleotide repeat mutation? Give some examples of diseases caused by this.

Ans. Normally, nucleotide triplets may repeat for a few times. If this repeat increases for much more than normal times it disrupts the normal function of the gene. Usually, the repeat amplification becomes more prominent in each subsequent generation making the trait more pronounced.

Examples: 1. Fragile X syndrome, inheritance X-recessive (triplet involved-CGG).

2. Huntington disease, inheritance autosomal dominant (triplet involved-CAG).
3. Myotonic dystrophy, inheritance autosomal dominant (triplet involved-CTG).
4. Friedreich's ataxia, inheritance autosomal recessive (triplet involved-GAA).

44. What are mitochondrial gene mutation disorders?

Ans. Not inherited like mendelian. All inherited from mother (ovum) because sperms do not have mitochondria. ATP biosynthesis is hampered affecting organs with high ATP requirement like CNS, heart and skeletal muscles. Example-Leber hereditary optic atrophy.

45. What are multifactorial inheritance (polygenic-familial)?

Ans. Diseases due to disorders of genes (2 or more of small effect) plus environmental factors (familial diseases). Many of our traits like body height, intelligence do not follow classical rules of mendelian inheritance. These traits depend upon interaction of multiple genes (polygenic) with environmental factors. The degree of clinical symptoms is directly proportional to the number of mutant genes. Therefore, close relatives have a greater chance of developing symptoms as they have more mutant genes (familial). Risk for first-degree relative is approximately 2% and for identical twins is approximately 20%. *Examples of multifactorial inheritance are:*

1. Hypertension
2. Noninsulin-dependent diabetes mellitus (NIDDM).
3. Congenital heart diseases.
4. Cleft lip and cleft palate.
5. Gout.
6. Schizophrenia.
7. Breast tumors.
8. Atherosclerosis.
9. Congenital pyloric stenosis.
10. Neural tube defects (anencephaly, meningomyelocele, spina bifida).

46. What are some of the genetic disorders of the somatic cells?

Ans.
1. Philadelphia chromosome in CML: t (9;22).
2. Acute promyelocytic leukemia: t (15; 17).
3. Burkitt's lymphoma: t (8; 14).
4. Follicular lymphoma: t (14; 18).
5. Ewing's sarcoma: t (11; 22).

47. What are the environmental causes of congenital diseases?

Ans. A. Physical B. Chemical C. Microbiologic.

A. *Physical causes:*

1. Radiation (e.g. X-ray) during first trimester of pregnancy.

B. *Chemical causes:*

1. Maternal alcohol consumption: Alcohol consumption by mother during pregnancy causes **fetal alcohol syndrome** consisting of: growth retardation, abnormal facies, heart defects, mental retardation.
2. Maternal smoking: Causes growth retardation.
3. Maternal diabetes mellitus: Large baby, predisposition to development of hyaline membrane disease—HMD.
4. Maternal folate deficiency.
5. Maternal drug consumption:
   a. Aspirin (fetal kernicterus, neonatal hemorrhage).
   b. Busulphan.
   c. Cocaine (affects fetal neurologic development adversely).
   d. Dicoumarol—anticoagulants.
   e. Cyclophosphamide.
   f. Flagyl.
   g. Thalidomide—malformed limbs **(phacomelia)**.
   h. Retinoic acid.
   i. *DES*—High incidence of clear cell adenocarcinoma of vagina of the female baby.
   j. Antithyroid drugs **(goiter)**.
   k. Progestins (masculanization of female, e.g. hypertrophy of clitoris, fusion of labia, hypoplasia of uterus and vagina).
   l. Lithium (Ebstein's anomaly). (*see* page 174).
   m. Mercury.
6. Oxygen.
7. Antibodies from mother against fetal RBCs (Rh incompatibility).
8. Maternal iodine deficiency **(cretinism)**.

C. *Microbiologic causes:*

1. "TORCHS": Toxoplasmosis, rubella, cytomegalovirus, herpes, syphilis:

   Toxoplasmosis: Infection of the fetus in 3rd trimester: Mental retardation, microcephaly, hydrocephalus, chorioretinitis, dystrophic calcification of the brain.

   Rubella: During first trimester congenital heart disease (septal defects and PDA-patent ducuts arteriosus), cataract, glaucoma, deafness, microcephaly, mental retardation.

   Cytomegalovirus: Microcephaly, hydrocephalus, mental retardation, cerebral calcification, hepatosplenomegaly.

Herpes: Acquired in utero or at birth from birth canal infection: Viremia, encephalitis, conjunctivitis.

Herpes of the mother's birth canal is an absolute indication (i.e. a must) for delivery by cesarean section delivery.

Syphilis: Transplacental infection when mother has early active syphilis. Abnormal teeth **(Hutchinson's teeth)**, bone defects, nerve deafness, blindness from interstitial keratitis.

2. Gonorrhea: Conjunctivitis.
3. *Lymphogranuloma venereum:* Conjunctivitis.

48. What are some of the congenital diseases due to unknown causes?

Ans. 1. *CVS:* 90% of congenital heart diseases (only in 10% of congenital heart diseases contributing factors are known, e.g. due to maternal rubella in the 1st trimester, or chromosomal abnormalities, e.g. Turners syndrome (XO), or trisomy 13, 15, 18, 21.

2. *RS:* Tracheo-esophageal fistula.
3. *US:* Atresia of the urethra, valve formation in urethra or ureter, aberrant renal artery, renal ptosis.
4. *GIS:* Cleft lip, cleft palate, esophageal atresia, tracheoesophageal fistula, esophageal achalasia (megaesophagus-similar to megacolon). In small intestine: atresia or stenosis, Meckel's diverticulum, omphalocele. In large intestine-malrotation, Hirschprung disease (megacolon).
5. *CNS:* Vascular malformations of the nervous system (Arteriovenous malformations, cavernous angiomas, capillary telangiectasias, venous angiomas of meninges and spinal cord), Arnold-Chiari malformation, Dandy-Walker malformation, meningomyelocele, cyclopia, etc.
6. *ES:* Thyroglossal duct cyst.
7. *REP.S:* Hypospadias, epispadias, cryptorchidism.
8. *MSS:* Supernumerary digits (fingers or toes).

7

Environmental Diseases

OVERVIEW

1. Etiologic classification of environmental diseases.
2. Diseases due to physical causes.
3. Diseases due to physiochemical causes and chemical causes including nutritional causes.

Major categories of environmental diseases are due to physical, chemical, physiochemical and infectious causes.

Major types of physical causes are mechanical, thermal (high and low), electrical, radiation (ultraviolet and ionizing radiation), atmospheric pressure-related, and sound.

Major types of physiochemical diseases are pneumoconiosis, caused mostly by coal, asbestos, silica, etc.

Major types of chemical causes are natural, man-made and body-made.

Major causes of nutritional disorders are related to energy/calories, water, carbohydrates, fats, proteins, vitamins, and minerals.

Major types of infectious causes are prions, viruses, chlamydia, rickettsia, mycoplasma, bacteria, fungi, protozoa, and helminths.

1. What are the main categories of environmental diseases?

Ans. 1. Physical.
2. Chemical/physiochemical (pneumoconiosis).
3. Infectious.

Physical Injuries

2. What are the physical causes of diseases?

Ans. 1. Mechanical.
2. Thermal: High/low.
3. Electrical.
4. Radiation.
5. Pressure.

3. What are the mechanical injuries?

Ans. a. *Abrasion:* Wound with removal of only epidermal layer of skin or epithelial layer of internal tissue/organ.
b. *Contusion (bruise):* Blunt injury with damage to blood vessels with extravasation of blood into tissues.
c. *Laceration:* Blunt injury with tear of tissue with irregular edges.
d. *Incised wound:* Sharp instrument wound with smooth edges.
e. *Puncture wound:* Wound caused by a long narrow instrument.
f. *Penetrating wound:* Puncture wound which pierces the tissue.
g. *Perforating wound:* Puncture wound which goes through and through a tissue causing an exit wound also.
h. *Gunshot wound:* Entrance wound is smaller than the exit wound.

4. What are the thermal injuries?

Ans. 1. High 2. Low.

5. What are the high thermal injuries?

Ans. 1. Burns—1st, 2nd, 3rd degree.
2. Heat cramps.
3. Heat exhaustion.
4. Heat stroke (heat shock).

Burn, 1st degree: Involves epidermis only.
Burn, 2nd degree: Involves epidermis and superficial dermis.
Burn, 3rd degree: Involves epidermis, dermis and dermal appendages.

Heat cramps: Cramps of voluntary muscles due to loss of electrolytes due to sweating. Core body temperature is normal.

Heat exhaustion: Acute collapse due to water depletion hypovolemia which resolves within short time when CVS compensates for the hypovolemia.

Heat stroke (heat shock): Severe life-threatening heat injury due to failure of thermoregulatory mechanisms, cessation of sweating. Rise of core body temperature, generalized peripheral vasodilation with peripheral pooling of blood and decreased effective circulating blood volume. **Hence, can be called "heat shock" (author's term).**

6. What are the low thermal injuries (hypothermia)?

Ans. 1. Systemic effect of severe hypothermia consists of loss of consciousness, cardiac arrhythmias and death.

2. *Frost bite:* This is local effect of severe hypothermia consisting of vasoconstriction, ischemia, thrombosis and possibly gangrene of the affected parts, e.g. fingers, toes, etc.

7. What are the electrical injuries?

Ans. Electrical injury causes cardiac arrhythmias, cardiac arrest, respiratory arrest, and burns.

8. What are the radiation injuries?

Ans. a. *Ultraviolet light:* In acute mild cases causes sunburn with erythema and superficial desquamation. In acute severe cases causes blisters. In chronic cases causes **actinic keratosis**, which is a **premalignant** skin lesion; and malignant skin lesions such as **basal cell carcinoma**, **squamous cell carcinoma** and **melanoma**.

b. *Ionizing radiation: Terms:* Roentgen: Unit of radiation in air to which one is exposed. RAD (radiation-absorbed dose) unit of radiation absorbed by the tissue. Source could be X-ray, radioactive waste, nuclear accidents, etc. Radiation causes skin changes such as dermatitis, ulcers, malignancies; lung changes such as adult respiratory distress syndrome, septal fibrosis, hyaline thickening of blood vessels, bronchiolar metaplasia; gastrointestinal inflammation and ulcers, mucosal denudation; hematopoietic changes such as marrow depression, leukemia, acute marrow failure.

9. What are the atmospheric pressure-related injuries?

Ans. These are:

1. High altitude illness 2. Air embolism 3. Decompression (caisson) disease.

10. What is high altitude illness?

Ans. This happens to mountain climbers above 4000 meters altitude. The low oxygen tension at this altitude causes mental obtundation and increased capillary permeability with pulmonary and cerebral edema.

11. What is air embolism?

Ans. This can happen as a complication of hyperbaric oxygen therapy, positive-pressure ventilation, scuba diving. Increased intra-alveolar pressure causes entry of air into interstitium and small blood vessels and may lead to pulmonary, mediastinal and subcutaneous emphysema. Combining of small air bubbles in cerebral or coronary arteries may result in stroke or myocardial ischemia.

12. What is caisson (decompression) disease?

Ans. Caisson is a watertight chamber used in underwater construction work. There, due to increased atmospheric pressure oxygen and nitrogen dissolve in blood and tissues. When the caisson is brought up out of the water too fast this dissolved gas comes out of the blood and forms tiny bubbles in blood and tissues. These bubbles around the joints cause joint pains called **bends**, within lungs cause respiratory difficulties and substernal pain called **chokes**. Few days later embolic occlusion of the bones can cause **aseptic necrois of the heads of femur and humerus** called **caisson disease of the bone**.

Chemical Injuries

13. What are the chemical causes of injury?

Ans. Any chemical agent can cause injury depending upon the situation. These can be classified as follows:

A. Natural.

B. Body-made.

C. Man-made

A. *Natural:*

1. Nutritional deficiency or excess (calorie, proteins, fats, carbohydrates, vitamins, minerals, water).
2. Alcohol, tobacco, beetle nuts, venoms (snake, spider, scorpion, etc), cyanide, lead.

B. *Body-made:*

1. Chemical mediators of inflammation.
2. Products of metabolism (ammonia, bilirubin, urea, creatinne, uric acid, free radicals, etc).
3. Enzymes.
4. Hormones.

C. *Man-made:*

1. Drugs used in medicine (aspirin, acetaminophen, antibiotics, sulphonamides, chemotherapeutic-antineoplastic drugs).
2. Drugs used as substances of abuse.

3. Industrials or pollutants from industries, occupationals (asbestos, beryllium, coal, silica, carbon monoxide (CO), carbon tetrachloride CCl_4), insecticides, fungicides, herbicide, etc.), methyl alcohol, cocaine, heroine.

14. What are diseases caused by chronic alcoholism?

Ans. *Chronic alcoholism causes:* Hepatitis, cirrhosis, pancreatitis, gastritis, oral and esophageal carcinoma, vitamin B_1 (thiamine) deficiency causing cardiomyopathy **(wet beriberi)**, peripheral neuropathy **(dry beriberi)**, encephalopathy **(Wernicke-Korsakoff psychosis)**.

15. What is fetal alcohol syndrome?

Ans. *DEF:* This is a syndrome affecting babies of chronically alcoholic mother both before and after birth. *C/Fs*: Deficiency of growth before and after birth both mental and physical. Also, eyes and head are small.

16. What happens in arsenic poisoning?

Ans. Cancer of skin, liver, lung.

17. What happens in methyl alcohol (methanol) poisoning?

Ans. Causes metabolic acidosis due to formation of formaldehyde and formic acid. It causes **blindness** by damaging the cells of retina, optic nerve and CNS.

18. What are harmful effects of acute carbon monoxide (CO)?

Ans. *DEF/DES:* CO binds with hemoglobin with formation of carboxyhemoglobin. Carboxyhemoglobin causes decreased binding of the oxygen with the hemoglobin in the lungs (decreased formation of oxyhemoglobin) and decreased release of the hemoglobin-bound oxygen in the tissues (interference with oxygen dissociation—oxygen dissociation curve shifts to the left). CO is **colorless, tasteless and odorless resulting in acutely exposed unaware patient** loss of consciousness and **death within a very short time (minutes)**. Fatal cases show **cherry-red color of skin, blood, viscera, and muscles**.

19. What are harmful effects of carbon tetrachloride (CCl_4)?

Ans. Causes centrilobular necrosis and fatty change in the liver.

20. What are harmful effects of cocaine?

Ans. Causes mood changes consisting of elevation, irritability, anxiety, depression, which may lead to suicide; cardiac arrhythmias which could be fatal, hypertension which could cause cerebral hemorrhage; and with intranasal use—nasal congestion, ulceration, septal perforation; with intravenous use—HIV or hepatitis B infections, infective endocarditis, epiletic seizures, respiratory arrest, myocardial infarction; in newborns of addicted mothers—multiple small cerebral infarcts.

21. What are harmful effects of cyanide?

Ans. Causes death within minutes by stopping cellular oxidation due to inhibition of intracellular cytochrome oxidase. **Breath smells like bitter almond which is helpful in diagnosis.**

22. What happens in heroin poisoning?

Ans. Severe pulmonary edema. HIV, hepatitis B, infective endocarditis death from respiratory or cardiac arrest.

23. What happens in poisoning by lye?

Ans. When swallowed it causes damage to the wall of the esophagus causing scarring with formation of stricture.

24. What is plumbism?

Ans. *DEF:* Poisoning by lead is called plumbism. *DES:* Exposure is by ingestion from lead-containing paints or inhaled from car emissions. It results in: Hypochromic microcytic anemia, due to decreased heme synthesis mediated by inhibition of delta-aminolevulinic acid (ALA) dehydrase and by decreased incorporation of iron into heme.
C/Fs: Hypochromic microcytic anemia with **basophilic stippling of RBCs**, encephalopathy from edema, neuronal degeneration with delirium, coma and death, neuropathy from demyelination with wrist and foot drop, **Fanconi's syndrome** (glycosuria, aminoaciduria, hyperphosphaturia) with impaired proximal renal tubular absorption of phosphate, glucose and amino acids; **lead line** at the junction of teeth and gums and epiphyseal areas of the bones (seen by X-ray) due to deposition of lead.

25. What are the harmful effects of sulfonamides?

Ans. Sulfonamides cause immune complex disease by acting as haptens and stimulating antibody production; calculi formation by crytallization in the renal collecting system (therefore, patients should be advised to drink plenty of oral fluids while taking sulfonamides to prevent this crystallization and calculi formation); hemolytic anemia in people with G6PD (glucose-6-phosphate-dehydrogenase) deficiency.

26. What are the harmful effects of aspirin?

Ans. Aspirin causes gastrointestinal bleeding due to aspirin gastritis or inhibition of platelet cyclooxygenase with thromboxane A2 deficiency and impaired platelet plug formation. Reye's syndrome in children following acute viral febrile illness with fatty change in liver and encephalopathy. Allergic reactions consisting of urticaria, asthma, nasal polyps, angioneurotic edema. In acute toxicity respiratory stimulation leads to respiratory alkalosis. Kidneys compensate for this by increased excretion of bicarbonate and potassium resulting in compensatory metabolic acidosis. Vomiting, dehydration, hypokalemia may cause **death**. Chronic toxicity causes tinnitus (ringing in the ears), hearing difficulty.

27. What are the harmful effects of acetaminophen?

Ans. Hepatic necrosis by free radicals after exhausting the glutathione peroxidase free radical-removing system. *C/Fs*: Nausea, vomiting, abdominal pain, shock, hepatic failure.

28. What are the harmful effects of tobacco smoking?

Ans. 1. Cancers of oral cavity, larynx, lungs, pleura, esophagus, pancreas, urinary bladder.
2. COPD.
3. Atherosclerosis.
4. MI.
5. Peptic ulcer.

29. What are the effects of marijuana?

Ans. It is a hallucinogen, which produces relaxation and sensation of feeling high.

30. What are the harmful effects of oral contraceptives?

Ans. 1. *Neoplasms:* Cancer of cervix, hepatic adenoma.
2. *Cardiovascular:* Thromboembolism hypertension.

31. What is pneumoconiosis?

Ans. *See* chapter 10.

32. What are the harmful effects of mercury?

Ans. Mercury inactivates cytochrome oxidase, binds with cell membrane proteins causing cell membrane damage leading to increased permeability. *C/Fs*: GIT ulceration, acute renal tubular necrosis, cerebral edema (acute poisoning), atrophy (chronic poisoning) with dementia (**mad as hatter**—hat makers in the past used to use mercury to paint the hat ribbon and used to lick the tip of the brush to make it pointed thereby exposing themselves to mercury).

Foods (Nutrition)

33. What are essential nutrients for our body?

Ans. We need 6 essential nutrients for our body to survive and function. These are:
1. Protein
2. Carbohydrate
3. Fat
4. Vitamins
5. Minerals
6. Water and
7. Adequate amount of calories.

34. What roles do these play in our body?

Ans. In production of energy and maintenance of various body structures and functions.

35. What happens with increased carbohydrate, fats and calories than required by the body in the diet?

Ans. Increased carbohydrates, fats or calories cause obesity (body weight more than 20% than ideal weight for the general population), diabetes mellitus, atherosclerosis and predispose to hypertension.

36. What are the causes of decreased nutrition?

Ans.
1. Diet deficiency.
2. Malabsorption.
3. Increased loss.
4. Decrease in use or storage by the body.
5. Increased demand by the body.

37. What are the causes of dietary deficiency?

Ans.
1. Poverty.
2. Ignorance.
3. Alcohol consumption.
4. Chronic illness.

38. What happens when there is decreased protein, calories and energy required by the body in the diet?

Ans. This is called PEM (protein energy malnutrition). When the child's weight is below 80% than an average child, the child is considered to be **malnourished**. When it is below 60% than average the child is considered to have **marasmus**. When protein deprivation is more than deprivation of total calories the child is considered to have **kwashiorkor**.

39. What is marasmus?

Ans. *DEF:* Malnutrition when the weight loss is 60% of normal weight for age and sex due to deficiency in both calories and protein. *DES:* Occurs in children below 1 year of age, who do not get breast-feeding and adequate supplemental nutrition. It causes retarded growth , loss of muscle and subcutaneous fat. It is the **compensated phase** of protein-calorie malnutrition where body's dietary deficiencies are compensated by catabolism of tissues such as fat and skeletal muscles.

40. What is kwashiorkor?

Ans. *DEF:* Malnutrition when protein deprivation is more than the total calories. *DES:* In Ghana language it means second child displaces the first child or **rejected first child**, i.e. the first child nutrition suffers because the second child is born. This has

worse prognosis than marasmus. It is the **decompensated phase** of the protein-calorie malnutrition where compensatory mechanisms fail, metabolism slows down and there is decreased synthesis of enzymes and proteins resulting in malabsorption (due to decreased digestive enzymes), edema (due to decreased albumin) hepatomegaly with fatty liver (due to defective lipid metabolism), atrophy of small intestinal villi, anemia (due to decreased iron, B_{12}, folic acid absorption and decreased erythropoietin production). It occurs in children above one year of age. Causes retarded growth and muscle wasting only with preservation of subcutaneous fat.

41. What are vitamins?

Ans. These are essential food elements for our body. These are of 2 types:

1. Fat soluble (A, D, E, K); and
2. Water soluble (B, folic acid and C).

42. What happens with deficiency of vitamin A?

Ans.

1. **Night blindness**.
2. **Xerophthalmia:** Dryness of the conjunctiva and cornea.
3. **Keratomalacia:** Dryness, softening and later necrosis of cornea.
4. Metaplasia of columnar epithelium to squamous epithelium.
5. **Bitot spots** (small plaque of opaque metaplastic squamous cells on cornea).
6. Decreased immunity.

43. What is the physiology of vitamin D?

Ans. Vitamin D is taken from food or made from skin precursors under sunlight. It combines with albumin and goes to liver. From there to kidneys where its most active form is formed. The active vitamin D's actions are absorption of calcium and phosphorus from small intestine, from bone and distal renal tubules.

44. What is pathology of vitamin D?

Ans. Deficiency of vitamin D causes increased unmineralized bone matrix, increased disordered cartilage. This results in rickets in children and osteomalacia in adults.

Rickets: Condition due to vitamin D deficiency in children where there is defective mineralization of the developing bones with deformities. Frontal bossing, rachitic rosary, pigeon chest, bowing of legs, lumbar lordosis, craniotabes, Harrison groove is seen.

Osteomalacia: Condition due to vitamin D deficiency in adults where there is decreased mineralization of the developed bones **(osteopenia)**. Hypocalcemic tetany (*see* chapter 16).

45. What is the role of vitamin E in our body?

Ans. *Physiology:* It decreases free radicals in body. It is available in green leafy vegetables, nuts, vegetable oils.

Pathology: Its deficiency causes degeneration of posterior columns of spinal cord, atrophy of nerve cells in dorsal root ganglia, degeneration of spinocerebellar tract resulting in ataxia, decreased position and pain sensation, absent tendon reflexes **(spinocerebellar syndrome)**.

46. What is the role of vitamin K in our body?

Ans. *Physiology:* Vitamin K is necessary for liver to make clotting factors II, VII, IX, X. Vitamin K is available in diet and also made by intestinal bacteria. It is recyded by liver.

Pathology: It is decreased in fat malabsorption, decreased intestinal bacteria. In neonates due to decreased liver reserve. It is not abundant in breast milk. Also, reduced in liver diseases. This leads to bleeding diathesis.

47. What is the role of vitamin B_1 (thiamine) in our body?

Ans. *Physiology:* Available in unpolished rice. It is cofactor for many enzymes in carbohydrate metabolism.

Pathology: Its deficiency causes:

1. Beriberi (wet and dry)
2. Wernicke-Korsakoff syndrome.

48. What is beriberi—wet (CCF) and dry (peripheral neuropathy)?

Ans. In Sinhalese, beriberi means: **I cannot/I cannot**.

49. What is dry beriberi?

Ans. Symmetric peripheral polyneuropathy with degeneration of myelin of axons of motor and sensory nerves causing foot and wrist drop and sensory changes.

50. What is wet beriberi?

Ans. Blood vessels are dilated. Cardiac output is increased. All 4 chambers of the heart become dilated and flabby. High output cardiac failure.

51. What is the effect of vitamin B_1 deficiency on the brain?

Ans. Hemorrhage in the mammillary bodies. Causes **Wernicke encephalopathy** and **Korsakoff's psychosis**.

52. What is Wernicke encephalopathy?

Ans. Brain disease due to vit. B_1 (thiamine) deficiency where the mind, the eyes, and the gait all are unsteady: **(mind-confused, eyes-nystagmus, gait-ataxia)**. *PROG*: Good response with early treatment by vitamin B_1. If not so treated patient **may die**.

53. What is Korsakoff's psychosis?

Ans. Brain disease due to vit. B_1 deficiency. When Wernicke's encephalopathy is not treated urgently it **can lead to permanent memory deficit**, where either new memories are not formed or old memories cannot be recalled and person makes up stories to cover up the gap in his memory **(confabulation)**.

54. What is the role of vitamin B_2 (riboflavin) in our body?

Ans. Riboflavin plays a role in oxidation–reduction. It is available in meat, dairy products and vegetables. Its deficiency causes cheilosis, glossitis, dermatitis, keratitis.

55. What is the role of vitamin B_3 (niacin or nicotinic acid) in our body?

Ans. It is a coenzyme. It is found in grains. Also, made from tryptophan. Its deficiency disease is called **pellagra**, consisting of: **D**iarrhea, **D**ermatitis, **D**ementia and **Death** **(D^4)**. Dermatitis (in Italian, Pella = skin, Gra = dry).

56. What is the role of vitamin B_6 (pyridoxine) in our body?

Ans. It is a coenzyme. It is found in most foods. Isoniazid (INH) (antituberculosis drug) interferes with mycobacterium tuberculosis' metabolism of B_6 and also in our body. Therefore, with INH treatment for tuberculosis pyridoxine should be given. Its deficiency causes diseases such as dermatitis, glossitis, cheilosis, peripheral neuropathy.

57. What is the role of folate (folic acid) in our body?

Ans. Folate or folic acid belongs to vitamin B group. It is coenzyme in DNA synthesis. Its deficiency causes reduced DNA. RNA is normal. Therefore, nucleus is not normal but cytoplasm is normal. Its deficiency causes anemia both of decreased production and increased destruction. It is available in many fruits and vegetables. Its deficiency is due to poor diet, increased demand as in pregnancy, decreased absorption from ileum due to diseases (malabsorption disorders) or surgery (resection). Its deficiency causes megaloblastic anemia. In the bone marrow there are megaloblasts, large megakaryocytes and large myelocytes.

58. What is the role of vitamin B_{12} (cyanocobalamin) in our body?

Ans. Vitamin B_{12} combined with intrinsic factor from stomach mucosa is absorbed in the ileum. Its deficiency causes **megaloblastic anemia, subacute combined degeneration of the spinal cord** where there is demyelination of dorsal tracts with ataxia and lateral tracts with spastic paresis. Also, it can cause **megaloblastic madness**.

59. What is the role of vitamin C (ascorbic acid) in our body?

Ans. Vitamin C acts as antioxidant. It is necessary for collagen synthesis. Its deficiency causes weakness of the blood vessel walls due to decreased collagen. Also, it causes decreased osteoid in the bones. Its deficiency causes bleeding (scurvy): Bleeding in gums, joints and subperiosteal regions of the bones.

60. What is the role of minerals in our body?

Ans. There are 2 categories of minerals in our body:

1. In large amounts, e.g. calcium and phosphorus.
2. Trace elements.

61. What are the minerals in large amounts in our body. What is their role in our body?

Ans. *Calcium* and *phosphorus.* Deficiency of these cause rickets and osteomalacia. Hypocalcemia may also cause tetany, convulsions, long QT interval on ECG.

62. What are the trace elements in our body? What is their role in our body?

Ans.
1. *Iron:* Component of hemoglobin and many iron-containing metalloenzymes. Deficiency causes hypochromic microcytic anemia.
2. *Zinc:* Component of enzymes, mainly oxidases. Deficiency causes growth retardation, infertility.
3. *Iodine:* Component of thyroid hormone. Deficiency causes hypothyroidism and goiter.
4. *Selenium:* Component of glutathione peroxidase. Deficiency causes myopathy and rarely cardiomyopathy.
5. *Copper:* Component of cytochrome C oxidase, tyrosinases. Deficiency causes muscle weakness, neurologic defects, hypopigmentation.
6. *Manganese:* Component of metalloenzymes, e.g. oxidoreductases, hydrolases, lipases. Deficiency causes no well-defined known syndrome.
7. *Fluoride:* Deficiency causes dental caries. Mechanism unknown.

Infectious Diseases

63. What are the infectious causes of diseases of our body?

Ans.
1. Prions.
2. Viruses.
3. Mycoplasma.
4. Chlamydia.
5. Rickettsia.
6. Bacteria.
7. Fungi.
8. Protozoa.
9. Helminths.

Various diseases caused by them are described in pertinent systems in Section 2.

Section 2
Systemic Pathology

8 Diseases of the Hematopoietic System (HS)

OVERVIEW

1. Diseases of the organs of the hemapoietic system.
2. Non-neoplastic diseases of the RBCs.
3. Non-neoplastic diseases of the WBCs.
4. Neoplasms of the formed elements of the blood (WBCs, RBCs, platelets).
5. Bleeding disorders.

Organs of the hematopoietic system are:

1. Bone marrow.
2. Thymus.
3. Spleen.
4. Lymph nodes.
5. Liver.

Major diseases of the bone marrow are: **Aplasia**, either congenital (Fanconi's anemia), or acquired either idiopathic or due to drugs and chemicals (antimetabolites, benzene, chloramphenicol), radiation, viruses (hepatitis C, EBV, HIV), aplastic crisis in certain hemolytic anemias (paroxysmal nocturnal hemoglobinuria, sickle cell anemia), **myeloid neoplasms** (acute myelogenous leukemia, chronic myeloproliferative disorders, myelodysplastic syndromes), and **myelophthisis** (marrow replacement by fibrosis, lipid storage diseases, tuberculosis, leukemia, lymphoma, multiple myeloma, metastatic cancers from breast, lung, prostate, thyroid, etc.

Major diseases of the thymus are: Hyperplasia and thymoma.

Splenomegaly is enlargement of the spleen more than the normal weight of 150 gm usually due to:

A. Infections.
B. Congestion.
C. Neoplasia.
D. Hematologic disorders.
E. Autoimmune diseases.
F. Miscellaneous conditions.

Hypersplenism is a triad of:

1. Splenomegaly.
2. Cytopenia.
3. Splenectomy correcting the cytopenia.

Lymphadenopathy is usually due to:

A. Infections.
B. Immunologic causes.
C. Malignancies.
D. Lipid storage diseases.
E. Miscellaneous conditions.

Disorders of RBCs are:

1. Anemia.
2. Polycythemia.

Anemia is defined as reduction in the oxygen-carrying capacity of blood due to reduction of the total circulating RBC mass to below normal levels, reflected as reduced RBCs, hemoglobin, hematocrit. *S/S* of anemia are due to hypoxia. Anemia can be classified on the following basis:

A. Morphologic.
B. Etiologic.

A. Morphology-based anemia are:
   1. Microcytic hypochromic.
   2. Normocytic normochromic.
   3. Macrocytic.

B. Etiology-based anemia are:
   1. Increased loss—internally (by hemolysis) or externally (by hemorrhage).
   2. Decreased production.

Polycythemia is opposite of anemia consisting of increased RBCs, hemoglobin and hematocrit. It can be:

1. Apparent due to reduced plasma volume; or
2. Real due to increase in RBCs, which could have:
   a. Normal erythropoietin level as in polycythemia vera or
   b. Increased erythropoietin level either appropriately, e.g. high altitude or cyanosis or inappropriately as in renal cell carcinoma (RCC), hepatocellular carcinoma (HCC), etc.

Variants of RBCs seen in the peripheral blood could be several based on:

1. Color.
2. Size.
3. Shape.
4. Contents.

Blood groups are based on antigens present on the RBC surface and antibodies present in the serum. Main antigens are A, B, and Rh antigens. Based on this the blood groups are A, B, AB, and O, all of these could be Rh positive or negative. Significance of blood group lies in blood transfusion: as a rule a person should receive the blood transfusion with the same type of blood as his/her own. In urgent situations type O blood **(universal donor)** can be used for patients with other blood types. Person with AB blood group can receive type A, B, and O blood **(universal recipient)**. Rh negative patient should only receive Rh negative blood. Rh positive patient can receive either Rh positive or Rh negative blood.

WBCs are of five types:

1. Neutrophils.
2. Eosinophils.
3. Basophils.
4. Monocytes.
5. Lymphocytes.

Disorders of WBCs are:

1. *Disorder of structure* (morphologic alterations).
2. *Decrease in number* (leukopenia).
3. *Increase in number:*
   a. Reactive.
   b. Neoplastic.
   a. *Reactive consists of* leukocytosis, leukemoid reaction consisting of severe leukocytosis, when accompanied by nucleated RBCs in peripheral blood called **leukoery-throblastic reaction**.
   b. *Neoplastic consists of* various leukemias.

Neoplasms of formed elements of blood (WBCs, RBCs, platelets) are of following types:

1. Lymphoid (B, T, NK cells).
2. Myeloid (granulocytic, monocytic, thrombocytic, erythroid).
3. Histiocytic (histiocytic lymphoma).

Lymphoid neoplasms are:

1. Non-Hodgkin's lymphoma.
2. Lymphocytic leukemias.
3. Hodgkin's lymphoma.

Non-Hodgkin's lymphomas are defined as malignant neoplastic proliferation of lymphoid cells as discrete tissue masses in lymph nodes, spleen or other sites.

Lymphocytic leukemias are defined as malignant neoplasms of lymphoid cells with widespread involvement of the bone marrow usually with large number of tumor cells in peripheral blood.

Hodgkin's lymphomas are defined as malignant neoplasm of the lymphoid tissue with characteristic Reed-Sternberg giant-cell, which most likely is a B lymphocyte, within a background of reactive lymphocytes, plasma cells, histiocytes, granulocytes–mainly eosinophils.

Myeloid neoplasms are:

1. Acute myelogenous leukemia **(AML)**.
2. Chronic myeloproliferative syndromes **(CMS)**.
3. Myelodysplastic syndrome **(MDS)**.

AML is a heterogenous group of malignant neoplastic disorder where myeloid progenitor cells (blasts) collect in the bone marrow. *Its WHO classification includes*:

1. With recurrent chromosomal rearrangements.
2. With multilineage dysplasia.
3. Treatment-related.
4. Not otherwise specified (NOS) or French American British (FAB) classification consisting of M0 to M7.

CMS is a malignant neoplastic proliferation of myeloid stem cells. Its types are:

1. Chronic myeloid leukemia (CML).
2. Polycythemia vera (PV).
3. Myelofibrosis with myeloid metaplasia (MMM).
4. Essential thrombocytosis (ET).

MDS consists of mutation of multipotent stem cell affecting all three lineages of bone marrow cells (RBC, WBC, platelets).

Bleeding disorders are due to:

1. Blood vessel disorders.
2. Platelet disorders of number, structure or function.
3. Clotting disorders.

Some of the blood vessel disorders consist of:

1. Scurvy.
2. Henoch-Schonlein purpura.

Some of the platelet disorders consist of:

1. Thrombocytopenia.
2. Idiopathic thrombocytopenic purpura (ITP).
3. Thrombotic thrombocytopenic purpura (TTP).
4. Hemolytic uremia syndrome (HUS).

Some of the clotting disorders consist of:

1. *Hereditary:*
   A. Hemophilia A.
   B. Hemophilia B.
   C. von Willebrand disease.
2. *Acquired:* Liver diseases.

Some of the tests for bleeding disorders are:

1. Complete blood count.
2. Peripheral smear examination.
3. Prothrombin time (PT).
4. Partial thromboplastin time (PTT).
5. Factor assays.

1. What are the organs of the hematopoietic system?

Ans. Bone marrow, thymus, spleen, lymph nodes and liver.

Thymus

2. What are the disorders of thymus?

Ans. 1. Hyperplasia 2. Thymomas.

3. What is hyperplasia of thymus?

Ans. *DEF:* Appearance of lymphoid follicles in the medulla. (Normal thymus does not have lymphoid follicles).

Seen in: Myasthenia gravis, SLE, rheumatoid arthritis (RA).

4. What is thymoma?

Ans. *DEF:* Neoplasia of the epithelial cells. (Not of the lymphocytic cells).

Classification:

1. Benign (75%).
2. Malignant (25%).

   C/Fs: Asymptomatic or cough, dyspnea, superior vena cava syndrome. Myasthenia gravis.

Spleen

5. What is splenomegaly?

Ans. Normal spleen weighs approximately 150 grams. Spleen size larger than this is considered splenomegaly.

6. What is the classification of splenomegaly?

Ans. On etiologic basis splenomegaly can be classified as due to:

A. *Infections:* Infectious mononucleosis (EB virus), typhoid, malaria, TB, infective endocarditis, sepsis.

B. *Congestion:* Cirrhosis, portal hypertension, portal vein thrombosis.

C. *Neoplasia:* CLL, hairy cell leukemia, CML, lymphomas (Hodgkin's and Non-Hodgkin's) polycythemia rubra vera, histiocytosis, acute leukemias.

D. *Hematologic:* Hemolytic anemias, (thalassemic, autoimmune), extramedullary erythropoiesis, myeloid metaplasia with myelofibrosis, hereditary spherocytosis.

E. *Miscellaneous:* Sarcoidosis, amyloidosis, Gaucher's disease, Niemann-Pick disease.

F. *Autoimmune:* RA (Still's disease, Felty's syndrome) SLE, ITP.

7. What is hypersplenism?

Ans. *DEF:* Excessive removal by an enlarged spleen of one or more of the formed elements of blood leading to anemia, leukopenia or thrombocytopenia. Its three features are:

1. Splenomegaly
2. Cytopenia.
3. Corrected with splenectomy.

Primary hypersplenism: Above with normal-size spleen without any apparent cause.

Lymph Nodes

8. What is the classification of lymph node enlargement (lymphadenopathy)?

Ans. This can be classified according to causes and whether acute or chronic.

9. What are the causes of lymphadenopathy?

Ans.

I. Infectious.
II. Immunologic.
III. Malignant neoplastic.
IV. Lipid storage.
V. Miscellaneous.

10. What are the infectious diseases causing lymphadenopathy?

Ans. A. *Viral:* Infectious mononucleosis, AIDS, rubella, varicella zoster.

B. *Bacterial:* Streptococci, staphylococci, salmonella, brucella, listeria, pasteurella, hemophilus, cat-scratch disease, mycobacterium tuberculosis, M. leprae, spirochetal diseases.

C. Chlamydial infections.

D. Fungal infections.

E. Parasitic infections.

11. What are the immunologic diseases causing lymphadenopathy?

Ans. A. SLE B. Rheumatoid arthritis.

12. What are the malignant neoplastic diseases causing lymphadenopathy?

Ans. a. *Primary:* Hodgkin's lymphoma, non-Hodgkin's lymphoma, leukemias.

b. *Secondary:* From various sites.

13. What are the lipid storage diseases affecting the lymph nodes?

Ans. 1. Gaucher's disease 2. Niemann-Pick disease.

14. What are the miscellaneous diseases causing lymphadenopathy?

Ans. a. Sarcoidosis.

b. Sinus histiocytosis.

c. Mucocutaneous lymph node syndrome (Kawasaki's disease).

15. What is cat-scratch disease?

Ans. *ETIO:* Caused by *Bartonella henselae*. Extracellular. Can be seen by silver stain or EM. Seen mostly below 18 years of age. *C/Fs*: Regional lymph nodes of axilla and neck are affected with enlarged tender lymph nodes seen approximately in 2 weeks after scratch by a cat. Spontaneous regression in 2–4 months. Sometimes leads to osteomyelitis, thrombocytopenia, encephalitis. *MORPHO:* Granuloma with central necrosis with PMNs infiltration.

RBCs

16. What are normal RBC indices?

Ans. 1. MCV (Mean cell volume) (normal 80 to 95 fL-femtoliter)—denotes RBC size.

Measured as: $$\frac{\text{PCV} \times 10}{\text{No. of RBCs (million/microliter)}}$$

Increased in: Megaloblastic anemia (B_{12} or folate deficiency), macrocytic anemia (acute bleeding due to release of large reticulocytes in peripheral blood, alcoholism due to RBC membrane abnormalities. In these conditions bone marrow is not megaloblastic). Thus, all macrocytic anemias are not megaloblastic; but all megaloblastic anemias are macrocytic. Decreased in: Iron deficiency anemia, thalassemia.

2. MCH (Mean cell hemoglobin) (normal 27 to 30 picogram-pg/RBC)—denotes amount of hemoglobin in a single RBC.

Measured as: $$\frac{\text{Hemoglobin-gm/dL} \times 10}{\text{RBCs million/microliter}}$$

Increased in: Macrocytosis, decreased in microcytosis.

3. MCHC (mean cell hemoglobin concentration) (normal 33 to 37%)—denotes Hb concentration in one RBC.

$$\frac{\text{Hbgm/dL} \times 100}{\text{PCV}}$$

Increased in spherocytosis, decreased in iron deficiency anemia, thalassemia.

4. *RDW (RBC distribution width):* Denotes difference in sizes of RBC in a person's blood (anisocytosis) normal 13%.

17. What are the disorders of RBCs?

Ans. 1. Anemia 2. Polycythemia.

18. What is anemia?

Ans. *DEF:* Reduction in the oxygen-transporting capacity of blood due to reduction of the total circulating RBC mass to below normal levels. Reflected as reduced red blood cells (RBCs), hemoglobin (Hb) and hematocrit (Hct) (PCV) (Normal RBC count in males 4.4 to 6 millions/c mm; in females 3.5 to 5 millions/c mm) (Normal Hb in males 13 to 17 gm/dl, in females 12 to 15 gm/dl) (Normal Hct in males 39 to 49%, in females 33 to 43%). Anemia is **not** a disease but a manifestation of some other disease(s). Its symptoms arise from hypoxia, e.g. weakness, vertigo, headache, tinnitus, fatigue, drowsiness, etc. Its signs are from cardiovascular-pulmonary compensatory responses to the hypoxia, e.g. tachycardia, tachypnea, etc.

19. What are the basis of classifying anemia?

Ans. Two basis:

1. Morphologic
2. Etiologic.

20. What is the classification of anemia by morphologic basis?

Ans. 1. RBC size (normocytic, microcytic, macrocytic).

2. RBC hemoglobinization (normochromic, hypochromic).

Types of anemia by this basis are:

1. Hypochromic microcytic anemia, e.g. iron deficiency anemia, thalassemia.
2. Normochromic normocytic anemia, e.g. chronic renal failure, chronic diseases, hypothyroidism, adrenal insufficiency, myelofibrosis.
3. Macrocytic anemia, e.g. megaloblastic anemia due to vitamin B_{12}/folic acid deficiency, alcoholism, cirrhosis. *Note:* Macrocytic is **not** hyperchromatic because normal-sized RBCs have hemoglobin concentration at saturation point.

21. What is the classification of anemia by etiologic basis?

Ans. 1. Blood loss anemia.

2. Hemolytic anemia.
3. Decreased production anemia.

22. What are blood loss anemias?

Ans. *Acute:* Causes: Trauma, massive GIT bleeding, urinary tract bleeding, uterine bleeding. Findings: In the beginning the tests may show no abnormalities as the loss of RBCs is equal to plasma. Within a few hours tissue fluid enters the circulation and RBC count, Hb and Hct will be low. Since there is no change in the RBCs the indices will show normochromic normocytic anemia. If body/bone marrow iron store is normal marrow will produce extra compensatory RBCs and blood picture will become normal.

Chronic: Causes: Chronic bleeding from GIT, e.g. peptic ulcer disease, gastric cancer, colon cancer, hookworm infestation, intestinal bleeding, hemorrhoids, from urinary tract, from excess menstrual loss, etc. Findings: Similar to iron deficiency anemia since marrow iron stores are used up.

23. What are hemolytic anemias?

Ans. *DEF:* Shortened life-span of RBCs (normal 120 days). Marrow cannot keep pace with RBC destruction.

General: Destruction of RBCs can occur within blood vessels **(intravascular hemolysis)**, e.g. in DIC due to mechanical trauma, in hemolytic transfusion reaction or in malaria, etc. Destruction of RBCs can also occur outside the blood vessels **(extravascular hemolysis)** in the mononuclear phagocytic system (previously called reticuloendothelial system—RE system) of spleen and liver. Normally the RBCs are very flexible and pass through the splenic sinusoids. When RBCs become less flexible due to injury or altered Hb or other causes they cannot pass through splenic sinusoid and are engulfed by the monocytes and destroyed.

24. What are the disorders of RBC membrane cytoskeleton?

Ans. 1. Spherocytosis 2. Elliptocytosis.

25. What is spherocytosis?

Ans. Types:

1. Acquired 2. Hereditary.

26. What is acquired spherocytosis?

Ans. Seen in immune hemolytic anemia. Here the RBCs are coated by antibodies (opsonization). Macrophages try to eat (engulf) them and sometimes are only able to bite off portion of the RBC membrane. This reduces the surface area of the RBC. This forces the RBC to assume the smallest possible diameter for a given volume, i.e. a sphere. This spherical RBC is less flexible and is caught in the splenic sinusoids and engulfed by macrophages and destroyed (double jeopardy).

27. What is hereditary spherocytosis?

Ans. *DEF:* Inherited disorder of RBCs where RBCs are in a less flexible spherical form making them susceptible to be destroyed in the spleen by the macrophages.

ETIO: Autosomal dominant inheritance.

PATHOG: Abnormality of the protein structure of the RBC membrane. Main cytoskeletal membrane protein is lacking causing instability of the RBC membrane leading to damage due to mechanical stresses during circulation with loss of portions of the cell membrane forcing the RBC to assume the smallest possible diameter for a given volume, i.e. a sphere. This sphere is less flexible and thus caught in the splenic sinusoids and subsequently destroyed by the splenic macrophages. **Therefore, splenectomy corrects the anemia** even though the basic problem of spherocytosis remains.

MORPHO: In peripheral blood, RBCs appear spherical and do not have central pallor due to spherical shape. Reticulocytes (polychromatic RBCs) are increased. Bone marrow is hypercellular. Spleen is enlarged. Spleen microscopically has congestion of its cords with increased enlarged macrophages. Also, there is hemosiderosis.
C/Fs: Anemia, splenomegaly, jaundice. Anemia usually is moderate. Parvovirus infection of the marrow erythroblasts may precipitate an **aplastic crisis**.
Test: Erythrocyte osmotic fragility to hypotonic saline is increased.

28. What is the osmotic fragility test?

Ans. *Normal:* Hemolysis begins at 0.45% and is complete at 0.35%.
Increased in:

1. Hereditary spherocytosis (begins at 0.65% and complete at 0.45%).
2. Elliptocytosis with hemolytic anemia.
3. Acquired hemolytic anemia.
4. Hemolysis with ABO and Rh incompatibility.
5. Hemolysis with burns.
6. Drugs.
7. Pernicious anemia.
8. Malaria.

Decreased in:

1. Iron deficiency anemia.
2. Thalassemia.
3. Sickle cell anemia.

29. What is hereditary elliptocytosis (ovalocytosis)?

Ans. Inherited, autosomal dominant disease with elongated, oval RBCs. Does not always cause anemia. But may cause hemolytic anemia with splenomegaly.

30. What are the disorders of enzyme deficiencies of RBCs leading to hemolytic anemias?

Ans. Erythrocyte and its membrane are vulnerable to injury due to enzyme deficiencies. Two of these are:

1. Pyruvate kinase deficiency.
2. Glucose-6-phosphate dehydrogenase (G-6-PD) deficiency.

31. What is the pyruvate kinase deficiency of RBCs?

Ans. Deficiency of glycolytic enzyme pyruvate kinase is the most common cause of hereditary non-spherocytic hemolytic anemia. Inheritance: Autosomal recessive.
C/Fs: Heterozygotes are normal. Homozygotes have chronic anemia.

32. What is the glucose-6-phosphate dehydrogenase (G-6-PD) deficiency?

Ans. In this condition, RBCs are susceptible to injury by oxidants which are normally inactivated by intracellular reduced glutathione (GSH). Due to deficiencies of enzymes which produce GSH, regeneration of GSH is hampered and hydrogen peroxide collects and denatures Hb which precipitates in RBC as inclusion bodies called **Heinz bodies** which damage RBC membrane and cause intravascular hemolysis and also make RBCs, less flexible thereby predispose them to be caught in splenic sinusoids where macrophages remove these Heinz bodies turning RBCs into **bite cells** further making them vulnerable to be caught and phagocytosed (double jeopardy!) *C/Fs:* Usually there is no symptoms. But, when a person is exposed to reducing agents, e.g. primaquine, sulfonamides, nitrofurantoin, vitamin K derivatives then GSH is oxidized to glutathione and accumulated hydrogen peroxide denatures hemoglobin with precipitation. Because the G6PD gene is located on X chromosome all the RBCs of affected males are deficient in enzyme activity and are prone to oxidant injury, whereas carrier females are asymptomatic.

33. What are the two common disorders of hemoglobin synthesis?

Ans. 1. Thalassemia 2. Sickle cell anemia.

34. What is thalassemia (mediterranean anemia)?

Ans. *DEF:* (Gr. thalassa = sea, originally observed in people around mediterranean sea), however, it is now known to be worldwide). It is heterogenous group of autosomal codominant inherited disorder where there is decreased (quantitative) production of either alpha chain **(alpha thalassemia)** or beta chain **(beta thalassemia)** of the hemoglobin causing reduced structurally normal hemoglobin synthesis **(decreased RBC production anemia)** and precipitation of hemoglobin due to compensatory increase in the non-deficient chain with hemolysis of RBCs in peripheral blood **(hemolytic anemia** by damaging the cell membrane, and making RBCs less flexible and vulnerable to be caught in the splenic sinusoids and engulfed by macrophages), and similarly of erythroblasts in the marrow **(ineffective erythropoiesis)**. Alpha chains are coded **by 2 alpha globin genes located on chromosome 16. Beta chains are coded by a single gene located on chromosome 11**.

Types: 2 types:

1. Heterozygous type (thalassemia minor or trait)—Asymptomatic or mildly symptomatic.
2. Homozygous type (thalassemia major)—Severe hemolytic anemia.

35. What is beta thalassemia?

Ans. *DEF:* Defect in synthesis of beta chain of the hemoglobin. *PATHOG*: In beta thalassemias the genes are muted (changed) and only rarely deleted or absent (Unlike alpha thalassemias where the genes are deleted).

Types: 1. Thalassemia major with severe hemolytic anemia,

2. Intermedia with intermediate severity.
3. Minor.

MORPHO: *In peripheral blood:* RBCs are microcytic hypochromic. Some RBCs due to larger surface area than the volume (due to low hemoglobin) have pooling of Hgb in the centre, giving them a target-like appearance **(target-cells)**. Also, peripheral blood has poikilocytosis, anisocytosis, reticulocytosis. *In marrow:* There is hypercellularity with shift towards primitive forms. Due to hyperactivity marrow even encroaches/invades bony cortex, impairs bone growth and produces skeletal abnormalities. Spleen and liver are enlarged due to extramedullary erythropoiesis and R-E cell hyperplasia due to excess RBC phagocytosis and destruction and hemosiderosis. Late stages may also have secondary hemochromatosis.

36. What is thalassemia major (Cooley's anemia)?

Ans. This is due to homozygous state. Growth is retarded from birth. Due to severe anemia repeated blood transfusions are required. Secondary hemochromatosis causes myocardial damage leading to cardiac failure and death by teenage. Peripheral blood smear shows severe microcytic, hypochromic anemia, anisocytosis, poikilocytosis and reticulocytosis.

37. What is thalassemia minor?

Ans. Patients may be asymptomatic. Anemia is usually mild microcytic hypochromic. Life expectancy is normal.

38. What is thalassemia intermedia?

Ans. *DEF:* Thalassemia of moderate severity with hemoglobin level of 7 to 10 gm/dl. These patients do not require regular blood transfusion. This clinical syndrome can be caused by many genetic defects, e.g. beta thalassemia trait of unusual severity ("dominant" beta thalassemia); hemoglobin H (3 gene deletion of alpha thalassemia.

39. What is alpha thalassemia?

Ans. *DEF:* Alpha chain synthesis is defective. *PATHOG*: Deletion of 1 or more of the 4 alpha genes on chromosome 16.

C/Fs:

1. 1 gene deleted—silent career state: Asymptomatic.
2. 2 genes deleted—alpha thalassemia trait: Like beta thalassemia minor.
3. 3 genes deleted—HbH disease: Like beta thalassemia intermedia.
4. 4 genes deleted—hydrops fetalis: Intrauterine death.

40. What is sickle cell anemia (SS anemia)?

Ans. *DEF:* Anemia due to inherited autosomal recessive defect in the **structure** of hemoglobin where valine replaces glutamic acid as the 6th amino acid on beta globin chain due to mutation in beta chain gene on chromosome 11 (as opposed to reduced or absent quantity of Hb in thalassemia). Its types are as follows:

1. Homozygous—sickle cell anemia.
2. Heterozygous—sickle cell trait (generally asymptomatic).

   PATHOG: On deoxygenation, HbS molecule undergoes polymerization (crystallization) giving it a crescentic or sickle shape. Initially, with oxygenation it becomes normal in shape; but, with each episode of sickling the membrane is damaged a little more when finally, it is damaged so much that sickle shape becomes permanent.

   Sickling causes 2 major problems:

   1. Sickled cells are rigid and hence caught in splenic sinusoids and engulfed and destroyed by macrophages, reducing their life-span to approximately 1/6 of normal (120 days).
   2. Sickled cells do not flow well within the blood vessels and block the small vessels causing generalized obstruction of small blood vessels resulting in ischemic damage to multiple organs. *MORPHO:* In peripheral smear RBCs are of sickle shape. Bone marrow is hypercellular with encroachment to cortical bone-skull bone giving a **crew-cut** appearance. Spleen and liver may show extramedullary hemopoiesis. Heart, liver and renal tubules may show fatty changes due to severe anemia and vascular stasis. In children, spleen is moderately enlarged due to jammed sickled RBCs. In adults, due to repeated hypoxic injury spleen is shrunken and fibrotic **(autosplenectomy)**. Vascular thrombosis can cause infarction of organs, e.g. bones, liver, kidney, retina. Thrombosis in pulmonary vessels may cause pulmonary hypertension and cor pulmonale. Increased bilirubin may cause bile gallstones. Thrombosis of leg vessels cause leg ulcers.

      C/Fs: **Severe hemolytic anemia**, with reticulocytosis, and hyperbilirubinemia. Also patient suffers with acute crises, e.g.

      1. **Vaso-occlusive crises (pain crises)** due to infection or dehydration-pain in abdomen **(appearing as acute abdomen)**, in bone, in joints; Ishemia of CNS may cause stroke.
      2. **Aplastic crisis** of the bone marrow due to parvovirus infection.
      3. **Acute chest syndrome** due to lung infections. Also, patients are susceptible to infections, specially to Salmonella osteomyelitis infection due to unknown reasons. Patient with sickle cell trait is usually asymptomatic unless there is extreme hypoxia.

41. What is paroxysmal nocturnal hemoglobinuria (PNH)?

Ans. *DEF:* Acquired disorder of the myeloid stem cell due to mutant gene called PIG-A causing proliferation of abnormal clone of myeloid stem cell producing RBCs, granulocytes and platelets which are very sensitive to the lytic activity of complement resulting in hemolysis due to lack of complement-regulating surface proteins.

PNH is a descriptive term for the clinical manifestation of red cell breakdown with release of hemoglobin into the urine that is manifested most prominently by dark-colored urine in the morning. The term "nocturnal" refers to the belief that hemolysis is induced by activation of complement by acidosis during sleep at night. Now, it is known that **hemolysis happens continuously during day or night** and the change in color seen in the morning is due to the concentration of urine during the night. PNH currently is **reclassified** from purely an acquired hemolytic anemia **to a hematopoietic stem cell mutation defect** because of new knowledge that **surface proteins are missing not only in the red cell membrane but also in all blood cells, including the platelet and white cells.**

C/Fs: Hemolysis is intravascular. Intravascular thrombosis is also common due to platelet disorder. Due to neutropenia there is susceptibility to infection. Since this is an acquired disorder of myeloid stem cell, during the course it may transform into other disorder, e.g. acute leukemia or aplastic anemia.

The clinical syndrome can present in 3 types of symptoms including:

1. An **acquired** intracorpuscular hemolytic anemia due to the abnormal susceptibility of the red cell membrane to the hemolytic activity of complement.
2. Thrombosis in large vessels, such as hepatic, abdominal, cerebral and subdermal veins; and
3. A deficiency in hematopoiesis that may be mild or severe, such as pancytopenia in aplastic anemia state.

The classic description of the manifestations of PNH is the presence of dark urine during the night with partial clearing during the day; however, hemoglobinuria may occur every day in severe cases, more frequently in episodes lasting 3–10 days, or, in some cases, not at all. Thrombosis of the veins usually manifests as a sudden catastrophic complication, with severe abdominal pain and rapidly enlarging liver and ascites **(Budd-Chiari syndrome)**. Deficient hematopoiesis may occur due to diminished blood cell production with a hypoplastic bone marrow. Aplastic anemia may develop in 1 in 10 patients.

42. What are the hemolytic anemia due to extracorpuscular abnormalities?

Ans. Antibody-mediated:

Isohemagglutinins:

1. Transfusion reactions.
2. Erythroblastosis fetalis (Rh incompatibility—fetus Rh +, Mom Rh –).

Autoantibodies: 2 types:

1. *Warm antibody.*

   ETIO:

   a. Lymphoma b. SLE c. Drugs (Aldomet, penicillin).

2. *Cold antibody.*

   ETIO:

   a. Lymphoma.

b. Mycoplasma infection.

c. Infectious mononucleosis.

43. What is the Coomb's antiglobulin test?

Ans. *Purpose:* Diagnosis of immunohemolytic anemia by demonstration of anti-RBC antibodies either coated on patient's RBCs (direct Coomb's test) or in patient's serum (indirect Coomb's test).

Method: Direct Coomb's test: Patient's RBCs are incubated with an animal's serum containing antihuman antibodies (developed by injecting human antibodies in the animal). If patient's RBCs are coated with antibodies there will be agglutination. This is positive result.

Indirect Coomb's test: Patient's serum is incubated with normal human RBCs. If patient's serum has anti-RBC antibodies they will coat these RBCs. On these RBCs a direct Coomb's test is done as above.

44. What is hemolytic disease of the newborn?

Ans. When the mother is RhD blood group negative and fetus positive, due to inheritance from father, the transplacentally transmitted small anti-Rh IgG antibodies generated in mother against fetal RBCs cause hemolysis of fetal RBCs due to complement-mediated type II hypersensitivity reaction. This is less severe with ABO incompatibility due to large anti-AB IgM antibodies which cannot cross placenta. There is no disease with first pregnancy due to production of IgM antibodies, but during subsequent pregnancies IgG antibodies are produced in mother which cross placenta and cause hemolysis of fetal RBCs which is worse with every subsequent pregnancy. Due to this the newborn suffers from hemolytic anemia, jaundice, liver failure, CCF, edema. If hyperbilirubinemia is severe, brain of the new born is affected **(kernicterus)**. If anemia is severe, the resultant hypoxic injury to liver and heart leads to severe widespread edema **(hydrops fetalis)**. Compensatory increased erythropoiesis results in release of RBC precursors (reticulocytes, erythroblasts) in the peripheral blood **(erythroblastosis fetalis)**.

45. What is hemolytic anemia from mechanical trauma?

Ans. *DEF:* Hemolysis within the blood vessels and heart due to mechanical trauma. *ETIO:* Artificial mechanical valves, microangiopathic hemolytic anemia (DIC, malignant HTN, SLE, thrombotic thrombocytopenic purpura (TTP), hemolytic-uremic syndrome, disseminated cancer. *Features:* In the peripheral blood, **burr cells, helmet cells and triangle cells may be seen**.

46. What is hemolytic anemia from infection?

Ans. *Malaria:* Mosquito injects sporozoites in man. These go to liver. After multiplication in liver merozoites are liberated. These go to RBCs. There gametocytes are developed. Also trophozoites are formed which further produce merozoites, which escape RBCs by destroying them and enter liver cells or new RBCs repeating the cycle of RBC destruction.

47. What are the anemias of impaired red cell production?

Ans. 1. Iron deficiency anemia.
2. Megaloblastic anemia.
3. Aplastic anemia.
4. Myelophthisic anemia.

48. What is iron deficiency anemia?

Ans. *ETIO:*

1. *Increased iron requirement:* During pregnancy (due to increased demands of fetus); children (increased demands of growth).
2. *Dietary deficiency:* In infants, since human milk is low in iron, and newborns storage iron is depleted in 6 months, at 6 months of age iron supplement is required; or diet adequate but absorption decreased, e.g. due to gastrectomy.
3. *Chronic blood loss:* Major cause of anemia in adults. Most commonly due to GIT bleeding or menorrhagia.

MORPHO: Peripheral blood smear has RBCs which are microcytic and hypochromic. Marrow is only slightly hyperactive due to limitation of iron availability with slightly increased volume with normoblastic hyperplasia.

LAB:

1. Decreased Hb, Hct, RBC count.
2. Decreased serum ferritin.
3. Increased total iron-binding capacity (TIBC).
4. Decreased hemosiderin in marrow as seen by special iron stain.

C/Fs: Fatigue, dyspnea on exertion. Pallor of conjunctiva, mucus membranes and nail bed. Angina in patients with coronary artery atherosclerosis. Atrophic glossitis, dysphagia and esophageal webs **(Plummer-Vinson syndrome)**. **Koilonychia** (spooning of the nails).

49. What is macrocytosis?

Ans. *DEF:* MCV greater than 100 fL.

Types:

a. Megaloblastic
b. Non-megaloblastic

ETIO:

a. Megaloblastic
   1. Vitamin B_{12} deficiency
   2. Folate deficiency

b. Non-megaloblastic
  1. Reticulocytosis due to hemorrhage/hemolysis.
  2. Alcohol
  3. HIV treatment
  4. Hypothyroidism
  5. Liver disease
  6. Primary bone marrow dysplasias (myelodysplasia, myeloproliferative).

PATHOG:

a. *Megaloblastic:* Vitamin B_{12} and folate deficiencies lead to defective RNA and DNA synthesis resulting in delayed nuclear division without any defect of cytoplasm maturation resulting in large cells. Treatment of HIV with reverse transcriptase inhibitors interfere with DNA production.

b. *Macrocytic:* Reticulocytosis (larger than RBCs) due to hemolysis/hemorrhage. Alcohol toxicity causes macrocytosis due to causing RBC membrane defect; and also chronic alcoholism leads to vitamin B_{12} and folate deficiency. Mechanism of other conditions is not understood.

MORPHO:

a. *Megaloblastic:* Peripheral smear shows macro-ovalocytes and hypersegmented neutrophils.

b. *Non-megaloblastic:* Round macrocytes.

LAB:

1. Serum B_{12} level
2. RBC folate level (serum folate level may be misleading)
3. Reticulocyte count.

50. What are megaloblastic anemias?

Ans. 1. Vitamin B_{12} deficiency   2. Folate deficiency

General features: Large erythroid precursor cells (megaloblasts) in the marrow. Due to deficiency in vit. B_{12} or folate. Leading to decreased DNA synthesis resulting in delayed nuclear division and with no problem with cytoplasm maturation the cells are thus large. Many of these large cells are destroyed in the marrow without being released in the peripheral blood **(reduced erythropoiesis)**. Also, the cells which are released in the peripheral blood are more vulnerable to destruction in the splenic sinusoids **(hemolytic component of the anemia)**. *LAB: Peripheral blood:* Pancytopenia, macrocytosis, hypersegmented PMNs (>5 lobes). *Bone marrow:* Megaloblastic hyperplasia. Serum vit. B_{12} or folate reduced (depending on whether due to B_{12} or folate deficiency).

51. What is megaloblastic anemia due to vit. B_{12} deficiency?

Ans. *ETIO:*

1. Decreased or defective gastric intrinsic factor **(pernicious anemia)**.

2. Gastric resection
   a. Peptic digestion releases dietary vit. B_{12} from the salivary R binders-impaired;
   b. Intrinsic factor binds this released B_{12}, which is transported to distal ileum-impaired.
3. Disorders of distal ileum (B_{12} is absorbed in distal ileum-impaired).
4. *Blind loop syndrome:* Bacterial overgrowth in surgically created blind loop results in depletion of B_{12}.
5. Broad spectrum antibiotics-same mechanism of bacterial overgrowth.
6. *Diphyllobothrium latum* infestation.

52. What is pernicious anemia?

Ans. Most common of all the above causes of B_{12} deficiency anemia. Due to autoimmunity with anti-intrinsic factor and anti-parietal cell antibodies. *C/Fs*: Onset is gradual. Symptoms are similar to that of iron deficiency anemia with fatigue, dyspnea on exertion, angina in patients with coronary atherosclerosis. In B_{12} deficiency there is also **Subacute combined degeneration of the spinal cord** affecting posterolateral regions due to myelin vacuolation since B_{12} is necessary for maintenance of myelin. There is ataxia, impaired position and vibration sense. There is also tingling numbness and burning of hands and feet. Also, patient may become confused (megaloblastic madness). **Increased incidence of gastric carcinoma**.

DIAG:

1. Pancytopenia, hypersegmented neutrophils in peripheral blood.
2. Megaloblastic hyperplasia of the marrow.
3. Low serum B_{12} levels.
4. Normal serum folate levels.
5. Histamine-fast gastric achlorhydria due to loss of gastric parietal cells.
6. Inability to absorb an oral dose of cobalamin, corrected by parenteral intrinsic factor **(Schilling test)**.
7. After parenteral administration of B_{12} increased reticulocyte response in 2–3 days.

53. What is folate deficiency anemia?

Ans. It is a megaloblastic anemia.

ETIO:

1. Diet deficiency.
2. Pregnancy.
3. Intestinal malabsorption due to sprue, *Giardia lamblia* infestation, dilantin and folic acid antagonist chemotherapy.

C/Fs: Similar to above. Except no neurologic abnormalities (which is seen in B_{12} deficiency) and not prone to gastric cancer (as in pernicious anemia).

DIAG: Serum folate levels are low.

54. What is sideroblastic anemia?

Ans. Due to the failure of synthesis of hem, iron is seen as ring around nucleus of normoblast by Prussian blue stain in conditions such as lead poisoning, chronic diseases, etc.

55. What is aplastic anemia?

Ans. *DEF:* Pancytopenia (anemia, thrombocytopenia, leukopenia) with hypocellularity (aplasia) of the bone marrow.

ETIO:

1. Toxic drugs and chemicals (alkylating agents, antimetabolites, benzene, phenylbutazone, chloramphenicol), radiation.
2. *Viral infections:* Hepatitis C, HIV.
3. Aplastic crisis in certain hemolytic anemias, e.g. PNH sickle cell anemia.

MORPHO: Marrow is hypocellular. Peripheral blood has pancytopenia. *C/Fs*: Gradual onset. *S/S* of anemia: Weakness, fatigue, etc. of thrombocytopenia: petechiae, ecchymoses of granulocytopenia, frequent infections.

56. What is myelophthisic anemia?

Ans. *ETIO:* Extensive replacement of marrow by:

1. Neoplasm or other lesions, e.g. metastatic cancers from breast, lung, prostate, thyroid; due to multiple myeloma, lymphoma, leukemia. Advanced TB, lipid storage disorders.
2. Marrow fibrosis. Features: RBCs of abnormal shapes and immature RBCs are present in peripheral blood.

57. What are laboratory tests for diagnosis and *D/D* of anemias?

Ans.

1. Hb, Hct, RBC, reticulocyte count.
2. Smear.
3. Serology-Coomb's test.
4. Hemoglobin electrophoresis.
5. Biochemical-serum iron, ferritin, B_{12}, folate levels.
6. Aspiration of the marrow.
7. Osmotic fragility.

58. What is polycythemia (erythrocytosis)?

Ans. *DEF/DES:* Increase in concentration of RBCs and Hb level.

CLASSI: I. With reduced plasma volume: Dehydration/hemoconcentration.

II. With normal plasma volume:

A. With normal erythropoietin level: Polycythemia vera-due to abnormal proliferation of myeloid stem cells.

B. With increased erythropoietin level:
1. With erythropoietin level appropriately increased: High altitude, cyanotic heart diseases, lung diseases.
2. With erythropoietin level inappropriately increased: Renal cell carcinoma, hepatoma, cerebellar hemangioblastoma.

C/Fs: CVS: Increased incidence of atherosclerosis and thromboembolism leading to MI, stroke, hepatic and mesenteric vein thrombosis, TIAs, visual disturbances. Tendency to hemorrhage (unknown mechanism). Splenomegaly.

59. What are different variants of RBCs seen in peripheral blood?

Ans. These are according to:

1. Color.
2. Size.
3. Shape.
4. Contents:
   1. *Acanthocytes (spur cells):* Irregularly speculated. Seen in abetalipoproteinemia, cirrhosis, hepatic necrosis.
   2. *Burr cells:* Regularly speculated. Seen in uremia.
   3. *Elliptocytes:* Elliptical. Seen in hereditary elliptocytosis.
   4. *Sickled cells:* Sickle-shaped. Seen in sickle cell anemia.
   5. *Spherocytes:* Small spherical without central pallor. Seen in hereditary spherocytosis, extravascular hemolysis as in autoimmune hemolytic anemia, G6PD deficiency.
   6. *Target cells:* Central and outer rim staining with intervening ring of pallor. Seen in thalassemia, hemoglobin C, sickle C disease, liver diseases.
   7. *Tear drop cells:* Shape of tear drop. Seen in myelofibrosis and other infiltrative processes of marrow, e.g. carcinoma.
   8. *Rouleaux:* In stacks. Seen in multiple myeloma, macroglobulinemia.
   9. *Howell-Jolly bodies:* 2 micrometer basophilic cytoplasmic inclusions. Seen in asplenic patients.
   10. *Heinz bodies (aggregates of denatured hemoglobin):* G6PD deficiency after oxidant stress, e.g. infection, certain drugs. Unstable hemoglobin variants.
   11. *Basophilic stippling (aggregated ribosomes seen as multiple basophilic cytoplasmic bodies):* Lead poisoning, thalassemia, myelofibrosis.
   12. *Pappenheimer bodies (iron):* Resemble basophilic stippling, but also stain with iron stains, e.g. Prussian blue. Seen in sideroblastic anemias, lead poisoning.
   13. *Schistocytes (fragmented RBCs):* Microangiopathic hemolytic anemia (DIC, thrombotic thrombocytopenic purpura TTP).
   14. *Cabot's ring bodies (nuclear remnants):* Lead toxicity, pernicious anemia, hemolytic anemia.

15. *Parasites:* Intracytoplasmic malaria, babesia, bartonella.
16. *Reticulocytes:* RBCs which are one stage before final maturation. Seen in peripheral smear within 2 days from release from bone marrow. These are slightly larger (7.5 micron) than normal RBCs (7 micron). These are light-bluish in color (due to RNA in the cytoplasm). These can be better visualized by staining with basic dye supravitally (meaning staining before making blood film) whereby RNA precipitates as reticulum. Normal range is 0.2 to 2%. These are increased in increased erythropoiesis, e.g. hemolytic diseases, severe hemorrhage, treatment of pernicious anemia by vitamin B_{12}, etc.

60. What are blood groups?

Ans. RBCs have antigens on their surface and correspondingly different antibodies are present in the serum. On this basis blood group of an individual is determined. Main antigens are A, B and Rh.

ABO Blood Groups

Based on A and B, 4 ABO blood groups are determined by testing for the presence or absence of A and B antigens on the RBCs using anti-A and anti-B reagents **(cell typing** or **forward typing)**; and, by testing for anti-A and anti-B in the serum using reagents A and B RBCs **(serum** or **reverse typing)**. Based on these, 4 blood groups are determined as follows:

1. O
2. A
3. B
4. AB

1. Individual having O blood group has no antigens on RBC surface. So, his RBCs do not react with either anti-A or anti B or anti-AB serum. And, his serum has both anti-A and anti-B antibodies. So, his serum reacts positively with both RBCs containing antigen A and B.
2. Individual having A blood group has only antigen A on his RBC surface. So his RBCs do not react with anti-B serum. And only react with anti-A serum. And, his serum contains anti-B antibody. So, his serum reacts with RBCs containing B antigen.
3. Individual having B blood group has only B antigen on his RBCs. So his RBCs do not react with anti-A serum. And only react with anti-B serum. His serum contains anti-A antibody. So, his serum reacts with RBCs containing A antigen.
4. Individual having AB blood group has both A and B antigens on their RBCs. So his RBCs react with serum containing anti-A, anti-B and anti-AB antibodies. His serum contains no antibodies. So, his serum does not react with RBCs containing A and/or B antigens.

61. What is Rh typing?

Ans. Besides A and B antigens other important RBC antigen is Rh (D) antigen. If it is present on a person's RBC, he is called Rh-positive. If not, then Rh-negative.

Method: Clotted blood is optimal for determining antigens on the RBCs and antibodies in the serum. Also, blood from a skin puncture may be added directly to isotonic saline for RBC typing.

62. What is the significance of blood groups?

Ans. As a rule, a person should receive the blood for transfusion with the same type of blood as his own. In urgent situations, type O RBCs may be used for patients of other blood types. Rh-negative patient should only receive Rh-negative blood. Rh-positive patient can receive either Rh-positive or Rh-negative blood.

63. What are the hazards of blood transfusion?

Ans. a. *Hemolytic:* Fever, chills, flushing, chest pain, flank pain, hypotension, shock, hemoglobinemia, hemoglobinuria, DIC, renal failure, anuria.

b. *Anaphylactic:* Flushing of skin, abrupt hypertension followed by hypotension, substernal chest pain, dyspnea, nausea, abdominal cramps.

c. *Bacterial contamination:* Fever, chills, hypotension, tachycardia, shock (skin warm), hemoglobinemia, hemoglobinuria.

d. *Circulatory volume overload:* Anxiety, restlessness, coughing, tachycardia, dyspnea, cyanosis.

WBCs

64. What are some of the causes of neutrophilia (absolute count > 10,000/c mm)?

Ans. *Infections:* By various pyogenic bacteria (e.g. Ac. appendicitis, salpingitis, otitis, tonsillitis, pharyngitis, pneumonia, etc.) and also by various fungi and spirochetes. Toxic and traumatic causes, e.g. uremia, eclampsia, gout, diabetic acidosis, myocardial infarction, burns, neoplastic diseases, etc. Hematologic disorders, e.g. myeloproliferative disorders, myelogenous leukemia, postsplenectomy.

65. What are some of the causes of neutropenia/agranulocytosis (absolute count <2500/c mm)?

Ans. *ETIO* and *PATHOG* 2 categories:

1. *Decreased production:*

   Aplastic anemia, B_{12} and folate deficiencies, myelofibrosis, malignant infiltrates. Due to drugs causing idiosyncratic reaction, e.g. chloramphenicol, sulfonamides, chlorpromazine **(not dose-related)** or causing bone marrow suppression, e.g. chemotherapeutic drugs **(dose-related)**.

2. *Increased destruction:*

   Severe bacterial, fungal or rickettsial infections or hypersplenism; idiopathic or by drugs, e.g. aminopyrine; due to sequestration.

3. *Miscellaneous:* Typhoid, paratyphoid, brucellosis (possibly due to toxic suppression of the marrow), kala-azar, rheumatoid arthritis **(Felty's syndrome** = RA+ splenomegaly + neutropenia). Megaloblastic anemia, etc.

66. What are the morphologic alterations of neutrophils?

Ans. **Shift to left:** Less number of lobes of the nucleus. Seen in severe infection because marrow is trying to produce these cells and release them in the circulation rapidly and so releases them prematurely.

Shift to right: Increased number of lobes in the nucleus (e.g. > 5 in macrocytic anemia due to decreased DNA synthesis leading to reduction in division of cells).

Toxic granulation: Toxic granules are dark blue to purple. They are peroxidase positive. These are seen in severe infections or toxic conditions.

Dohle inclusion bodies: Present in the cytoplasm. 1–2 micron, pale blue with Wright's stain. They are remnants of free ribosomes or rough endoplasmic reticulum. They are seen in scarlet fever, and in many other infections and toxic conditions. Therefore, they are present with toxic granulations.

Pelger-Huet anomaly: Autosomal dominant condition. Neutrophils have bilobed nuclei. Ineffective for defense purposes predisposing to infections.

Pseudo-Pelger-Huet: Associated with myelodysplastic syndrome and some leukemias.

Chediak-Higashi syndrome: Autosomal recessive. Cells have giant granules which are abnormal lysosomes with decreased lysosomal function, thereby predisposing to infections.

Auer rods: Eosinophilic rod-like cytoplasmic inclusions. Seen in AML.

67. What are some of the causes of eosinophilia (absolute count >500/c mm)?

Ans. Allergic conditions, e.g. bronchial asthma and seasonal rhinitis (hay fever). These immune reactions are mediated by IgE which result in mast cells and basophil degranulation with release of ECF-A. Allergic reactions to drugs.

Parasitic infections: E.g. trichinosis, **visceral larva migrans** (dog and cat worms). **Loeffler syndrome** (temporary pulmonary eosinophilia with peripheral eosinophilia, with cough, fever, SOB, idiopathic or due to larval infiltration of lung by *Ascaris lumbricoides, Ancylostoma duodenale, Necator americanas, Strongyloides stercoralis*), **Loeffler endocarditis** (restrictive cardiomyopathy with eosinophilic infiltrate and peripheral eosinophilia with a **rapid fatal course**). Decreased glucocorticoids in blood **(Addison's disease)**.

68. What are some of the causes of eosinopenia (absolute count <50/c mm)?

Ans. Any situation which causes acute stress resulting in adrenal glucocorticoid and epinephrine secretion. Also, in Cushing's syndrome due to increased glucocorticoids in the blood.

69. What are some of the causes of basophilia (absolute count >100/c mm)?

Ans. 1. Allergic reactions.

2. Chronic granulocytic leukemia.
3. Myeloid metaplasia.
4. Polycythemia vera.
5. Postsplenectomy.
6. Postirradiation.
7. Chronic hemolytic anemia.
8. Hypothyroidism.

70. What are some of the causes of basopenia?

Ans. 1. Basophils and eosinophils have diurnal variations, i.e. level is lowest in morning and highest during night.
2. Chronic treatment with steroids.
3. Cushing's syndrome.
4. Acute infection or stress.
5. Hyperthyroidism.

71. What are some of the causes of monocytosis (absolute count >800/c mm)?

Ans. 1. Subacute bacterial endocarditis.
2. Mycotic, rickettsial (typhus), protozoal (malaria, kala-azar, trypanosomiasis), and viral infections, TB.
3. Sarcoidosis.
4. Rheumatoid-arthritis (RA), SLE.

72. What are some of the causes of monocytopenia (absolute count <100/c mm)?

Ans. 1. Hairy cell leukemia.
2. Aplastic anemia.
3. Steroids.
4. Immunosuppressive or chemotherapeutic drugs.

73. What are some of the causes of lymphocytosis (absolute count >5000/c mm)?

Ans. 1. Almost all viral infections, e.g. infectious mononucleosis, cytomegalovirus, herpes virus, measles, mumps.
2. Pertusis.
3. Toxoplasmosis.
4. Adrenal insufficiency.

74. What are some of the causes of lymphocytopenia (absolute count <1000/c mm)?

Ans. 1. Increased levels of adrenocortical hormones.
2. Chemotherapeutic drugs.

3. AIDS.
4. Chronic illness, e.g. SLE, CCF, uremia.

75. What is leukemoid reaction?

Ans. 1. Severe leukocytosis (>50,000/c mm) with immature neutrophils in peripheral blood due to severe infections, severe hemolysis, malignancies, e.g. cancer of breast, lungs, kidneys. D/D with CML: Leucocyte alkaline phosphatase **(LAP)** increased in leukemoid reaction and severely reduced or **absent in CML**. Also, **philadelphia chromosome** and **massive splenomegaly is seen in CML** but not in leukemoid reaction.

2. Severe lymphocytosis may be seen in severe viral illnesses, e.g. chickenpox or pertusis. D/D with lymphocytic leukemia: In lymphocytic leukemia the lymphocytes are homogenous in appearance whereas reactive lymphocytes which are seen in non-leukemic lymphocytosis are heterogenous.

76. What is leukoerythroblastotic reaction? What is leucoblastotic reaction?

Ans. Leukoerythroblastotic reaction is similar to leukemoid reaction plus there are nucleated RBCs in peripheral blood smear. Also, tear drop RBCs are seen in peripheral blood. *ETIO:* Severe hemorrhage, hemolysis, bone marrow infiltration by fibrosis, granulomas, neoplasm. **Leucoblastotic reaction** is the presence in the peripheral blood of immature forms of neutrophils which are more immature than bands.

77. What is infectious mononucleosis?

Ans. *DEF/DES:* An acute self-limited viral disease of young adults. *ETIO*: EBV (member of herpes virus family). It has an affinity for B lymphocytes. After intimate oral contact, kissing, the virus which is present in saliva, penetrates the recipient's nasopharyngeal, oropharyngeal and salivary epithelial cells, spreads to underlying oropharyngeal lymphoid tissue, specifically to B lymphocytes. B-cells produce antibodies, one of which is used for diagnostic purpose is the **Heterophil anti-sheep RBC antibody**. First the IgM and later IgG antibodies are produced. Also, cytotoxic CD8+ T-cells and natural killer (NK) cells participate to control the proliferation of the B-cells. Virus specific T-cells appear as **atypical lymphocytes** seen in the peripheral blood smear. *C/Fs*: Onset: Acute. *S/S*: Sore throat, fever, malaise, lymphadenopathy, splenomegaly, hepatitis with disorder of LFTs, skin rash.

Tests/DIAG:

1. Peripheral blood smear has atypical lymphocytes.
2. Monospot test, consisting of detecting anti-sheep RBC antibodies (IgM)-positive heterophil test **(Paul-Bunnell reaction)**. Condition resolves spontaneously in 4–6 weeks. *COMPLI:* These can involve any organ in the body. Mainly worsening of the hepatitis with sometimes even hepatic failure. CNS, kidney, marrow, lungs, eyes, heart, spleen **(Fatal rupture of spleen)**. *MORPHO*: Peripheral blood has absolute lymphocytosis with TLC 12–18000 per microliter with lymphocytes 60%, many of these are large 12–16 micrometer in diameter, with increased cytoplasm

with clear vacuoles and oval, folded nucleus. *Lymph nodes:* Enlarged lymph nodes all over the body, mainly in posterior cervical, axillary and groin regions. *MICRO:* Lymphoid tissue has many atypical lymphocytes in the paracortical (T-cell) area. Some enlargement of follicles due to proliferation of B-cells is also present. Sometimes cells similar to Reed-Sternberg cells may be seen.

Spleen: Enlarged, 300–500 gm. *MICRO:* Similar to lymph nodes with a heavy infiltration of atypical lymphocytes. Spleen is susceptible to rupture due to weakening of the trabeculae and capsule from infiltration by lymphocytes.

Liver: Mild hepatitis with mild temporary abnormality of LFTs. *MICRO:* Atypical lymphocytes are present in portal areas and sinusoids and focally in small groups with small areas of necrosis.

78. What are hematological malignancies?

Ans. These are leukemias and lymphomas of the myeloid and lymphoid systems of our body which somewhat occur in an inter-related spectrum of malignant diseases.

79. What are the etiologic factors which contribute to white cell neoplasia?

Ans. A. *Microbial and environmental agents:*

1. EBV.
2. HTLV-1.
3. HHV-8.
4. *H. pylori* in gastric marginal zone lymphoma.
5. Gluten sensitive enteropathy in intestinal T-cell lymphoma.

B. *Genetic:* Bloom syndrome, Fanconi syndrome, ataxia telangiectasia–increased risk of Ac. Leukemia. Down syndrome (trisomy 21) and neurofibromatosis type I-increased risk of childhood leukemia.

C. *Chromosomal translocations and oncogenes:* t(15;17)-M3 (Ac. promyelocytic leukemia) t(9;22)-philadelphia chromosome—(ALL, AML, CML).

D. *Iatrogenic:* Radiotherapy, chemotherapy increase the risk of AML, NHL, MDS.

80. What are the categories of hematological proliferative diseases?

Ans. 1. Lymphoid (T, B, NK cells) neoplasms.

2. Myeloid (Granulocytic, monocytic, thrombocytic, erythroid) neoplasms.
3. Histiocytosis (Langerhans cell histiocytosis).

Lymphoid neoplasms: Arise from multipotent stem cells which give rise to T, B, NK cells. All are malignant:

Types:

A. *Non-Hodgkin's lymphoma:*

DEF: Neoplastic proliferation of lymphoid cells as discrete tissue masses in lymph nodes, spleen or other sites.

B. *Lymphocytic leukemias:*

DEF: Neoplasms present with widespread involvement of bone marrow usually with large numbers of tumor cells in peripheral blood.

C. *Hodgkin's lymphoma:*

DEF: Hodgkin's lymphoma is now thought to be a lymphoma of B-cell origin, the diagnosis of which is made by biopsy of lymph node or extranodal lymphoid tissue showing Reed-Sternberg cell within the cellular background of lymphocytes, eosinophils, histiocytes, neutrophils, plasma cells, fibroblasts, and collagen fibres.

Classification of Hodgkin's lymphoma:

1. Lymphocytic predominant.
2. Lymphocytic-rich.
3. Lymphocyte-depleted.
4. Mixed cellularity.
5. Nodular sclerosis.

Myeloid neoplasms: Arise from multipotent stem cells which give rise to myeloid lineage cells—granulocytes, monocytes, erythrocytes and platelets.
Types:

a. AML (acute myelogenous leukemia).
b. Myelodysplastic syndrome (MDS).
c. Chronic myeloproliferative syndromes (CMS).

Histiocytosis (Langerhans cell histiocytosis)

a. Eosinophilic granuloma.
b. Hand-Schuller Christian disease.
c. Letterer-Siwe disease.

81. What is the classification of non-Hodgkin's lymphomas and lymphoid leukemias. Revised American-European lymphoma (REAL)/World Health Organization (WHO) (1995)?

Ans. 1. Precursor B-cell Ac. lymphoblastic leukemia (ALL)/lymphoma.
2. Precursor T-cell Ac. lymphoblastic leukemia (ALL)/lymphoma.

Neoplasms of mature B-cells

1. Burkitt lymphoma.
2. Diffuse large B-cell lymphoma.
3. Extranodal maginal zone lymphoma (MALToma).
4. Follicular lymphoma.
5. Hairy cell leukemia.
6. Mantle cell lymphoma.
7. Multiple myeloma/solitary (plasmacytoma).
8. Small lymphocytic lymphoma (chronic lymphocytic leukemia) (CLL).

Neoplasms of mature T-cells or NK-cells

1. Adult T-cell leukemia/lymphoma.
2. Anaplastic large cell lymphoma.
3. Extranodal NK/T-cell lymphoma.
4. Mycosis fungoides/Sezary syndrome.
5. T-cell granular lymphocytic leukemia.

82. What is the classification of myeloid neoplasms?

Ans. a. *AML:* Collection of immature myeloid cells in BM with suppression of normal hematopoiesis.

1. AML with recurrent chromosomal rearrangements.
2. AML with multilineage dysplasia.
3. AML therapy-related.
4. AML, NOS (FAB).

FAB Classification of AML

1. M0-minimally differentiated.
2. M1-without maturation AML.
3. M2-with maturation AML.
4. M3-Ac. promyelocytic leukemia.
5. M4-Ac. myelo-monocytic leukemia.
6. M5-Ac. monocytic leukemia.
7. M6-Ac. erythroleukemia.
8. M7-Ac. megakaryocytic leukemia.

b. *Myelodysplastic syndromes (MDS):* Maturation defects with ineffective hematopoiesis with cytopenias with risk of transformation to AML.

1. Idiopathic/primary
2. Secondary to treatment (therapy-related)

c. *Chronic myeloproliferative syndromes (CMS):*

1. CML (chronic myelogenous leukemia).
2. Polycythemia vera.
3. Essential thrombocytosis.
4. Primary myelofibrosis.

83. What are the tests for classification of leukemias and lymphomas?

Ans.

1. Acid-base reactions of cellular organelles/components (Leishman's stain).
2. Cytosol enzymes (cytochemistry) (special stains). [Myeloperoxidase (MPO), Sudan black B specific esterase—positive in myelocytes/non-specific esterase—positive in monocytes/PAS—positive in lymphocytes].
3. Surface antigens (CD = Cluster differentiation/designation) (immunochemistry/immunophenotype) (TdT = Terminal deoxynucleotidyl transferase).

4. Chromosome analysis (karyotyping, cytogenetics):
   a. t(18;14)—Seen in ALL with a mature B-cell phenotype (has a very poor prognosis).
   b. t(15;17)—Seen in M3 (Ac. promyelocytic leukemia): Here a transcriptional unit called PML on chromosome 15 fuses with a gene on chromosome 17 [retinoic acid receptor—alpha (RAR-alpha)]—This fusion blocks myeloid differentiation. This block can be overcome by high doses of all-transretinoic acid A (vit. A analog).
   c. t(9;22)-(philadelphia chromosome-Ph chromosome)—Seen in CML-Here c-abl proto-oncogene on chromosome 9 is transposed to an area on chromosome 22 besides an oncogene forming a fusion gene (bcr-c-abl) which codes for a protein, which activates cells for neoplastic proliferation.
   d. Trisomy 21—Seen in ALL and AML.
5. EM (Electron microscope).

84. What is cluster differentiation/designation?

Ans. Cluster = A cluster (group) of many different antibodies react with different epitopes (antibody-binding sites) on molecules on the surface of cells. Differentiation = These epitopes on cell-surface molecules are different depending on the type and stage of differentiation of cells. Hence, the term "differentiation molecule". Therefore, cluster differentiation = specific target molecule on cell surface (based on the differentiation and stage of cell) which are recognized by a cluster (group) of antibodies. CD-34 (pluripotent hematopoietic cell). CD-45 (leucocyte common antigen present on ALL WBCs).

TdT and CDs help in D/D of various cells as follows:

- Enzyme terminal deoxynucleotidyl transferase (TdT) is present on ALL T and B immature lymphocytes (lymphoblasts) and absent in all myelocytes (myeloblasts). This helps to distinguish immature lymphocytes (lymphoblasts) from immature myelocytes (myeloblasts).

CDs positive in lymphocytes:

- CD-2, 3, 4, 7, 8 in T-cells (CD-4-helper/CD-8-suppressor/cytotoxic).
- CD-10, 19, 20 and surface Ig in B-cells.
- CD-16, 56 in NK-cells.
- CD-15, 30 in Hodgkin's cells.

CDs positive in granuocytes/monocytes:

- CD-14 in monocyte, CD-15 in granulocytes.

85. What are the main categories of malignant proliferations of white cells?

Ans. 1. Lymphoid neoplasms.
2. Myeloid neoplasms.

86. What are the categories of the lymphoid neoplasms?

Ans. 1. Hodgkin's lymphoma.
2. Non-Hodgkin's lymphoma/lymphoid leukemia.

87. What are some diagnostic features of Hodgkin's lymphoma and non-Hodgkin's lymphoma?

Ans. *Diagnosis of Hodgkin's lymphoma is made by:* Biopsy of lymph node or extranodal lymphoid tissue showing Reed-Sternberg cell within cellular background of lymphocytes, eosinophils, histiocytes, neutrophils, plasma cells, fibroblasts and collagen fibres. *Diagnosis of non-Hodgkin's lymphoma is made by:* a combination of abnormal cellular architecture, abnormal phenotype and lymphoid monoclonality.

88. How are Hodgkin's lymphoma and non-Hodgkin's lymphoma classified?

Ans. WHO classification of Hodgkin's lymphoma divides it into 2 groups:

A. Classical:

1. Nodular sclerosis
2. Mixed cellularity
3. Lymphocyte-rich
4. Lymphocyte-depleted

B. Nodular lymphocyte-predominant.

Non-Hodgkin's lymphomas are classified based on: The cell of lineage, i.e. B, T, or natural killer cells.

89. What are the non-Hodgkin's lymphomas/lymphoid leukemias?

Ans. *DEF of lymphoma:* Malignant neoplasms of lymphoid system where neoplastic lymphoid cells are **seen as discrete masses**. 2/3 arise in lymph nodes and 1/3 in lymphoid tissue in various organs.

DEF of lymphoid leukemia: Malignant lymphoid neoplasms presenting with **widespread involvement of bone marrow**; and usually with large number of tumor cells in **peripheral blood**.

The difference between lymphoma and lymphoid leukemia in various cases is in tissue distribution when initially seen, because in these in course of time lymphoma cells spread to blood and leukemia cells to solid lymphoid tissues.

90. What are precursor B- and T-cell acute lymphoblastic leukemia (ALL) and lymphoma?

Ans. B-lymphocyte precursors arise in bone marrow. Similarly their lymphomas arise in bone marrow involving it and also peripheral blood (leukemia-ALL). T-lymphocyte precursors are in thymus. Similarly their lymphomas are in thymus and mediastinum and also involve peripheral blood (leukemia-ALL). ALL are similar in many ways to AML (acute myeloblastic leukemia). However, ALL is seen in children and young adults and overall prognosis is good, whereas median age in AML is 50 years and overall prognosis is poor.

Similarities in ALL and AML are:

1. The cells have long generation time making them take over the bone marrow replacing the normal cells causing anemia, thrombocytopenia and susceptibility to infections.
2. Generalized lymphadenopathy, splenomegaly, hepatomegaly—more in ALL than AML.
3. CNS involvement—more in ALL than AML.

91. What is diffuse small lymphocytic lymphoma?

Ans. *Diffuse small lymphocytic lymphoma:* Almost all are B-cell. They have pan-B antigen (CD19). *C/Fs:* Age: Mainly old age-related CLL. Generalized lymphadenopathy with mild to moderate splenomegaly and hepatopmegaly. Survival is prolonged. Hypogammaglobulinemia is present with susceptibility to infections. Some patients have autoimmune hemolytic anemia and thrombocytopenia. *MORPHO:* Cells are uniform, small, with dark round nuclei, and little cytoplasm. These patients have morphologic and clinical similarities with CLL. Marrow is involved in almost all patients and 1/2 patients have neoplastic cells in the peripheral blood appearing like CLL.

92. What is chronic lymphocytic leukemia (CLL)?

Ans. *Incidence:* 60 years and above. Oldest age group out of all leukemias. *S/S*: Accidental diagnosis. Palpable lymph nodes, fewest symptoms. *DIAG:* TLC—increased in all cases and could be 100,000/microliter. DLC—small lymphocytes (B-cells), mild normochromic, normocytic anemia, platelets—decreased, lymph nodes are enlarged, spleen is moderately enlarged, liver may be enlarged, hypogammaglobulinemia is present, autoimmunity with warm autoantibody hemolytic anemia is seen. *PROG*: Good, longest survival average 10 years.

93. What is diffuse large cell lymphoma?

Ans. Most are B-cell; 10% T-cell. *C/Fs:* Age: average 60 yearss. EBV virus lymphomas and lymphomas in patients with AIDS are of this type. Onset is acute consisting of a mass at a single nodal region or extranodal region, e.g. GIT, skin, bone, brain, Waldeyer's ring. **Aggressive without treatment, but respond well to aggressive treatment with even cure**. *MORPHO:* Cells are large. Nuclei are round with large one or two nucleoli. Cytoplasm is dark and stains positive (pink) with methyl green pyronine stain.

94. What is follicular lymphoma?

Ans. *C/Fs:* Age: Older people. Present as painless generalized lymphadenopathy. Bone marrow involvement is common, visceral involvement is uncommon. Median survival 10 years. Do not respond to treatment. Sometimes, these progress to high grade diffuse lymphoma. *MORPHO:* Normal architecture of lymph node is replaced by nodules of type B lymphoma cells which appear like activated B-cells in the lymphoid follicles.

95. What is small noncleaved (Burkitt's) lymphoma?

Ans. Three types:

a. Endemic (African).

b. Nonendemic (sporadic).

c. HIV patients:

Cells are of B-cell origin with pan-B marker CD-19. *C/Fs:* Age-kids and young adults. Presentation in African type: Is with involvement of maxilla or mandible. North American type: Is with involvement of bowel or retroperitoneal lymphoid tissue with tumor formation. High grade, **perhaps the fastest growing human neoplasm**, but with aggressive treatment long-term survival can be seen in 50% cases. *MORPHO*: Cells are of intermediate size with oval nuclei and 2–3 nucleoli. Cytoplasm appears pink by methyl green pyronine stain. Mitotic figures are many. There are a large number of necrotic tumor cells engulfed by macrophages with clear space around them giving a **starry sky** appearence.

96. What is hairy cell leukemia?

Ans. Cell involved is B-cell. **Positive for tartrate-resistant acid phosphatase**. Cells have hair-like projections. *C/Fs:* Splenomegaly (massive), hepatomegaly (less common and less enlarged), lymphadenopathy (rare). Pancytopenia. Monocytopenia with predisposition to atypical mycobacterial infection. Prognosis: Good.

97. What are plasma cell dyscrasias, disorders of neoplasms?

Ans. These are a group of neoplasms of plasma cells, which are the final differentiated B lymphocytes, which produce monoclonal immunoglobulin (M protein) due to neoplastic proliferation of monoclonal plasma cells. Some of the conditions included in this are: Multiple myeloma, solitary plasmacytoma, Waldenstrom's macroglobulinemia, lympho plasmacytic lymphoma, heavy chain disease, primary amyloidosis having AL (Amyloid light chain).

98. What is multiple myeloma?

Ans. *DEF:* Malignant plasma cell disease with neopiastic plasma cells in the bone marrow with many lytic lesions of the skeleton. *DES:* Normally, plasma cells produce immunoglobulins to fight infection. But, in multiple myeloma, the monoclonal plasma cells produce M protein (abnormal IgG in 60% cases, IgA in 30% cases and rarely IgM, IgD or IgE). In 10% cases not the whole immunoglobulin molecule is produced but only kappa or lambda light chains are produced, which due to their low molecular weight are excreted in the urine and are called **Bence Jones proteins**. In these patients where there is **Bence Jones proteinuria** with increased serum protein the disease is called **light chain disease**. But, in 80% cases malignant plasma cells secrete both complete immunoglobulins plus the light chains **(Bence Jones proteins)**.

Also, they produce cytokines that stimulate osteoclasts and suppress osteoblasts. *MORPHO:* Bones have lytic lesions mainly involving vertebrae, skull, ribs pelvis, femur clavicle and scapula. These begin in marrow and spread to destroy cancellous and cortical bone predisposing to pathological fractures. By X-ray the lesions appear as punched out defects of 2–4 cm. Microscopically, marrow has increased number of plasma cells in focal to diffuse distribution which may appear normal or immature. Plasma cell infiltrate may also be seen in spleen, liver, kidneys, lungs and lymph nodes. *Renal involvement:* Interstitial infiltrate of plasma cells is present. Bence Jones protein casts are present in convoluted tubules and collecting ducts. AL amyloid might be also present. Hypercalcemia can cause metastatic calcification. *PATHOG* and *C/Fs:* Age—50 yrs. Increased serum **M protein** causes hyperviscosity; light chain proteins cause end-organ damage mainly in the kidneys; invasive bone lesions cause bone pain and pathological fractures, vertebral compression fractures can cause paresthesias of the lower limbs, osteoporosis and hypercalcemia; hypercalcemia can cause confusion, constipation, polydypsia, lethargy, somnolence, anorexia, nausea; bone marrow invasion causes anemia; anemia causes weakness and lethargy; impaired antibodies and leucopenia causes recurrent infections. *DIAG:* X-ray-punched out lesions. Serum and urine protein electrophoresis with monoclonal gammopathy. *PROG:* Progressive disease with median survival 2–4 yrs.

99. What is Waldenstrom's macroglobulinemia?

Ans. It is a hyperviscosity syndrome due to increased production of monoclonal IgM commonly seen as a component of lymphoplasmacytic lymphoma which is a malignant neoplasm of B lymphocytes/plasma cells. It is usually seen in approximately 60-year-old males. *MORPHO*: Diffuse infiltrates of plasma cells is present in bone marrow, lymph nodes and spleen. *C/Fs:* Hyperviscosity can cause CHF, retinal ischemia with visual disturbances, cerebral ischemia with neurologic distrubances. Plasmapheresis may be helpful. Average survival is 5 years.

100. What is mantle cell lymphoma?

Ans. Tumor cells are present besides the germinal centers in lymph nodes or diffusely efface normal lymph node architecture. *C/Fs:* 50-year-old males. Generalized lymphadenopathy, bone marrow and liver involvement. *PROG*: Poor. Median survival—3–4 years.

101. What are extranodal marginal zone lymphoma (MALTomas)?

Ans. MALT = Mucosa-associated lymphoid tissue/marginal zone-associated lymphoid tissue. These are low grade B-cell lymphomas. They are called MALTomas because these are commonly seen in mucosa-associated lymphoid tissue, e.g. small and large intestines, lungs, salivary glands. Also, because tumor cells look like B-cells which are seen in the margins of B-cell follicle. These are commonly seen with Sjogren syndrome or *H. pylori* infection in the stomach.

102. What are the neoplasms of mature T- and NK-cells?

Ans. 1. Adult T-cell lymphoma/leukemia.

2. Mycosis fungoides/Sezary syndrome.

103. What is adult T-cell lymphoma/leukemia?

Ans. Seen in patients infected with human T-cell leukemia virus type 1 (HTLV-1) (endemic in Southern Japan and Caribbean). *MORPHO:* Multilobular nuclei **(flower cells, cloverleaf)**. *C/Fs:* Skin involvement, generalized lymphadenopathy, hepatosplenomegaly, lymphocytosis, hypercalcemia. *PROG*: Poor. Median survival is < 1 year.

104. What are mycosis fungoides and Sezary syndrome (cutaneous T-cell lymphomas)?

Ans. Mycosis fungoides is an uncommon T-cell lymphoma of the skin, grossly showing patches and plaques and microscopically showing atypical lymphocytes with cerebriform nuclei in epidermis and superficial dermis. Usually, it has benign course of 10 years or more. Sometimes, it can progress to a nodular (tumor) stage and also involve systemic organs. And in elderly males it can, sometimes, spread to lymph nodes and peripheral blood (known as **Sezary syndrome**).

105. What is Hodgkin's lymphoma?

Ans. *DEF/DES:* Malignant neoplasm of B lymphocytes with characteristic Reed Sternberg giant cell, within a background of reactive lymphocytes, plasma cells, histiocytes, granulocytes (mainly eosinophils).

Types:

A. Classical:

1. Nodular sclerosis.
2. Mixed cellularity.
3. Lymphocyte-rich.
4. Lymphocyte-depleted.

B. Nodular lymphocyte predominant.

Prognosis does not depend on these morphologic features but on the clinical stage.

1. *Nodular sclerosis:* R-S cell **lacunar variant**. Collagen bands. Prognosis—excellent.
2. *Mixed cellularity:* **Classic R-S cells**. Prognosis—good.
3. *Lymphocyte-rich:* Rare. Majority cells—reactive lymphocytes. **Classic R-S cells**. Prognosis—excellent.
4. *Lymphocyte-depleted:* Very few lymphocytes. **Classic R-S cells**. Prognosis—worst of all types.
5. *Nodular lymphocyte predominant:* **Classic R-S cells almost absent**. **Popcorn cells present**. Prognosis—good.

106. What is the staging of Hodgkin's lymphoma? What is its clinical application?

Ans. Staging in Hodgkin's lymphoma guides therapy and prognosis. It is done as follows:

I. One lymph node region involved or 1 extranodal site (Ie).

II. Two lymph nodes involved in the same side of diaphragm.
III. Both sides of diaphragm (with spleen IIIs) (with extranodal IIIe) (both IIIes).
IV. Generalized.

Subclassification of above:

a. Absence of symptoms.
b. Presence of symptoms: Weight loss, fever, night sweats.

107. What is the *D/D* between Hodgkin's and non-Hodgkin's lymphomas?

Ans. *In non-Hodgkin's lymphomas:*

1. Multiple nodes are involved.
2. Waldeyer's ring is involved.
3. Extranodal involvement is present.
4. Non-continuous.
5. Systemic *S/S* not present.

In Hodgkin's lymphomas:

1. Single node area is involved.
2. Waldeyer's ring is not involved.
3. Extranodal involvement is not seen.
4. Spread is continuous.
5. Systemic *S/S* are present.

108. What are the myeloid neoplasms?

Ans. Arise from hematopoietic stem cells which give out myeloid lineage cells (granulocyte, monocyte, RBC, platelets). These mainly involve the bone marrow and to lesser extent the secondary hematopoietic organs: Liver, spleen, lymph nodes.

Three types:

1. *Acute myelogenous leukemia (AML):* Here there is accumulation of immature myeloid cells in the bone marrow.
2. *Chronic myeloproliferative syndromes (CMS):* Here there is increased production of terminally differentiated myeloid cells.
3. *Myelodysplastic syndromes (MDS):* Here there is ineffective hematopoiesis with cytopenias.

109. What is AML?

Ans. It is a heterogenous group of disorders where undifferentiated myeloid progenitor cells (blasts) collect in the bone marrow. Myeloid cells normally die through differentiation. Thus, the block in differentiation leads to collection of blasts in marrow. These blasts suppress normal marrow cells with marrow failure. Therefore, treatment requires killing these blast cells to allow normal marrow to proliferate; except in acute promyelocytic leukemia (M-3) where overcoming this block is the principle of treatment.

110. What is the WHO classification of AML?

Ans. a. With recurrent chromosomal rearrangements.

b. With multilineage dysplasia.

c. Treatment-related.

d. Not otherwise specified (NOS). French American British—(FAB) classification of 1976: M0 to M7: M0 to M3 by degree of maturation; M4 to M7 by lineage of blasts.

1. M0-Minimum differentiated AML—Myeloperoxidase negative. Antigens and EM appearance of myeloblasts.
2. M1-Without maturation AML, few myeloperoxidase + few granules, **auer rods,** no maturation beyond blasts. Auer rods are diagnostic of leukemic myeloblasts.
3. M2-With maturation AML, mature to PMNs, **auer rods** +.
4. M3-Ac. Promyelocytic-PML, **auer rods** ++, cells mostly promyelocytic, **t(15;17),** DIC.
5. M4-Ac. Myelomonocytic-AMML monoblasts +ve for non-specific esterase.
6. M5-Ac. Monocytic leukemia monoblasts, non-specific esterase +, peroxidase negative.
7. M6-Ac. Erythroleukemia—Wright Giemsa stain.
8. M7-Ac. Megakaryocytic—Identified by EM and reaction with antibodies to GPIIb/IIIa or vWF.

Incidence: Adults 20–40 years. *C/Fs*: Anemia, neutropenia, thrombocytopenia (bleeding) procoagulants released by leukemic cells in M3 (Ac. promyelocytic leukemia) may cause DIC. In M3 (PML): t (15;17) blocks cell differentiation. This knowledge is used for its therapy by treatment which overcomes this block, thereby cells mature and die and are replaced by normal marrow cells. *S/S*: Same as ALL, CNS involvement is less common than ALL. *DIAG*: TLC-increased in 50% cases could be >100,000/microliter, myeloblasts ++, anemia in >90%, normochromic normocytic, platelets decreased in 90% cases, splenomegaly in 50% cases, liver and lymph nodes enlarged occasionally. *DIAG:* Marrow >30% blasts, M1-M3: myeloperoxidase, sudan black B and specific esterase positive, M4-M5-non-specific esterase positive, M6-erythroleukemia, mainly immature erythroblastic morphology, M7 by EM.

D/D with lymphoblasts: CD 33 positive in myeloblasts and CD 15 positive in mature myeloid series–both negative in lymphoblasts.

PROG: Before treatment was available life expectancy was 4 months only. Now good. Cure 90%. Prognosis is poor in patients over 50 yrs of age and in PML.

111. What is aleukemic leukemia?

Ans. When there are no blasts present in the peripheral blood; but, only in the bone marrow. Also, *see* page 387.

112. What are chronic myeloproliferative syndromes (CMS)?

Ans. *DEF:* Neoplastic clonal proliferation of myeloid stem cells. These include:

1. CML (Chronic myeloid leukemia).
2. PV (Polycythemia vera).
3. Myelofibrosis with myeloid metaplasia (MMM) (malignant megakaryocytic leukemia with myelofibrosis with myeloid metaplasia with extramedullary hematopoiesis).
4. ET (essential thrombocythemia).

In CML: The **pluripotent stem cell**, which can give rise to both myeloid and lymphoid lineage of cells, is transformed into malignant neoplastic cell.

In PV, MMM and ET: **Multipotent stem cell** capable of giving rise to mature RBC, granulocyte, monocyte, platelets is transformed into malignant neoplastic cell. Since in CMS terminal differentiation of cells is not affected (as opposed to AML) the marrow is hypercellular and there is elevated peripheral blood count.

113. What are the common features of CMS?

Ans.
1. Peak incidence in middle-aged and elderly people.
2. Proliferation of one or more of the myeloid series.
3. Peripheral blood basophils increased.
4. Serum uric acid increased.
5. Marked splenomegaly.
6. Neoplastic stem cells seen in circulation and also in secondary hematopoietic organs, mainly spleen with extramedullary hematopoiesis.
7. In the end there is marrow fibrosis and peripheral blood cytopenias.
8. Progression in due course of time to AML—This always occurs with CML.

114. What is CML?

Ans. *Incidence:* 40+ yrs. of age. *ETIO:* Translocation 9 and 22 **(philadelphia chromosome)** which activates cells for neoplastic proliferation. *S/S*: Abdominal discomfort due to splenomegaly. *DIAG:* TLC-increased in 100%, DLC-basophilia, entire myeloid series seen. Anemia-mild, normochromic normocytic, platelets-increased, lymph nodes-enlarged sometimes, spleen-enlarged severe, liver may be enlarged, **leukocyte alkaline phosphatase-reduced/absent helps in *D/D* of leukemoid reaction and other 3 CMS where it is elevated**. *PROG:* In approximately 5 years blast crisis develops.

115. What is polycythemia vera?

Ans. *DEF:* Abnormal proliferaton of myeloid stem cells.

Features: 1. Peripheral blood erythrocytes severely increased (erythrocytosis).

2. Peripheral blood granulocytes and platelets moderately increased.

3. Serum erythropoietin level is decreased.

4. Hypercoagulability with increased thrombosis.
5. In late stage myelofibrosis with anemia.
6. Extramedullary hematopoiesis with increased white cells in peripheral blood mimicking CML.
7. Acute leukemia can be seen in approx. 5% cases, more commonly in patients who receive chemotherapy or radiotherapy. *DIAG*: Serum erythropoietin level is decreased. (In all other types of absolute polycythemia erythropoietin level is increased). *D/D:* Secondary polycythemia. (*see* above in section of disorders of RBCs).

116. What is myelofibrosis with myeloid metaplasia (MMM)/agnogenic myeloid metaplasia (AMM)?

Ans. *DEF*: Non-neoplastic proliferation of the fibrous tissue of the bone marrow (myelofibrosis) with extramedullary hematopoiesis in liver and spleen.
PATHOG: Thought to be primarily proliferation of megakaryocytes with production of platelet-derived growth factor and transforming growth factor leading to increased fibroblastic proliferation. Megakaryocytes are not destroyed from increased fibrosis resulting in increased megakaryocytes in the bone marrow and increased platelets in the peripheral blood.
C/Fs:

1. **Tear drop-shaped RBCs** in peripheral blood.
2. Abnormally large platelets in peripheral blood.
3. Anemia.
4. Splenomegaly.
5. Hyperuricemia and gout.
6. Immature granulocytes and nucleated RBCs in peripheral blood **(leukoery throblastosis)**.

117. What is essential thrombocythemia (ET)?

Ans. *DEF:* Severe increase in the megakaryocytes in the bone marrow and increase in platelets in the peripheral blood (over 1 million/microliter—normal is 150,000 to 350,000/microliter). Also there is bleeding and increased thrombosis.

118. What are the myelodysplastic syndromes (MDS)?

Ans. Here, there is mutation of the multipotent stem cell affecting all 3 lineages (RBC, WBC, platelets-erythroid, myeloid, megakaryocytic), with dysplastic (disordered) differentiation of all three:

1. *Erythroid:* Bone marrow has **ring sideroblasts:** Erythroblasts with iron-laden mitochondria—Seen as perinuclear granules with Pearl's Prussian blue stain. Megaloblastoid maturation.
2. *Granulocytic:* Neutrophils with decreased number of normal secondary granules and presence of toxic granules and Dohle bodies. **Pseudo-Pelger-HueT-cells**—PMNs have bi-lobed dumb-bell shaped nuclei seen in Pelger-Huet anomaly.

3. *Megakaryocytic:* Megakaryocytes have single nuclear lobe or multiple separate nuclei **(pawn ball megakaryocytes)**. This term has been used to describe a peculiar type of abnormal cell that can be found in the bone marrow of patients with MDS. The appearance of these cells resembles the **three-ball pawnbroker's symbol**.

Peripheral blood: Myeloblasts, giant platelets, poikilocytes, macrocytes, PMNs with **pseudo-Pelger-Huet anomaly**. MDS is broadly classified according to WHO and FAB (French, American, British) as:

1. Refractory anemia (RA).
2. Refractory anemia and ring sideroblasts (RARS).
3. RA with excess blasts (RAEB).

C/Fs: Seen in elderly with *S/S*: Anemia, infection or bleeding as a result of pancytopenia. 1/3 develop acute myeloblastic leukemia (AML).

119. What is Langerhans cell histiocytosis?

Ans. It consists of idiopathic proliferation of a special type of histiocyte (macrophage) having intracytoplasmic **Birbeck granules** seen by EM as in Langerhans cells in the epidermis and hence the name. Three conditions have this common features and are thus included in this condition.

1. *Eosinophilic granuloma of bone:* This usually presents as solitary slow-growing osteolytic radiolucent lesion of bone in children with benign course and resolution. LM shows many eosinophils, foamy histiocytes and gian T-cells.
2. *Hand-Schuller-Christian disease:* This presents with fever, rash, upper, respiratory infections, mild hepatosplenomegaly, lymphadenopathy and sometimes with a **triad of exophthalmos, skull bone lesions** and **diabetes insipidus** due to involvement of the posterior pituitary stalk of hypothalamus.
3. *Letterer-Siwe disease:* This presents in infants with fever and multi-system involvement by Langerhans histiocytes involving lymph nodes, liver, spleen, skin, bone and has a downhill course with rapid death.

Bleeding Disorders

120. What are the bleeding disorders?

Ans. Three types:

1. Increased fragility of BVs 2. Platelet abnormalities—quantitative or qualitative.
3. Coagulation disorders.

Blood Vessels Disorders

121. What is the increased fragility of blood vessels?

Ans. *Seen in:* Vitamin C deficiency (scurvy), infections (meningococcemia, infective endocarditis, typhoid, rickettsia, hypersensitivity (Henoch-Schonlein purpura).

C/Fs: spontaneous petechiae and ecchymoses in skin and mucus membrane. *TESTS*: Normal BT, platelet count, PT and PTT (*see* page 152–53).

Scurvy

Due to vitamin C deficiency. Vit. C is essential for the activity of fibroblasts, osteoblasts and odontoblasts. Deficiency of vit. C affects collagen synthesis, particularly in BV walls leading to fragility of BVs and hemorrhages. *C/Fs:* Purpura, ecchymoses, skin and gingival mucosa, subperiosteal hematoma, bleeding in joint spaces. Due to effect on osteoblast activity, skeletal changes are seen in developing infants and children consisting of **defective osteoid matrix formation (mineralization is normal)**. The cartilage is not replaced by osteoid with weakening of bones leading to bowing of long bones of legs and deformity of sternum and rib cage. Wound-healing is also impaired due to defective collagen synthesis.

Henoch-Schonlein purpura

Deposition of IgA in the BV wall leads to a systemic syndrome involving skin (purpura), GIT bleeding with abdominal pain, joint bleeding with arthritis, and bleeding in kidneys with hematuria.

Platelet Disorders

122. What are the platelet disorders?

Ans. 1. Thrombocytopenia.

2. Platelet functional disorder, e.g. uremia, aspirin effect, von Willebrand disease.

C/Fs: Petechiae, ecchymoses, epistaxis, menorrhagia. BT is always prolonged. If due to thrombocytopenia, platelet counts low. PT and PTT—Normal.

Thrombocytopenia

DEF: Decreased platelets with spontaneous bleeding, a prolonged BT and normal PT and PTT. By definition thrombocytopenia = 100,000/c mm or less. Post traumatic **bleeding seen** in platelets 20,000 to 50,000. **Non-traumatic (spontaneous) bleeding seen** in platelet count 20,000.

ETIO: 1. *Decreased production:* Aplastic anemia, marrow infiltration by leukemia, metastatic disease, infections, e.g. measles, HIV, drug-induced, e.g. alcohol, thiazides, cytotoxic drugs. Ineffective erythropoiesis, e.g. megaloblastic anemia, PNH (paroxysmal nocturnal hemoglobinuria).

2. *Increased destruction/loss:*
   a. Loss in spleen due to hypersplenism.
   b. Autoimmune, e.g. ITP (idiopathic thrombocytopenic purpura), SLE isoimmune, e.g. post-transfusion, drug associated, e.g. quinidine, heparin, sulfas, infections, e.g. infectious mononucleosis, HIV, CMV.
   c. TTP (thrombotic thrombocytopenic purpura), DIC (disseminated intravascular coagulation), giant hemangiomas, microangiopathic hemolytic anemias. Bone marrow has compensatory increase in megakaryocytes—helps to *D/D* with thrombocytopenia due to decreased production.

ITP (Idiopathic thrombocytopenic purpura): ETIO: Autoimmune. Occasionally with SLE. *PATHOG:* Spleen produces antiplatelet IgG antibodies and also the site of destruction of these IgG-coated platelets. **Therefore, in majority of cases splenectomy is curative**. *C/Fs:* Onset gradual with petechiae, easy bruisability, epistaxis, gum bleeding. Sometimes serious bleeding, e.g. intracerebral or subarachnoid can be present. *DIAG:* Marrow is hypercellular with increased megakaryocytes, which helps in *D/D* with thrombocytopenia due to marrow failure.

TTP (Thrombotic thrombocytopenic purpura): ETIO: Unknown. *PATHOG:* Endothelial injury with activation of intravascular coagulation with generalized formation of thrombi made of platelet and fibrin. Also, deficiency of enzyme which breaks high-weight vWF allows collection of vWF, activation of which causes collection of platelets and formation of thrombi. This leads to thrombocytopenia and narrowing of BVs by thrombi to cause microangiopathic hemolytic anemia. *C/Fs:* Temperature, thrombocytopenia, temporary neurologic deficits, hemolytic anemia-microangiopathic, renal failure. Common in females. *DIAG, C/Fs:* Thrombocytopenia, normal PT and PTT.

HUS (Hemolytic uremia syndrome): Similar to TTP, but onset in childhood, neurological symptoms absent or mild, renal failure dominant, cause of endothelial injury is gastroenteritis due to some strains of *E. coli*.

Coagulation Disorders

123. What are the coagulation disorders?

Ans. Two types:

1. Hereditary 2. Acquired.

1. *Hereditary:* Affects every clotting factor. Common are factor VIII, IX and von Willebrand factor deficiencies.
2. *Acquired:*
   a. *Liver disease:* Liver synthesizes several clotting factors.
   b. *Vit. K deficiency:* Vit. K is necessary for synthesis of factors II, VII, IX and X.
   c. DIC (Both platelets and clotting factors are consumed).

124. What is factor VIII deficiency/hemophilia A/classic hemophilia?

Ans. *Inheritance:* X-recessive. Occurs in males, or homozygous females.

PATHOG: Reduced amount or activity of factor VIII. *C/Fs:* **Most common hereditary disease with serious bleeding**. Easy bruising. Massive hemorrhage after minor trauma. Bleeding in the joints with hemarthrosis with deformities of the joints. There is no petechiae.

DIAG: PTT is prolonged. BT, platelet counts and PT are normal.

TRT: Factor VIII infusion obtained from fresh human plasma.

125. What is factor IX deficiency/hemophilia B/Christmas disease?

Ans. *Inheritance:* X-recessive. *C/Fs:* Indistinguishable from hemophilia A. Only way to do so is by factor assay.

126. What is von Willebrand disease?

Ans. *DEF:* **It is the most common inherited bleeding disorder**. *Inheritance:* Autosomal dominant.

PATHOG:

1. Platelet adhesion to ECM is done by interaction with vWF (produced by endothelial cells and circulates in plasma), which acts as a bridge between platelet and exposed collagen. Therefore, there is defective platelet adhesion.
2. vWF stabilizes factor VIII by binding to it, deficiency of vWF leads to deficiency of factor VIII.

   Hence, deficiency of vWF leads to combined defect:

   a. Involving platelet function.

   b. Coagulation pathway.

C/Fs: Mild bleeding in skin and mucosa. *DIAG:* Bleeding time and PTT prolonged.

127. What is disseminated intravascular coagulation (DIC) (consumption coagulopathy)?

Ans. DIC is not a disease; but, a complication of any condition which causes generalized activation of coagulation pathway whereby platelets and coagulation proteins are consumed due to formation of many thrombi. Hence, the term consumption coagulopathy which leads to generalized bleeding. So, the thrombotic disorder evolves into a serious bleeding disorder.!!. More information in Chapter 5.

128. What are the tests for bleeding disorders?

Ans.
1. *Complete blood count:* It can show thrombocytopenia.
2. *Peripheral smear:* It can show abnormally shaped platelets.
3. *PT:* It measures the factors of extrinsic and common pathways (factors I, II, V, VII, X). Deficiencies of these factors, mainly factor VII will prolong PT. Vitamin K is required for the synthesis of the critical factors of these pathways (factors II, VII, IX, X). Therefore, patients with vitamin K deficiency may have prolonged PT. Vitamin K deficiency is seen in fat malabsorption (vitamin K is fat soluble), liver diseases (due to decreased synthesis). Oral anticoagulant warfarin acts by interacting with vit. K activity. Therefore, PT is used in the management of patients receiving warfarin.
4. *APTT:* It measures factors of intrinsic and common pathways. Deficiencies of these factors, including factor VIII (hemophilia A) and factor IX (hemophilia B) will prolong APTT. Also, in patients with von Willebrand disease APTT may be prolonged because factor VIII could be low in them. Also, inhibitors

(autoantibodies which attach to a factor and make it useless for clot formation) can also prolong APTT. Most common inhibitors are:

a. Factor VIII inhibitors; and

b. "Lupus anticoagulant" (incorrectly called anticoagulant because it more commonly causes thrombosis in our body and not bleeding).

APTT is used in management of patients receiving heparin therapy.

5. Factor assays.
6. *Bleeding time:* Normal by Duke, Ivy <6 minutes; Template <10 minutes.

   Increased in thrombocytopenia (ITP, TTP, DIC), von Willebrand's disease, defective platelet function, aspirin treatment.
7. *Clotting time:* Normal by Lee white 6–7 minutes.

   Increased in clotting factors deficiency (except factors VII and XIII), heparin treatment.

9 Diseases of the Cardiovascular System (CVS)

OVERVIEW

Blood Vessels

a. *Arteries:*
   1. Congenital anomalies.
   2. Arteriosclerosis.
   3. Hypertension.
   4. Aneurysm.
   5. Dissection.
   6. Inflammation.

b. *Veins:*
   1. Vericose veins.
   2. Thrombophlebitis/phlebothrombosis.
   3. Obstruction of SVC and IVC

c. *Lymphatics:*
   1. Lymphangitis.
   2. Lymphedema.

d. *Neoplasms:*
   1. Benign.
   2. Intermediate.
   3. Malignant.

Heart

1. Congenital anomalies.
2. CCF.
3. Hypertensive heart disease (systemic and pulmonary—cor pulmonale).
4. Ischemic heart diseases.
5. Endocardial/valvular diseases.
6. Primary myocardial diseases.
7. Pericardial diseases.
8. Neoplasms.

Diseases of the Blood Vessels

Arterial diseases

Arterial diseases consist of:

Congenital vascular anomalies, e.g.

1. Berry aneurysm of the circle of Willis, which can present as rupture with 50% mortality and considerable morbidity in the remainder of the cases.
2. Arteriovenous fistula, which could cause hemorrhage (could cause death when in the brain) or high output cardiac failure due to increased work load.
3. Cavernous or capillary hemangiomas, e.g. port wine stain, associated with Sturge-Weber syndrome or von Hippel-Lindau syndrome.

Arteriosclerosis are of 3 types:

1. Atherosclerosis which could have complications, e.g. calcification, ulceration, thrombosis and hemorrhage. Also, embolization, aneurysm development, dissection and rupture.
2. Arteriolosclerosis is of 2 types:
   a. Hyaline seen in elderly, mild hypertension and diabetes mellitus and
   b. Hyperplastic, necrotizing arteriolitis with fibrinoid necrosis in malignant hypertension (rapidly accelerated severe, i.e. >120 mmHg. diastolic).
3. Medial calcific sclerosis which does not cause any illness.

Hypertension is **secondary** in ~ 5% cases, recognition of the causes of which could lead to correct management and cure; and in ~95% cases **essential** without a known cause where proper management with good control is necessary to prevent complications such as stroke, retinopathy, ischemic heart diseases, nephropathy, dissection, etc.

Aneurysm is abnormal dilation of an artery or a vein, caused by various causes.

Dissection of arteries is splitting of their wall by blood flow between their layers. 90% are due to hypertension and ~10% due to congenital abnormality.

Vasculitis could be due to infection or immunologic reactions.

Venous diseases

Common venous diseases consist of:

1. Varicose veins (dilated tortuous veins).
2. Phlebothrombosis/ thrombophlebitis.
3. Superior vena cava syndrome.
4. Inferior vena cava syndrome.

Lymphatic diseases

Common lymphatic diseases are lymphangitis and lymphedema.

Vascular neoplasms

These are of 3 types:

1. Benign, e.g. hemangiomas, glomus tumor.
2. Intermediate grade, e.g. Kaposi sarcoma, hemangioendothelioma.
3. Malignant, e.g. hemangiopericytoma and angiosarcoma.

Diseases of the Heart

Congenital heart diseases are:

1. With a shunt, either left to right (e.g. VSD, ASD, PDA) or right to left (e.g. tetralogy of fallot, transposition of great arteries.
2. With obstruction, e.g. coarctation of aorta.

Congestive cardiac failure (CCF) is defined as inadequate pump function of the heart.

Common causes of the left-sided heart failure are:

1. Systemic hypertension (commonest cause).
2. Ischemic heart disease.
3. Mitral or aortic valve diseases.
4. Primary diseases of the myocardium.

Common causes of the right-sided heart failure are:

1. Left ventricular failure (commonest cause).
2. Intrinsic primary diseases of the lung resulting in pulmonary hypertension (pulmonary heart disease—**cor pulmonale**).
3. Pulmonic or tricuspid valve disease.
4. Congenital heart diseases with left to right shunt, e.g. PDA, ASD, VSD. CCF leads to congestion of the lungs, liver, edema eventually progressive failure can result in cyanosis, acidosis, ventricular arrhythmia and death.

Hypertensive heart disease is defined as left ventricular hypertrophy in a person who has chronic hypertension and does not have other conditions which could cause it.

Ischemic heart disease (IHD) is defined as decreased blood supply to the heart required for maintenance of its normal structure and function. It may present as:

a. Angina pectoris (chest pain) of three types:
    1. Typical or stable angina.
    2. Prinzmetal's or variant angina pectoris.
    3. Unstable or crescendo or preinfarction angina pectoris.
b. Acute myocardial infarction (MI).
c. Sudden cardiac death.
d. Arrhythmias
e. CCF

Unstable angina pectoris, acute myocardial infarction and sudden cardiac death are called **acute coronary syndromes**.

Main pathogenic factors affecting coronary artery are:

1. Severe atherosclerosis.
2. Acute change in the atherosclerotic plaque.
3. Thrombosis.
4. Vasospasm.

Other contributing factors are:

1. Increased myocardial demand: Hypertrophy in hypertension.
2. Emboli.
3. Acute hypotensive episode.

Myocardial infarction (MI) is defined as irreversible ischemia with necrosis of myocardium due to blockage of the blood supply.

Complications of MI are:

1. Arrhythmia in ~ 90% cases.
2. Left ventricular failure with pulmonary edema.
3. Cardiogenic shock.
4. Myocardial rupture.
5. Papillary muscle rupture.
6. Mural thrombosis.
7. Pericarditis.
8. **Dressler's syndrome** (autoimmune reaction to injured myocardium usually seen within two weeks to a few months consisting of fever, pericardial effusion with pain).

Tests to confirm MI are:

1. ECG.
2. Creatinine kinase MB fraction.
3. Cardiac troponin I **(cTnI)**.

Valvular heart diseases cause **stenosis** or **incompetence**.

Some of the common causes of acquired valvular heart diseases are:

1. Degeneration, e.g. calcitic aortic stenosis.
2. Immunologic, e.g. rheumatic endocarditis.
3. Infective, e.g. bacterial endocarditis.

Acute rheumatic carditis develops during acute rheumatic fever which occurs 2 to 6 weeks after group A beta hemolytic streptococcal pharyngitis. It is not due to direct infection but is due to an immunologic reaction due to cross reaction between streptococcal protein and our heart proteins. It affects all three layers of the heart (pancarditis).

Its outcome can be:

1. Complete resolution without any sequelae.
2. Acute CCF and death.
3. Chronic rheumatic heart disease, which is myocardial damage due to valvular injury including irreversible deformity.

Bacterial endocarditis is defined as infection of the cardiac valves or mural surface of the endocardium resulting in formation of an adherent mass of thrombotic debris and organisms termed vegetation. *It is of two types:*

1. Acute.
2. Subacute.

Acute bacterial endocarditis (ABE) is of rapid onset with fever, rigors. It is caused by high virulence organisms such as *Staphylococcus aureus* affecting normal valves.

Subacute bacterial endocarditis (SBE) is of gradual onset caused by low virulence organisms such as *Streptococcus viridans, Staphylococcus epidermidis,* enterococci, HACEK group of bacteria (haemophilus, actinobacillus, cardiobacterium, eikenella, kingella) affecting congenitally abnormal or acquired diseased valves.

Non-bacterial thrombotic endocarditis is sterile deposition of fibrin, platelets deposited on valve leaflets predisposed by hypercoagulable conditions or trauma.

Libman-Sacks endocarditis is seen in SLE consisting of sterile vegetations.

Primary myocardial diseases are:

1. Myocarditis.
2. Cardiomyopathies.

Myocarditis is caused by infections (viruses, chlamydia, bacteria, fungi, protozoa, helminths).

Cardiomyopathies according to American heart association (2006) are of four types: **HARD**

1. **H**ypertrophic.
2. **A**rrhythmogenic right ventricular.
3. **R**estrictive.
4. **D**ilated.

Pericardial diseases are:

1. Pericarditis.
2. Pericardial effusions.

Pericarditis is caused by infection by viruses, mycobacterium tuberculosis, fungi or secondary to acute MI, uremia, SLE, metastatic malignancies, etc.

Pericardial effusions are:

1. Serous.
2. Serosanguinous.
3. Chylous.
4. Pure blood.

May result in cardiac tamponade and **death**.

Cardiac tumors are primary, e.g. myxoma, rhabdomyoma and metastatic which are more common than primary. Metastatic tumors are usually from lung, breast, melanoma, lymphomas, leukemia.

Diseases of the Blood Vessels

1. What are congenital anomalies of the blood vessels?

Ans. *A few of the congenital anomalies of the blood vessels are:*

1. *Berry aneurysms of the circle of Willis:* These are aneurysms in the arterial circulation of the brain. Their rupture is the most common cause of spontaneous, sudden subarachnoid hemorrhage. Most arise at arterial bifurcations of internal carotid artery circulation and a few within posterior (vertebrobasilar) circulation.
2. *Arteriovenous fistulas:* These are connections between arteries and veins due to defective development. The clinical features of these are:
   a. Bleeding, which can be fatal when it occurs in the brain.
   b. High output cardiac failure if the size of the fistula is large resulting in increased workload of the heart.
3. Cavernous or capillary hemangiomas, e.g. **Port wine stain**, which are flat congenital capillary hemangioma over the face. These can be associated with hereditary diseases such as **Sturge-Weber syndrome** where there are venous angiomatous masses in leptomeninges on the cerebral cortex or **von Hippel-Lindau syndrome** where there are cerebellar hemangioblastomas, renal cell carcinomas and pheochromocytomas.

Arterial Disorders

2. What is arteriosclerosis?

Ans. Arteriosclerosis is thickening of arteries with loss of elasticity.

3. What are the types of arteriosclerosis?

Ans. There are 3 types of arteriosclerosis. These are:

1. Atherosclerosis.
2. Arteriolosclerosis.
3. Monckeberg's medial calcific sclerosis.

4. What is atherosclerosis?

Ans. In Greek language "athera" means porridge. Atherosclerosis consists of intimal lesion made of fibro-fatty plaque with a central porridge-like core which is rich in lipid. This plaque is called atheroma. Internally, it protrudes into the lumen and makes it narrow thereby reducing the blood flow within the blood vessel and externally, it compresses the media thereby making the blood vessel wall weak, thereby causing aneurysm (dilation) or dissection (splitting of wall), or rupture with hemorrhage.

5. What are the risk factors which cause atherosclerosis?

Ans. Risk factors for atherosclerois are:

Non-modifiable:

1. Age—higher the age, the higher the risk.
2. Sex—male more prone until menopause, then equal between males and females. Before menopause estrogens help in this regard by keeping LDL level low by increasing the number of LDL receptors in the liver.
3. Familial predisposition—history of same.

Modifiable major:

1. Hyperlipidemia.
2. Hypertension.
3. Cigarette smoking.
4. Diabetes mellitus (DM).

Modifiable minor:

1. Sedantary lifestyle.
2. Stress.
3. Obesity.
4. High carbohydrate diet.

6. What is the pathogenesis of atherosclerosis (mechanism or steps in atherosclerosis formation)?

Ans. This consists of:

1. Endothelial injury.
2. Low density lipoprotein (LDL) deposition in intima at site of injury.
3. Monocytes migrate into intima, become macrophages and engulf LDLs forming **foam cells**.
4. Smooth muscle cells from the media proliferate and migrate into intima and engulf LDLs, thereby becoming foam cells and synthesize collagen and glycoproteins and convert a fatty streak into a fibro-fatty atheroma.

7. What is the step-wise morphology of atherosclerosis?

Ans.

1. Initially, **fatty streak** which mainly consists of intracellular lipid accumulation.
2. This develops into **fatty atheromatous plaque**, which consists of a superficial **fibrous cap** which is made of smooth muscle cells and collagen. Just beneath the fibrous cap and to its side (shoulder) there are smooth muscle cells, macrophages, and proliferating new blood vessels. Beneath this is a **central necrotic core** containing:

   a. Cell debris
   b. Cholesterol clefts
   c. Foam cells
   d. Calcium.

8. What are the morphologic complications of atherosclerotic plaque?

Ans. These are:

1. Calcification
2. Ulceration
3. Hemorrhage
4. Thrombosis
5. Embolization.

9. What are the clinical problems due to atherosclerosis?

Ans. These can be mainly divided into two:

1. Obstruction of the vascular lumen leading to:
   a. *In heart:* Ischemic heart disease (angina and myocardial infarction).
   b. *In brain:* Thrombotic strokes.
   c. *In kidneys:* Renal failure.
   d. *In limbs:* Ischemia.
2. Weakening of the vascular wall leading to:
   a. *In aorta:* Aneurysm, dissection or rupture.
   b. *In brain:* Rupture causing stroke.

10. What is arteriolosclerosis?

Ans. It is the thickening of the arterioles.

11. What are the types of arteriolosclerosis?

Ans. Arteriolosclerosis is of 2 types:

1. Hyaline.
2. Hyperplastic.

1. In hyaline arteriolosclerosis there is the thickening of wall of the arteriole with "hyaline" deposit. It is seen in the:
   a. Elderly.
   b. Benign hypertension, and
   c. DM.

   Its clinical features consist of decreased blood supply due to the narrowing of the lumen of the arteriole leading to ischemic atrophy of the organ, e.g. kidneys.
2. In hyperplastic arteriolosclerosis there is thickening of wall of arteriole with concentric, laminated **onion-skin**, hypertrophy and hyperplasia in circular multilayers of the smooth muscle cells (SMCs). In smaller arteries there can be **fibrinoid deposits and acute necrosis (fibrinoid necrosis)** of BV wall together with some inflammation known as **necrotizing arteriolitis**. It is seen in **malignant hypertension (diastolic more than 120)**. Its clinical features consist of ischemia of the various organs of the body, mainly kidneys and intestine with kidney failure and intestinal pathology.

12. What is Monckeberg's medial calcific sclerosis?

Ans. It is calcification in the media of muscular arteries. It is seen in people over 50 years. It causes no problems. Hence, it is of no clinical significance.

13. What is the definition of hypertension?

Ans. Hypertension is defined as an arterial pressure greater than 140/90 mmHg during at least 3 consecutive visits to the doctor's office.

14. What is the classification of hypertension according to the cause?

Ans. Hypertension is classified into 2 types. These are:

1. Primary (essential), and
2. Secondary.

1. *Primary (essential) hypertension:* This is seen in approximately **95% cases**. Its exact cause is not known. But, some predisposing factors are known, which are:
   a. Genetic factors—Family history of hypertension.
   b. Increased dietary sodium intake.
   c. Stress.
   d. Cigarette smoking.
   e. Obesity.
   f. Sedentary lifestyle.
2. *Secondary hypertension:* This is seen in approximately **5% of cases**. Its main causes are 5, which are:
   a. Renal.
   b. Endocrine.
   c. Cardiovascular.
   d. Neurologic.
   e. Miscellaneous.

A. Some of the renal causes are:
   a. Renal artery stenosis.
   b. Acute glomerulonephritis.
   c. Chronic renal disease.
   d. Polycystic kidney diseases

B. Some of the endocrine causes are:
   a. Primary aldosteronism (Conn's syndrome).
   b. Cushing's syndrome.
   c. Pheochromocytoma.
   d. Acromegaly.
   e. Hyperthyroidism.

C. Some of the cardiovascular causes are:
   a. Coarctation of aorta.

b. Polyarteritis nodosa (PAN).
c. Increased cardiac output.
d. Increased intravascular volume.

D. Some of the neurologic causes are: Increased intracranial pressure due to hydrocephalus, edema, neoplasm, abscess.

E. Miscellaneous causes are:
a. Toxemia of pregnancy.
b. Drug consumption, e.g. steroids, amphetamines, sympathomimetics.

15. What is the significance/importance of knowing about the secondary hypertension?

Ans. **Secondary hypertension** is potentially **curable**. **Primary hypertension** is **controllable** requiring lifelong treatment, but not curable.

16. What are the complications of hypertension?

Ans. Complications of hypertension are:
1. Left ventricular hypertrophy.
2. Congestive cardiac failure (CCF).
3. Ichemic heart disease.
4. Stroke.
5. Retinopathy.
6. Renal failure.
7. Peripheral vascular diseases with ischemia.

17. What is malignant hypertension?

Ans. It is severe (diastolic blood pressure > 120 mmHg), rapid rise of blood pressure. It can be a complication of either primary or secondary hypertension. It has rapid clinical course with early death from **CVA, renal failure, LVH, left ventricular failure, retinopathy with focal retina hemorrhage and papilledema**. **Malignant nephrosclerosis**: There is rapid renal failure with proteinuria, hematuria and uremia. Glomerular capillaries and arterioles rupture with multiple pinpoint hemorrhage over the kidney surface **(flea-bitten kidney)**. Kidneys are large and swollen. Vessels are hyperplastic and have **necrotizing vasculitis with fibrinoid necrosis**.

18. What is an aneurysm?

Ans. Aneurysm is an abnormal dilatation of an artery or a vein.

19. What is the cause of aneurysm?

Ans. The cause of an aneurysm is weakening of the vessel wall.

20. According to the cause what are the types of aneurysms?

Ans. These are:

1. Congenital defects, e.g. berry aneurysms of circle of Willis, rupture of which causes subarachnoid hemorrhage.
2. Local infections (mycotic aneurysms).
3. Trauma.
4. Systemic diseases **(atherosclerosis, cystic medial necrosis, syphilis)**.

21. What are berry aneurysms?

Ans. *See* page 159.

22. What are atherosclerotic aneurysms? What are the complications?

Ans. Atherosclerotic aneurysms are the most common aortic aneurysms. These are usually seen in males more than 50 years of age. Commonly in the abdominal aorta mostly below the renal arteries. *Their complications are:* **ROPE**

1. **R**upture—this is the most serious complication.
2. **O**cclusion of the branches.
3. **P**ressure injury to adjacent structures.
4. **E**mbolization of formed thrombus.

23. What are syphilitic aneurysms?

Ans. These occur during the tertiary stage of syphilis. These occur due to obliterative endarteritis of **vasa vasorum** of aorta causing ischemic weakening of media leading to slowly increasing dilation. Their main locations are thoracic aorta (ascending and transverse aortic arch and root). Their complications are:

1. Difficulty in swallowing, breathing, cough due to pressure-effect on esophagus airway and recurrent laryngeal nerve respectively.
2. Pain.
3. Cardiac disease, due to dilation of aortic root leading to aortic valvular insufficiency leading to heart failure and **eventual death**.

24. What is mycotic aneurysm?

Ans. It is an aneurysm in a vessel wall which is infected or caused by infection due to weakening of the vessel wall. Infection is usually bacterial but could be fungal. However, the term "mycotic" is traditionally used for all infected aneurysms.

25. What are dissections of arteries? What are their types? What is their significance?

Ans. Dissections of the arteries are **splitting of their wall** by the blood flow. This usually occurs in the media. The cause in majority of the cases is **hypertension**. In a few cases it is due to the congenital abnormality of the connective tissue, e.g. **Marfan syndrome**). These are of 2 types:

1. **Type A**—Involves both ascending and descending aorta. (Sub-typed by **DeBakey's** as:
   a. **Type I**—Involving both ascending and descending aorta and
   b. **Type II**—Involving only ascending aorta.
2. **Type B**—Involves only descending aorta (This is **DeBakey's type III**). Their significance is: These are **emergency conditions** requiring immediate reduction of blood pressure followed by emergency surgical repair for the ascending aortic dissection. They cause sudden severe chest pain, like MI and may rupture into pericardial sac causing hemopericardium, cardiac tamponade and **death**. They can cause obstruction of the carotid branches leading to **stroke**, or of the coronary branches leading to **MI**.

26. What is vasculitis?

Ans. Vasculitis is inflammation of the walls of the vessels (arteries, arterioles, capillaries and venules).

27. What are the classifications of the vasculitides?

Ans. Vasculitides can be classified by 2 ways:

I. According to cause:
   a. *Infectious:*
      1. Viruses (chickenpox).
      2. Rickettsia (rocky mountain spotted fever).
      3. Bacteria (neisseria, syphilis).
      4. Fungi (aspergillosis).
   b. *Immunologic:*
      1. Type II hypersensitivity (Goodpasture's syndrome, kawasaki disease).
      2. Type III hypersensitivity (systemic lupus erythematosus—SLE).
      3. Type IV hypersensitivity (temporal arteritis) (giant cell arteritis).
      4. Antineutrophilic cytoplasmic antibodies (ANCA) related:
         a. cANCA (Wegener's granulomatosis).
         b. pANCA (Microscopic polyangiitis, Churg-Strauss syndrome).

II. According to size of blood vessels (BVs):
   a. *Large-sized vessel vasculitis:*
      1. Takayasu arteritis (pulseless disease).
      2. Giant cell arteritis (temporal arteritis).
   b. *Medium-sized vessel vasculitis:*
      1. PAN (polyarteritis nodosa).
      2. Kawasaki disease.

C. *Small sized vessel vasculitis:*
   1. Microscopic polyarteritis (microscopic polyangiitis).
   2. Churg-Strauss syndrome.
   3. Wegener's granulomatosis.

28. What is Takayasu arteritis (pulseless disease)?

Ans. It is a granulomatous vasculitis of the large to medium-sized arteries. There is fibrous thickening of the aortic arch and its major branches with almost obliteration of the mouths of the great vessels. Its etiology is unknown. *C/Fs:* It is usually seen in Japan in females below 50 years of age. *S/S:* Ocular disturbances, hypertension, neurologic deficits, **markedly diminished upper limb pulses due to fibrous thickening of the aortic arch and its branches**. **(Therefore, it is called pulseless disease)**. *PROG:* Heart failure and stroke develop in approximately 5 years.

29. What is temporal arteritis (giant cell arteritis)?

Ans. It is granulomatous arteritis of the aorta and its major branches. It can affect various arteries, commonly the temporal and ophthalmic arteries. Its morphologic features are: chronic mononuclear cell infiltration, giant cells and granuloma formation, and narrowing of the lumen. *C/Fs:* Ophthalmic artery involvement with vision problems-**may cause permanent blindness, therefore, emergency treatment with antiinflammatory drugs is a must**. Also, severe headache and facial pain, fever, tiredness, weight loss, often increased ESR and leukocytosis.

30. What is polyarteritis nodosa (PAN)?

Ans. It is inflammation of the medium- and small-sized muscular arteries. Its main distribution is widely scattered. Frequency of involvement is: **kidneys (major cause of death)**, heart, liver, GIT, pancreas, testes, skeletal muscles, nervous system, skin **(lungs, aorta and its main branches not involved)**. There are **no immune complex deposition or ANCA** but, **approximately 1/3 patients have hepatitis B antigen in their serum**. Principal morphologic features are: acute necrotizing arteritis involving full thickness and partial circumference of vessel wall with fibrinoid necrosis, PMN and eosinophilic infiltrate. *C/Fs:* Fever, malaise, weight loss. Hematuria albuminuria and hypertension due to involvement of kidneys. Abdominal pain and melena due to involvement of GIT. Often seen in young males. Diagnosis is done by biopsy. Prognosis in untreated cases is **poor with death**.

Treatment: With immunosuppressive therapy (corticosteroids and cyclophosphamide) there is **90% cure**.

31. What is Kawasaki's arteritis (mucocutaneous lymph node syndrome)?

Ans. It is inflammation of the medium- and small-sized arteries. *C/Fs* consist of fever congestion of conjunctiva, erythema of the oral mucosa, skin of the palms and soles, rash and enlargement of the cervical lymph nodes (therefore, it is also called mucocutaneous lymph node syndrome). It is often seen in Japan for unknown reason. It affects children usually younger than 5 years. Its cause is unknown. Approximately 1/4 patients have involvement of coronary arteries leading to **myocardial infarction** and **sudden death**. Main morphological features are: acute and chronic inflammation, mainly with lymphocytes and macrophages and endothelial cell necrosis.

32. What is microscopic polyarteritis (hypersensitivity vasculitis)?

Ans. It is the inflammation of the venules, capillaries and arterioles. Its distribution is widespread, but mainly skin is involved. *MICRO*: Necrosis with PMN infiltration. In some cases the neutrophils break into small fragments. Therefore, this condition is also called **leukocytoclastic angiitis**. Common involved sites are: skin and mucus membranes (causing purpura), lungs (causing hemoptysis), kidneys (causing hematuria and proteinuria), GIT (causing abdominal pain or GIT bleeding), skeletal muscles (causing weakness). p-ANCA is positive.

33. What is Wegener's granulomatosis?

Ans. It consists of a group of 3 pathologies:

1. Necrotizing granulomas of upper respiratory tract (ear, nose, throat), the lower respiratory tract or both.
2. Necrotizing or granulomatous vasculitis of small arteries and veins, in lungs, and other parts of the body.
3. Necrotizing often crescentic glomerulonephritis.

C/Fs: ANCA is positive. Almost all patients respond well to treatment with immuno-suppression, however, without treatment almost all patients die within one year.

34. What is "limited" Wegener's granulomatosis?

Ans. Involvement limited to the respiratory tract is "limited" Wegener's granulomatosis.

35. What is thromboangiitis obliterans (Buerger's disease)?

Ans. It is an **inflammatory disease** of medium- and small-sized arteries with segmental **thrombosis (thromboangiitis)** with **blockage of blood flow (obliterans)**. Tibial and radial arteries are mainly involved. There is a strong corelationship with heavy smoking of cigarettes. *C/Fs:* **Intermittent claudication** (pain in legs with exertion due to hypoxia, which is relieved with rest). Ischemia leads to **gangrene** of the extremity requiring **amputation**.

36. What is Raynaud disease?

Ans. Raynaud disease is paroxysmal pallor or cyanosis of the digits of the hands or feet or tips of nose or ears due to increased vasomotor response to cold or emotion resulting in **severe vasospasm** of small arteries or arterioles. Seen mostly in young healthy females without a known cause.

37. What is Raynaud phenomenon?

Ans. Raynaud phenomenon is arterial insufficiency of extremities **due to arterial narrowing secondary to atherosclerosis, SLE, systemic sclerosis (scleroderma), Buerger's disease**.

Venous Disorders

38. What are vericose veins?

Ans. Vericose veins are abnormally dilated tortuous veins. Etiology is increased intraluminal pressure and loss of support of vessel wall.
Common sites:
1. Superficial veins of the legs-most common site-stasis dermatitis—Ulceration.
2. Hemorrhoids-hemorrhoidal plexus at anorectal junction.
3. Esophageal varices-due to portal hypertension from cirrhosis.

39. What is phlebothrombosis/thrombophlebitis?

Ans. Formation of thrombus in veins is phlebothrombosis. This causes inflammation of vein (thrombophlebitis).
ETIO:
1. Cardiac failure.
2. Prolonged bed rest or immobilization of a limb.
3. Postoperative and postpartal states.
4. Severe trauma, especially extensive burns.
5. *Cancers:* Particularly in abdominal cancers there is a tendency for development of venous thrombosis spontaneously, which disappears and appears at another site: "migratory thrombophlebitis" **(Trousseau's sign)**.
   COMPLI: Pulmonary embolism, infarct, sudden death.

40. What is superior vena cava syndrome?

Ans. It is the obstruction of the superior vena cava.
ETIO:
1. Ca lung 2. Mediastinal lymphoma. 3. Aortic aneurysm.
C/Fs: Cyanosis and dilation of veins of head, neck and arms. Commonly pulmonary veins are also compressed causing respiratory distress.

41. What is inferior vena cava syndrome?

Ans. It is the obstruction of the inferior vena cava.
ETIO: 1. Compression in abdomen, e.g. by neoplasms.
2. Hepatocellular carcinoma and renal cell carcinoma have tendency to grow within lumina of their respective veins extending into inferior vena cava causing obstruction.

3. Upward propagation of thrombus from femoral or iliac veins.

C/Fs: Marked edema of legs, distension of superficial collateral veins of lower abdomen, and when renal veins are involved, massive proteinuria.

Lymphatic Disorders

42. What is lymphangitis?

Ans. Infection of the lymphatics. *ETIO:* Any virulent pathogen, most common—group A beta hemolytic streptococci. (red streaks), local tenderness, lymphadenitis of drainage area. Eventual bacteremia/septicemia.

43. What is lymphedema?

Ans. It is edema due to impaired lymphatic flow.

Types:

1. Primary.
2. Secondary.

ETIO of secondary:

1. Postinflammatory scarring of lymphatic channels.
2. Spread of malignancy with obstruction of the lymphatic channels or lymph nodes.
3. Radical surgical procedures, e.g. removal of axillary lymph nodes in mastectomy.
4. Postradiation fibrosis.
5. Filariasis.

C/Fs: Dilation distal to obstruction with increase in interstitial fluid, leading to interstitial fibrosis, commonly subcutaneously. Thickened skin develops texture of orange peel **(peau d'orange)** often seen with breast cancer. Persistent edema can lead to infection (cellulitis) and chronic skin ulcers.

Vascular Tumors

44. What are common types of vascular tumors?

Ans. These are of 3 types:

a. Benign (hemangiomas).

b. Intermediate grade (Kaposis's sarcoma, hemangioendothelioma).

c. Malignant (hemangiopericytoma, angiosarcoma).

45. What are hemangiomas?

Ans. These are lesions composed of cavernous (L. caverna=hollow; consisting of hollow spaces) or capillary-like channels filled with either blood or lymph.

46. What more you know about cavernous hemangioma?

Ans. These may arise in B.V. or lymphatics. Often occur on skin and mucosal surfaces. Sometimes seen in liver, spleen, pancreas, brain. In brain they may cause pressure symptoms or rupture. **von Hippel-Lindau disease:** Autosomal dominant-cavernous hemangiomas in cerebellum, brainstem, retina and sometimes in pancreas and liver. Renal cell carcinoma may also be present.

47. What do you know about capillary hemangioma?

Ans. Consists of capillaries filled with blood, separated by small amount of connective tissue. They are reddish few mm to few cm in size. Usually seen in skin, subcutaneous tissue or mucus membranes of oral cavity and lips.

48. Kaposi's sarcoma are of how many types?

Ans. These are of 4 types:

1. *Classic:* Not aggressive mainly in lower limbs.
2. *Endemic (or African):* Not aggressive or very aggressive.
3. *In immunosuppressed transplant patients:* Not aggressive.
4. *Epidemic:* Mostly seen in AIDS patients. Aggressive and fatal in 2–5 yrs.

Stages:

Patches: Red to purple macules made of dilated blood vessels lined by normal looking endothelial cells.

Raised plaques: Made of dilated vascular channels lined by spindle cells with interspersed RBCs, hemosiderin-laden macrophages, lymphocytes, plasma cells. Pink hyaline globules seen in spindled cells and macrophages.

Nodules: Made of sheets of spindle cells, small vessels and slit-like spaces containing RBCs arranged in a **boxcar pattern**. Hemorrhage, hemosiderin pigment, macrophages with pink cytoplasmic globules are seen.

49. What is hemangioendothelioma?

Ans. This is intermediate-grade vascular neoplasm. Microscopically, vascular channels are easily recognized within masses of proliferating, well-differentiated endothelial cells.

50. What is angiosarcoma?

Ans. Malignant vascular neoplasm. Microscopically, masses of anaplastic spindle cells with a few, poorly formed vascular channels, lined by endothelial cells.

Diseases of the Heart
Congenital Heart Diseases

51. What are the etiologies of the congenital heart diseases?

Ans. Etiology is unknown (idiopathic) in 90% of the cases. In 10% of the cases it is due to:

1. *Genetic factors:* Trisomies 13, 15, 18, and 21 and Turner syndrome.
2. *Environmental factors:* Rubella infection in first trimester of pregnancy. Mothers taking alcohol or drugs like thalidomide or exposed to radiation during pregnancy.

52. What is the classification of the congenital heart diseases?

Ans. Congenital heart diseases can be classified mainly into 2 types:

I. With shunt.

II. With obstruction.

I. *With shunt:*

a. Shunt from left to right (acyanotic at birth):
   1. Ventricular septal defect (VSD).
   2. Atrial septal defect (ASD).
   3. Patent ductus arteriosus (PDA).

b. Shunt from right to left (cyanotic at birth):
   1. Tetralogy of Fallot.
   2. Transposition of great arteries.

II. *With obstruction:*
   1. Coarctation of the aorta.

53. What are some general features of congenital heart diseases?

Ans.

1. *Central cyanosis:* Either at birth, e.g. tetralogy of Fallot, transposition of the great vessels or later following reversal of the shunt originally from left to right to right to left **(Eisenmenger's syndrome)**, e.g. in VSD, ASD, PDA.
2. *Clubbing of the fingers:* Due to cyanosis.
3. *Pulmonary hypertension:* Due to left to right shunt causing increased pulmonary blood flow.
4. *Polycythemia:* Due to hypoxia.
5. *Paradoxical embolism:* Embolus going from the right heart to the left heart through ASD/VSD thereby into systemic circulation instead of following the normal path of going into the lungs.
6. Syncope due to severe outflow obstruction.
7. Growth retardation.
8. Bacterial endocarditis.

9. Arrhythmias.
10. CCF.
11. Sudden cardiac death.
12. Cardiac murmurs.

54. What is Eisenmenger's syndrome?

Ans. Uncorrected VSD, PDA, and ASD lead to progressive pulmonary hypertension. As pulmonary resistance increases, the shunt changes from L to R to R to L, which causes late cyanosis (blue kids), polycythemia and clubbing.

55. What do you know about ventricular septal defect?

Ans. VSD is approximately 1/3 of all the congenital cardiac malformations. Most of these occur in the upper membranous portion of the interventricular septum, are small **(maladie de Roger–Roger's disease)** and close spontaneously. Large ones can cause reversal of shunt to left to right, pulmonary hypertension, cyanosis CHF. Small VSDs also predispose to the development of bacterial endocarditis.

56. What do you know about patent ductus arteriosus (PDA)?

Ans. *Embryology:* Arterial channel between descending aorta and pulmonary artery. During intrauterine life blood flows through it from pulmonary artery to aorta bypassing the non-functional lungs. At birth, pulmonary resistance decreases, blood oxygen level increases and prostaglandin levels decrease leading to constriction of the ductus. In premature babies, in babies with respiratory problems, in babies whose ductus have insufficient elastic tissue, e.g. with maternal rubella the ductus remains patent. *MORPHO*: Blood flows from aorta to pulmonary artery and to the lungs and back to L. atrium and L. ventricle increasing L. atrial and L. ventricular workload causing hypertrophy and dilatation of both. Due to increased circulation of blood through pulmonary vessels pulmonary hypertension develops leading to R. ventricular and R. atrial dilatation and hypertrophy with reversal of shunt to R to L. *C/Fs:* Reversal of shunt from L to R to R to L causes cyanosis. Also, high pressure shunt predisposes to infective endocarditis. With L to R shunt there is a continuous **machinery murmur. Closure of the PDA can be facilitated by giving indomethacin**, and, **keeping it open by giving prostaglandin** in cases such as transposition of great vessels until corrective surgery is done.

57. What do you know about atrial septal defect (ASD)?

Ans. ASD is mainly of two types:

1. Ostium primum defect involving the lower portion of the interatrial septum.
2. Ostium secondum defect (approximately 90% of ASD) involving the upper portion of the interatrial septum. It involves the fossa ovalis; however, it is not the same as patent foramen ovale (PFO) which is only a normal variant, and not a true ASD. In early life it is usually asymptomatic. At about third decade due to reversal of shunt pulmonary hypertension, cyanosis and CHF develop.

58. What do you know about congenital malformation causing left to right shunt at birth?

Ans. **Cyanosis is present since birth (blue babies)**. Two common ones are:

1. Tetralogy of Fallot.
2. Transposition of great arteries.

59. What do you know about tetralogy of Fallot?

Ans. It consists of:

1. Narrowing of the right ventricular outflow (pulmonary stenosis).
2. Defect in the interventricular septum (VSD).
3. Aorta saddling both the ventricles (overriding of the aorta).
4. R. ventricle with R. ventricular hypertrophy.

MORPHO: Due to R. ventricular hypertrophy heart is enlarged and **boot-shaped** on X-ray. Right ventricular wall may be thicker than the L. ventricular wall.
C/Fs: Due to pulmonary stenosis and VSD there is a R to L shunt through VSD causing cyanosis. Risk of infective endocarditis. Most common cause of congenital cyanotic heart disease. Children intermittently adopt a squatting position which causes reduction of venous de-saturated blood and an increase in systemic vascular resistance resulting in decreased right to left shunt and better cerebral oxygenation.

60. What do you know about transposition of great arteries?

Ans. Aorta arises from R. ventricle and pulmonary artery arises from L. ventricle. This is incompatible with life unless there also is VSD, ASD, or PDA to allow oxygenated blood to reach aorta. *MORPHO:* Some degree of R. ventricular hypertrophy is present due to increased pressure of systemic circulation. Surgery is required to correct this. Until then prostaglandin can be given to maintain PDA or some procedure to allow blood flow between the right and left heart.

61. What is a cardiac congenital malformation with obstruction?

Ans. **It is coarctation of aorta.**
DEF: Narrowing of the aorta.
Types:

1. Infantile (preductal) (**be**fore duct, seen in **b**abies).
2. Adult (postductal). (More common) (**a**fter duct, seen in **a**dults).

1. *Preductal: MORPHO:* Ductus arteriosus is patent and blood supplies to aorta distal to the narrowing causing extra work on the right heart resulting in right ventricular hypertrophy and dilatation. *C/Fs:* Develop in neonates consisting of CHF and cyanosis of the lower part of the body due to perfusion by pre-lung blood via PDA. Femoral pulses are weak. *PROG*: Death within 2–4 weeks without surgery.
2. *Postductal: MORPHO:* The ductus arteriosus is closed. L. ventricle is hypertrophied due to extra workload. Aortic arch and its branches are dilated

due to back pressure. Collateral flow through the inter costal, phrenic, and epigastric arteries supply most of the blood to the distal aorta and these are dilated too. Notching of the undersurfaces of ribs is seen on X-ray due to erosion by dilated intercostal arteries. *C/Fs:* Since the blood to distal part of the body distal to coarctation comes from L. ventricle through collateral circulation oxygen content of the blood is normal and there is no cyanosis. So, the patients are older children and adults. Hypertension of upper extremities is present and blood pressure is low with weak pulses in lower extremities.

62. What is Ebstein's anomaly?

Ans. Congenitally malpositioned, malformed tricuspid valve causing regurgitation is called Ebstein's anomaly. Lithium taken during first trimester of pregnancy increases the risk of developing this anomaly. Right heart failure develops if not surgically repaired.

Congestive Cardiac Failure (CCF)

63. What is the definition of CCF?

Ans. Inadequate pump function of the heart.

64. What do these terms mean?

Ans. **High output failure**—Heart fails because of increased demand of blood by tissues, e.g. in anemia, thyrotoxicosis, Paget's disease of bone, A-V fistula, gram negative septicemia, beriberi.

Forward failure—Inadequate cardiac output.

Backward failure—Increased congestion in the venous system.

Compensated heart failure—Heart is able to cope and maintain output to meet the needs of body.

Frank-Starling relationship—Lengthened fibers initially contract more forcibly, thereby, increasing cardiac output.

Decompensated heart failure—Beyond a certain point further lengthening does not cause more forcible contraction, but weak contractions and thus decrease cardiac output.

Cor pulmonale (pulmonary heart disease)—Right side heart failure due to primary pulmonary/respiratory diseases.

Dyspnea—Breathlessness (SOB = Shortness of breath).

Edema—Increased fluid in the intercellular tissue.

Exertional dyspnea—SOB during exertion.

Orthopnea—SOB in supine position, because increased amount of blood returned to thorax in this position.

Paroxysmal nocturnal dyspnea—Patient is woken up from sleep with sudden, severe SOB with coughing, chocking and wheezing due to edema of the lungs.

Heart failure cells—Alveolar macrophages filled with hemosiderin.

Brown induration of the lungs—After long-term pulmonary edema fibrosis of the alveolar walls occurs which gives firm consistency to the lungs **(induration)** and the hemosiderin gives it **brown** color.

Nutmeg liver—After long-term congestion of liver, liver cells around central veins atrophy give it an appearance of nutmeg. (Congested veins appear dark in color and atrophied liver cells appear pale in color).

Cardiac cirrhosis—After long-term liver congestion and subsequent atrophy, liver may become fibrotic and develop diffuse fibrosis. Cirrhosis is a misnomer as there is no disruption of architecture of liver with new regenerating liver nodules, which is essential for "cirrhosis".

65. What are common causes of left-sided failure?

Ans. 1. Systemic hypertension.

2. Mitral or aortic valve disease.
3. Ischemic heart disease **(most common cause)**.
4. Primary diseases of myocardium.

66. What are common causes of right-sided failure?

Ans. 1. Left ventricular failure **(most common cause)**.

2. Intrinsic (primary) diseases of lung (pulmonary heart disease–**cor pulmonale**) (due to pulmonary hypertension).
3. Pulmonic or tricuspid valve disease.
4. Congenital heart diseases with L to R shunt, e.g. PDA, ASD, VSD.

67. What is the pathogenesis of CCF?

Ans. In Heart

1. In response to increased workload by increased sympathetic nervous system activity heart beats more forcefully and fast. Myocardium adapts by becoming hypertrophied and myocardial fibers become long which according to the Starling's law, initially contribute to more forceful contraction and cardiac output (CO); but later fail to do so and decompensated heart failure develops.

In Lungs

Due to above phenomenon there is congestion of pulmonary circulation causing pulmonary edema and congestion of BVs of the lungs, leading to pulmonary hypertension resulting in right-sided heart failure.

In Kidneys

Decreased cardiac output causes decreased blood flow to the kidneys, activating the renin-angiotensin system and causing secondary hyperaldosteronism resulting in increase in total blood volume and worsening of CCF.

68. What are the morphological features in heart, lungs and liver in CCF?

Ans. Heart

1. Cardiac chambers are dilated.
2. Initially cardiac muscle is hypertrophied-with progressive dilation it gets thinner.

Lungs: GROSS

1. Lungs are congested.
2. Cut surface exudes edema fluid.

MICRO:

a. Pulmonary alveolar capillaries are congested.
b. There is transudation of fluid. This is initially limited to perivascular spaces widening the alveolar septa.
c. Later on, it overflows inside the alveoli (pulmonary edema). This protein-poor fluid stains pale-pink.
d. With persistent elevation of the pulmonary venous pressure, the capillaries become tortuous, which rupture with hemorrhage into alveolar spaces.
e. Alveolar macrophages engulf (phagocytose) these RBCs and eventually become filled with hemosiderin. These hemosiderin-laden (pigment-filled) macrophages are called **heart failure cells**.
f. In long-standing cases **brown induration of the lungs** develops (*see* page 175).

Liver

1. Central veins (CVs) are congested. Cut surface has a **nutmeg-like** appearance. In late stage there is fibrosis traditionally but inappropriately called **cardiac cirrhosis**.

69. What are the *C/Fs* of left heart failure?

Ans.
1. Dyspnea—Due to pulmonary edema and decreased lung compliance due to pulmonary congestion.
2. Exertional dyspnea—Due to increased oxygen demand.
3. Orthopnea—Due to increased amount of blood in thorax (lungs) in supine position.
4. Paroxysmal nocturnal dyspnea—Same reason as above.
5. Tachycardia with a third (S3) heart sound.
6. Fine rales/crepitations heard at lung bases produced by air flow through edematous pulmonary alveoli.
7. Progressive ventricular dilation displaces papillary muscles laterally causing mitral regurgitation and a systolic murmur.
8. Chronic dilation of left atrium causes atrial muscle to fibrillate (atrial fibrillation) with an irregularly irregular heartbeat.

70. What are the *C/Fs* of right heart failure?

Ans.
1. *Systemic venous congestion:* Distended neck veins. Enlarged tender liver.

2. *Edema:* In the dependent areas of the body, e.g. feet and ankles which progressively become generalized and may also cause pleural effusion, pericardial effusion and ascites.

71. What can be the outcome of progressive CCF?

Ans. Eventually with progressive failure:

1. Cyanosis
2. Acidosis
3. Ventricular arrhythmia
4. Sudden death.

Hypertensive Heart Disease

72. What do you know about hypertensive heart disease?

Ans. *DEF:* Left ventricular hypertrophy in a person who has chronic hypertension and does not have other conditions which could cause left ventricular hypertrophy, e.g. aortic stenosis. *MORPHO*: *GROSS*: Left ventricular wall is concentrically hypertrophied requiring increased blood flow in the absence of which interstitial fibrosis develops due to ischemia. Also, when the heart cannot cope, failure supervenes leading to right ventricular hypertrophy with dilation. *MICRO:* Myocytes are enlarged. *C/Fs:* Without CCF asymptomatic. Later, when CCF develops patient develops *S/S* of CCF, and of ischemia and of other organs involvement, e.g. kidneys brain, etc. Also sudden cardiac death can occur. **Good control of hypertension can prevent hypertrophy or even regress it and prevent its complications**.

73. What do you know about cor pulmonale (pulmonary heart disease)?

Ans. *DEF:* Disease of right side of heart due to pulmonary hypertension caused by primary pulmonary parenchymal or vascular disease (**not** due to left ventricular failure/any other left side heart disease or congenital heart diseases).

ETIO: Acute: Large pulmonary embolus.

Chronic:

1. Chronic obstructive pulmonary disease (COPD).
2. Pulmonary fibrosis.
3. Pulmonary atelectasis (collapse).
4. Small recurrent emboli.
5. Cystic fibrosis.
6. Hypoxemia.
7. Kyphoscoliosis.
8. Severe obesity.
9. Neuromuscular disorders.

PATHOG: Right ventricular hypertrophy in early stage, later dilation, leading to right-sided heart failure. *MORPHO:* Right ventricular hypertrophied/dilated. Pulmonary arteries atherosclerotic.

Ischemic Heart Disease

74. What is the definition of ischemic heart disease?

Ans. *DEF:* Decrease in blood supply to the heart required for maintenance of its normal structure and function.

75. In how many ways ischemic heart disease may present in a patient?

Ans. IHD may present as:

a. Angina pectoris (chest pain): 3 types:
   1. Typical or stable angina pectoris.
   2. Prinzmetal or variant angina pectoris.
   3. Unstable or crescendo, preinfarction angina pectoris.

b. Acute myocardial infarction (MI).

c. Sudden cardiac death.

   Unstable angina pectoris, acute MI and sudden cardiac death are called **acute coronary syndromes**.

d. Cardiac arrhythmias.

e. Chronic ischemic heart disease with CCF.

76. What is the etiology of IHD?

Ans. *ETIO:*

1. Decreased blood flow to the heart, e.g. coronary atherosclerosis, thrombosis, embolism, spasm, stenosis, arteritis, hypotension, etc.
2. Decreased oxygenated blood, e.g. anemia, carboxy hemoglobinemia, etc.
3. Increased cardiac demand, e.g. thyrotoxicosis, myocardial hypertrophy, etc.

77. What is the pathogenesis of IHD?

Ans. *PATHOG:*

Four main pathogenetic factors affecting coronary artery: **APTS**

1. Severe atherosclerosis—**A**therosclerosis.
2. Acute change in the atherosclerotic plaque—**P**laque change.
3. Thrombosis—**T**hrombosis.
4. Vasospasm—**S**pasm.

Three other factors: **DIE**

1. **D**ecreased supply (Ac. hypotensive episode).
2. **I**ncreased myocardial demand: (hypertrophy in HTN).
3. **E**mboli.

Four main factors:

1. **Severe atherosclerosis:** Causing 75% or more narrowing–"critical stenosis". Patient is asymptomatic at rest but with exercise or stress develops chest pain.

2+3. **Ac. change in plaque-thrombosis:** Seen with 50–75% narrowing consisting of fissuring, hemorrhage, rupture, embolization, thrombosis (partial or complete). Complete leads to **myocardial infarction**. Partial obstruction causes **unstable angina** (angina upon less exertion, more severe and lasts longer, increased frequency). It can progress to myocardial infarction. Therefore, it is also called **preinfarction angina**.

4. **Vasospasm:** Some atherosclerosis is usually present, but spasm can also occur in normal vessel.

78. What do you know about angina pectoris?

Ans. *DEF:* Episodic chest pain due to inadequate oxygen supply to the heart caused by **reversible** ischemia. Relieved by nitroglycerin.

Types:

1. Stable angina
2. Unstable angina.
3. Prinzmetal's angina.

1. *Typical or stable angina:* Pain occurs upon exertion and is relieved by rest or by vasodilator drugs, due to severe atherosclerotic narrowing of coronary arteries. Commonest type of angina.
2. *Unstable or crescendo or preinfarction angina:* A patient with history of stable angina, when starts having angina at rest or with less exertion or the pain is prolonged or recurrent, it is called unstable angina. **It is warning for the development of myocardial infarction soon.**
3. *Prinzmetal's or variant angina:* Chest pain is at rest from the beginning. Here there is no atherosclerosis, but chest pain is thought to be due to spasm of coronary arteries.

79. What is the definition of myocardial infarction (MI)?

Ans. *DEF:* **Irreversible ischemia with necrosis of myocardium** due to blockage of the blood supply. **Early diagnosis and immediate treatment is of utmost importance for better outcome.**

80. What are the morphologic features chronologically of MI?

Ans. *GROSS:* First 12 hours no changes seen. First 24 hours there is slight pallor. In 3 days there is more pallor. In first week there is central pallor with softening and hyperemic border. In 2 months area appears firm and gray.

MICRO: In first hour there is no change. In first 2 hours the cytoplasm of the cardiac myocytes becomes foamy. In first 12 hours there is some edema and few PMNs. In first 24 hours there is coagulation necrosis with cytoplasmic eosinophilia, pyknosis of nuclei and PMNs increased. In first 3 days PMNs increase with early breakdown of PMNs. In 1 week there is granulation tissue and presence of macrophages. In 2 months fibrosis occurs.

81. What are the types of MI?

Ans. *Types:*

1. *Transmural:* When infarction involves full thickness of the ventricular wall from endocardium to epicardium.
2. *Subendocardial:* When infarction is limited to interior 1/3 of the myocardium.

82. What are the common sites of MI?

Ans. Commonest site is the apex and anterior wall of left ventricle due to occlusion of the anterior descending branch of left coronary artery. Second common site is posterior and lateral wall of the left ventricle due to occlusion of circumflex branch of the left coronary artery or right coronary artery. Infarction of the right ventricle or right or left atrium is not common.

83. What are the *C/Fs* of MI?

Ans. *Onset:* In 1/2 cases there may be angina prior to MI. Acute onset of severe, crushing substernal chest pain which may radiate to neck, jaw, epigastrium, shoulder or left arm. Pain is not relieved by nitroglycerin. Pain lasts many hours to days. Pulse is fast, weak. Sweating. SOB, patient may develop cardiogenic shock. In 1/4 patients. arrhythmia causes sudden death. In 1/4 patients (elderly or with DM), there may be no pain—**Silent MI**.

84. What are the tests to confirm MI?

Ans. *Tests:* ECG: Q waves, ST elevation, T inversion. *LAB:* CK-MB—Rises within 2–4 hours, peaks in 24 hours and becomes normal in 72 hours. Cardiac troponin T (cTnT) and cardiac troponin I (cTnI). **cTnI is only found in heart muscle, therefore, specific for MI. Increases early like CK-MB, but lasts longer (4–7 days)**.

85. What are different outcomes of MI?

Ans. 25% die of lethal arrhythmia before reaching hospital. Almost all remainder develop following complications either one or more than one:

86. What are complications of MI?

Ans. *COMPLI:* 1. Arrhythmia.

2. Left ventricular failure with pulmonary edema.
3. Cardiogenic shock.
4. Myocardial rupture.
5. Rupture of papillary muscle.
6. Mural thrombosis with possible embolization.
7. Pericarditis.
8. **Dressler's syndrome**—Autoimmune reaction to the injured myocardium consisting of fever, pericardial effusion with pain, usually seen within 2 weeks to a few months.

87. What is sudden cardiac death? What are its common causes?

Ans. Causes of sudden cardiac death

a. *CAD (IHD):* Atherosclerosis with thrombosis and ventricular fibrillation. Approximately 1/2 the patients with coronary/ischemic heart disease are asymptomatic and unaware of having CAD/IHD. Routine screening examinations could identify by CAD and possibly prevent some of the these sudden deaths.

b. *Myocardial diseases:* Cardiomyopathies, myocarditis.

c. *Valvular diseases:* AS, MVP, endocarditis.

d. Conduction system abnormalities.

Valvular Heart Diseases

88. What are the problems due to valvular heart diseases?

Ans. Valve disease causes stenosis (narrowing) with obstruction to the flow of blood or insufficiency (incompetence), with regurgitation of flow of blood within the heart or both.

Stenosis (narrowing): Failure of valve to open completely and impeding forward flow.

Incompetence (insufficiency): Failure of valve to close completely allowing reversed flow.

89. What are the common acquired causes of valvular heart diseases?

Ans. *Causes:* Three most common causes of valvular heart disease are:

1. Degeneration, e.g. calcific aortic stenosis with or without a bicuspid valve, mitral annular calcification, mitral valve prolapse.
2. Immunologic inflammatory response, e.g. rheumatic endocarditis.
3. Infective endocarditis (acute or subacute).

90. What do you know about aortic valve diseases?

Ans. Commonly affected with mitral valve in rheumatic heart disease, or bacterial endocarditis.

Stenosis: Often due to **calcification** of a congenital bicuspid valve, or in elderly people due to degeneration, or due to rheumatic heart disease. *GROSS:* Calcification causes thickening of the cusps of the valve and narrowing of orifice. Left ventricule is hypertrophied. *C/Fs:* Angina due to decreased circulation in hypertrophied myocardium. Syncope, CHF **(valve should be replaced before CHF develops)**.

Insufficiency: Due to rheumatic heart disease, syphilis with dilatation of the aortic ring.

91. What do you know about mitral valve diseases?

Ans. *Prolapse:* Most common valvular lesion, commonly in young females. Due to rheumatic carditis, myxoid degeneration of the valve due to unknown cause, ischemic heart diseases, Marfan's syndrome. Posterior valve leaflet is stretched and floppy with prolapse into left atrium during systole producing a systolic murmur with a midsystolic click. Usually benign. Can cause mitral insufficiency, arrhythmia. Predisposes to infective endocarditis. Very rarely can cause sudden death.

Stenosis: Majority due to rheumatic heart disease. *C/Fs:* May cause arrhythmia, predispose to infective endocarditis.

Insufficiency: Usually due to rheumatic heart disease. Can also be due to mitral valve prolapse (described above), myocardial infarction with papillary muscle rupture, infective endocarditis, left ventricular dilatation due to any cause.

92. What do you know about tricuspid valve diseases?

Ans. Affected in rheumatic heart disease, mostly with mitral valve. In carcinoid syndrome.

93. What do you know about pulmonary valve diseases?

Ans. Commonly congenital. Either alone or with other defects such as Fallot's tetralogy. Rarely in rheumatic heart disease with mitral valve. In carcinoid syndrome.

Rheumatic Fever and Rheumatic Carditis

94. What is rheumatic fever? What are Jones criteria?

Ans. Rheumatic fever is an acute inflammatory disease which occurs 2 to 5 weeks after a group A beta hemolytic streptococcal infection.

Five major (Jones) criteria:

1. Erythema marginatum.
2. Subcutaneous nodules.
3. Migratory large joint polyarthritis.
4. Carditis.
5. Sydenham chorea.

Minor criteria:

1. Fever.
2. Arthralgia.
3. Leukocytosis.
4. Prolonged P-R interval on EKG.
5. Raised ESR/C-reactive protein/antistreptolysin O (ASO) titre (> 250 u).
6. Previous rheumatic fever.
7. History of recent group. A streptococcal sore throat or scarlet fever.

Diagnosis is made on 2 or > major criteria or 1 major and 2 or more minor criteria.

95. What do you know about acute rheumatic carditis?

Ans. During acute rheumatic fever, which occurs 2–6 weeks after a group A beta hemolytic pharyngitis, acute rheumatic carditis develops.

PATHOG: It is **not** due to direct bacterial infection of the heart nor due to any bacterial toxin. It is due to cross reaction between streptococcal and cardiac proteins. Thus, body's immune reaction against the streptococcal antigen also acts against the cardiac tissues **(Molecular mimicry)**.

MORPHO: Acute inflammation involving all 3 layers of the heart called **pancarditis:** pericardium, myocardium and endocardium.

Pericarditis: Fibrinous **(bread and butter)** sometimes with serosanguinous pericardial effusion.

Myocarditis: Multiple foci of inflammation are present in connective tissue, usually perivascular, and are called **Aschoff bodies** which are granulomas containing a central focus of fibrinoid necrosis surrounded by mononuclear inflammatory infiltrate (lymphocytes, plasma cells, macrophages), large **histiocytes** having 2 or more nuclei with prominent nucleoli **(Aschoff cells)**, the one with 2 nuclei give an appearance of **owl's eye**. **Anitschkow cells**, which are spindle-shaped **histiocytes** with a longitudinal chromatin bar in the nucleus **(caterpillar nucleus)** are also present.

Endocarditis: Mitral>aortic>tricuspid>pulmonary. Affected valves are edematous and thickened and have foci of fibrinoid necrosis which promote formation of small vegetations, along lines of valve closure **(verrucous endocarditis)**. *Outcome:* The above acute changes may:

1. Resolve without any residual effects, or
2. Lead to acute CHF and **death**; or
3. Lead to chronic rheumatic heart disease.

96. What do you know about chronic rheumatic heart disease?

Ans. *DEF:* Rheumatic fever does **not** produce "smoldering" chronic cardiac inflammation. Actually, scars left from fibrosis following acute valvular damage contract and change over period of time causing irreversible deformity of valves leading to secondary hemodynamic difficulties of myocardium and cardiac chambers over number of years. *Pathogenesis and morphology:* **Fibrosis, scarring and irreversible deformity of cardiac valves is the main pathology of chronic rheumatic heart disease** involving one or more valves, left side valves more often involved than the right side. Scarring of the valve leaflets may cause reduction in diameter of valve orifice **(stenosis)** with mid-diastolic murmur or scarring may prevent proper closure of valve leaflets resulting in **regurgitation** of blood during diastole with pansystolic murmur. Sometimes, **both** are present. **Stenosis causes increased pressure load. Regurgitation causes increased volume load** (by heart having to pump **same** blood over and over again). The "poor pump" eventually gives up and fails (cardiac failure/heart failure).

Mitral Valve

Females>males. Stenosis>regurgitation. *Mitral stenosis:* Valve leaflets, and chordae tendineae are thick and rigid due to fibrosis which is also present across the commissures, causing slit-like narrowing of the valve orifice which appear **like buttonhole** or **like fish-mouth**. Chordae tendinae are also thick and short. Subendocardial collections of **Ashoff nodule** cause thickening, mainly in left atrium and are called **MacCallum plaques**. Left atrial endocardial surface is thick and rough predisposing to mural thrombi and emboli (systemic). *Lungs:* Congested causing back pressure into right ventricle and atrium leading to their hypertrophy and dilation.

Mitral Regurgitation

Valve leaflets are retracted. Regurgitation and repumping of same blood over and over again (volume overload-though no actual increase in blood volume) causes left ventricular dilation and hypertrophy.

Aortic Valve

Males>females. Mostly mitral valve is also involved.

Aortic Stenosis

Valve cusps are thickened, and adherent to each other making valve orifice very small causing increased pressure load on left ventricle with hypertrophy of left ventricle. Later left ventricle dilates leading to left ventricular failure.

Aortic Regurgitation

Valve leaflets retracted due to fibrosis. Leading to regurgitation of blood into left ventricle. Repumping of same blood over and over again leads to heart failure.

Outcome

Hypertrophy (of left atrium and right ventricle with MS), left ventricular hypertrophy also with aortic stenosis; dilation, CHF, arrhythmias (mainly AF), thromboembolic complications and infective endocarditis. **Timely surgical replacement of diseased valve prevents above problems with greatly improved outlook for patients with rheumatic heart disease.**

Bacterial Endocarditis

97. What do you know about bacterial endocarditis?

Ans. *DEF:* Infection of the cardiac valves and/or surface of the endocardium, resulting with development of adherent mass of thrombotic debris and organisms called vegetation.

Two types:

a. Acute bacterial endocarditis (ABE) b. Subacute bacterial endocarditis (SBE).

General

Acute: Fever with rigors, develops quickly. Caused by high virulence organism, e.g. *Staphylococcus aureus*. Large vegetations on previously normal valves. Mitral valve is most frequently affected. Tricuspid valve endocarditis in IV drug abuse.

Subacute: Develops slowly. Caused by low virulence organism, *Streptococcus viridans*, *Staphylococcus epidermidis*, enterococcci, HACEK group of bacteria (Haemophilus, Actinobacillus, Cardiobacterium, Eikenella, Kingella). May follow simple dental procedures. Smaller vegetations on congenitally abnormal or diseased valves.

Etiology

Acute: Usually infection by organisms of high virulence, e.g. *Staphylococcus aureus*, beta hemolytic streptococci, *E. coli*, *Pseudomonas aeruginosa*. Can cause infection of the normal valves. Disease is usually rapidly progressive without enough time to develop local inflammatory reaction.

Subacute: Usually, infection of previously abnormal valves by organisms of lower virulence, e.g. alpha hemolytic streptococci. Therefore, infection progresses slowly with enough time to develop local inflammatory reaction and granulation tissue formation.

Predisposing Conditions: (Soil-1 and 2/Seed-3):

1. Any condition that causes hemodynamic trauma to the endocardial surface such as high pressure shunts in the heart, e.g. small VSDs or chronic valvular diseases, e.g. chronic rheumatic heart diseases, degenerative calcific aortic stenosis, mitral valve prolapse, congenital heart disease.
2. Prosthetic valves and indwelling catheters where organisms can deposit.
3. IV drug abuse which provide a good source of organisms with access to the bloodstream.

Pathogenesis and Morphology

Source of organisms in blood is obvious, e.g. IV drug abuse or not obvious, e.g. mild mucosal injuries such as during brushing of teeth, which deposit on the cardiac valves causing infection of the valves.

In acute type: Large loose friable vegetations are made consisting of organisms, fibrin and cellular debris. Organisms are very virulent causing quick destruction of the valve cusps and chordae and spread suppuration to adjacent heart muscle forming **ring abscesses**.

In subacute type: Low virulence organism causes slow progression of disease and vegetations making them firm, which are made of fibrin, platelets and bacterial colonies. The damage to the valves is slow within minimal spread to the adjacent heart muscle with minute abscesses **(Bracht-Wachter lesions)**.

C/Fs: Low-grade fever, malaise, weight loss (in subacute); high fever, shaking, chills (in acute); cardiac murmurs, splenomegaly.

Complications

Acute: Systemic septic emboli more common because vegetations are friable and organisms are highly virulent resulting in infarcts and abscess all over body, e.g. in brain, kidneys, myocardium.

Subacute: Systemic emboli do develop, but due to less virulence of the organisms the infarcts usually do **not** develop infection and abscess formation. Also, antigen-antibody complexes cause focal glomerulonephritis.

Some Common Sites of Emboli

In skin immune complex deposition on pads of fingers and toes with painful papules **(Osler's nodes)**, septic microemboli on palms and soles with painless hemorrhagic small areas **(Janeway lesions)**. From right heart to lungs, from left heart to brain, retina **(Roth's spots hemorrhage with pale center)**, kidneys **(flea-bitten kidney)**, spleen, walls of blood vessels **(mycotic aneurysms)**.

Prognosis

Without aggressive treatment ABE- rapid course leading to death; SBE- slow course leading to **death**. **Aggressive treatment required to save lives**.

Non-Infective Endocarditis (NIE)

98. What do you know about non-bacterial thrombotic endocarditis?

Ans. Consists of sterile, 1/2 cm deposition of fibrin and platelets on the cardiac valves, usually in debilitated patients from cancer or sepsis and hence, it used to be called **marantic endocarditis**; but also is in healthy people making this term inappropriate. *ETIO: PATHOG:* Conditions which predispose thrombosis such as hypercoagulability, trauma. Hypercoagulable states, e.g. some cancers such as cancer of pancreas (as part of **Trousseau's syndrome**), acute promyelocytic leukemia (FAB classification-M3). Trauma, e.g. Swanz-Ganz pulmonary artery catheter. *MORPHO: GROSS:* Vegetations are sterile. Small 1–5 mm. Located one or more along the line of closure of leaflets or cusps of the valve. There is no valve damage. *MICRO:* Formed of thrombus without inflammation. *C/Fs:* May produce emboli with infarcts in brain, heart, or other sites.

99. What do you know about endocarditis of systemic lupus erythematosus (Libman-Sacks endocarditis)?

Ans. Seen in SLE. Valves involved are mitral, aortic and tricuspid. Vegetations are sterile. *MORPHO: GROSS:* Small:1-5 mm. One or more located on undersurfaces of A-V valves, on valvular endocardium, on cords, on mural endocardium of atria or ventricles. *MICRO:* Verrucae consist of finely granular, fibrinous eosinophilic material which may contain eosinophilic bodies. *C/Fs:* Fibrosis and deformity of the valves may occur as seen in chronic rheumatic carditis requiring surgery.

100. What do you know about carcinoid heart disease?

Ans. Carcinoid tumors release 5 HT (5-hydroxytryptamine—serotonin), histamine, bradykinin, etc. which cause episodic flushing of the skin, cramps, nausea, vomiting, diarrhea, intimal thickening on the inside surfaces of cardiac chambers and valve leaflets.

Serotonin is metabolized in the liver and lung. Therefore, only when there is liver involvement unmetabolized scrotonin can cause lesions only in the right side of the heart: tricuspid incompetence and pulmonary stenosis. Left side lesions develop if there is ASD or carcinoid tumor of the lung is present. *GROSS:* Fibrous thickening of the inner surface of right ventricle and valves. *MICRO:* Endocardial plaque-like thickenings made of smooth muscle cells and collagen fibers.

Primary Myocardial Diseases

101. What do you know about myocarditis?

Ans. *DEF:* Inflammation of myocardium causing injury to cardiac myocytes.

ETIO:

a. Infections: Viruses, e.g. coxsackievirus, cytomegalovirus, influenza, ECHO, HIV. Chlamydia, e.g. *C. psittaci*, Rickettsia, e.g. *R. typhi* (typhus fever). Bacteria, e.g. *Corynebacterium diphtheriae*, Borrelia (Lyme disease). Fungi, e.g. Candida. Protozoa, e.g. Trypanosoma (Chagas' disease), *T. gondii* (toxoplasmosis). Helminths, e.g. Trichinosis.

b. *Immune-mediated:* Poststreptococcal (rheumatic carditis). SLE.

c. *Drugs (cause hypersensitivity myocarditis):* Methyldopa, sulphonamides, ampicillin, furosemide.

d. *Unknown:* Sarcoidosis. Giant cell myocarditis.

MORPHO:

Viral: Myocardium is edematous. Myocyte degeneration and necrosis. Lymphocytic infiltrate. Viral inclusions, e.g. in CMV. *Parasitic:* Organisms seen, e.g. in Chagas' disease and *Toxoplasma gondii*. *Bacterial:* PMN infiltrate. Abscess formation. *Giant cell myocarditis:* Multi-nucleated giant cells. Lymphocytes, macrophages, eosinophils, scattered foci of necrosis. *C/Fs:* CHF, arrhythmia.

102. What do you know about cardiomyopathies?

Ans. *DEF:* The American Heart Association (AHA) defines cardiomyopathy as heterogenous group of diseases of the myocardium, usually with inappropriate ventricular hypertrophy and dilatation.

Classification-Types: In 2006, AHA classified cardiomyopathies as primary, i.e. genetic, mixed or acquired or secondary, i.e. infiltrative toxic, inflammatory. The four major types are:

1. Dilated (congestive).
2. Hypertrophic.
3. Restrictive (obliterative).
4. Arrhythmogenic right ventricular.

1. *Dilated (congestive):*
   ETIO: Alcohol, beriberi, cocaine, coxsackievirus, doxorubicin, peripartum. *MORPHO*: Heart dilates and looks like a balloon on chest X-ray. *C/Fs:* Most common. Both ventricles dilated with poor systolic function.
2. *Hypertrophic:*
   ETIO: It is inherited as AD trait in approximately half of the cases, unknown in other half. *MORPHO:* Hypertrophy often asymmetric and involving the interventricular septum. Walls of LV are thick and stiff causing increased diastolic pressure and chamber becomes **banana-shaped** on echocardiogram. *C/Fs:* Systolic function is normal, however, left ventricular outflow obstruction is present due to hypertrophy. Diastolic pressure is raised leading to dyspnea on exertion and angina. **It is the cause of sudden death in young athletes**.
3. *Restrictive (obliterative):*
   ETIO: Major causes are hemochromatosis sarcoidosis, amyloidosis, endocardial fibroelastosis, and eosinophilic endomyocardial fibrosis **(Loeffler endocarditis)**.
4. *Arrhythmogenic right ventricular:*
   Autosomal dominant (AD) disorder of muscle of right ventricle leading to ventricular arrhythmia, syncope, heart failure.

Pericardial Diseases

103. What do you know about pericardial diseases?

Ans. Pericarditis/pericardial effusions due to local (myocardial/mediastinal) or systemic (uremia) pathologies.

Pericarditis

ETIO: Primary: Infection: Viruses (most of the cases), TB, pyogenic bacteria, fungi. *Secondary:* Acute MI, cardiac surgery, radiation, uremia, rheumatic, SLE, metastatic malignancies.

MORPHO: Acute: Rheumatic, uremic. Viral-effusion is fibrinous, making the pericardial surface appear irregular and shaggy **(bread and butter)**. Bacterial-effusion is fibrinopurulent. Tuberculosis-effusion is caseous or sero sanguinous. Tuberculosis is one of the commonest causes of constrictive pericarditis.

Metastases-effusion is fibrinous/bloody with irregular nodular excrescences. Most cases heal/resolve without residual changes. When suppuration or caseation is extensive then healing is with fibrosis and scarring leading to:

Chronic: Fibrosis/scaring and when very severe it compresses, squeezes/constricts/restricts the heart so much that it cannot expand normally during diastole. This condition is called **constrictive pericarditis**. Tuberculosis is one of the commonest causes of constrictive pericarditis.

C/Fs: Acute: Pain, fever, pericardial friction rub. With rapid and significant collection of effusion **cardiac tamponade** develops with decrease in cardiac output leading to shock.

Chronic: Chronic low cardiac output, venous congestion.
Outcome:

1. **Cardiac tamponade, shock and death.**
2. May resolve without any residual changes.
3. May cause fibrosis, scarring, and constrictive pericarditis.

Pericardial effusions: Serous: CHF, hypoalbuminemia. *Serosanguinous:* Blunt chest trauma, malignancy. *Chylous:* Mediastinal lymphatic obstruction. *Hemopericardium:* Pure blood and not bloody fluid, e.g. open (penetrating) trauma to heart, ruptured MI, ruptured AA (aortic aneurysm). **Cardiac tamponade** and **death**.

104. What is cardiac tamponade?

Ans. Acute collection of fluid in the pericardial sac hindering/restricting filling of heart chambers, thereby diminishing cardiac output leading to **shock and death if not treated immediately**.

ETIO: Complication of acute MI, trauma, pericarditis, iatrogenic during invasive procedures.

Cardiac Tumors

105. What do you know about cardiac tumors?

Ans. Metastatic are far more common than primary cardiac tumors. These are mainly from lung, breast, melanomas, lymphomas, leukemias. *MORPHO*: Most often involve pericardium causing pericarditis and hemorrhagic pericardial effusion.

Myxoma

It is the commonest primary neoplasm of the heart in adults. It is benign.
GROSS: It is a soft mass, usually pedunculated, commonly in the left atrium. Its surface is irregular with focal thrombus formation. *MICRO:* It is made of irregular star-shaped cells and edematous connective tissue. *C/Fs:* Small pieces of surface-attached thrombi or the tumor may break and cause systemic embolization. The neoplasm may block the mitral value causing syncope or even **sudden death**. *TRT:* Resection is curative and if timely done could prevent sudden cardiac death.

Rhabdomyoma

It is the commonest primary tumor of the heart in children. *GROSS:* Soft mass on the ventricular wall growing into ventricular cavity. *MICRO:* Made of pinkish polygonal cells. By EM myofibrils are seen. *C/Fs:* May present with *S/S* of valvular obstruction. It may occur sporadically but usually it is associated with **tuberous sclerosis**. It is a benign neoplasm.

10 Diseases of the Respiratory System (RS)

OVERVIEW

1. Congenital diseases.
2. Upper respiratory tract diseases.
3. Infections of the lower respiratory tract.
4. Obstructive lung diseases.
5. Restrictive lung diseases.
6. Vascular lung diseases.
7. Neoplasms.
8. Diseases of the pleura.
9. Atelectasis.

One of the *congenital anomalies* is tracheoesophageal fistula.

Some of the **upper respiratory tract diseases** are common cold (acute coryza), acute pharyngitis, acute bacterial epiglottitis (which could cause airway obstruction and *death*), acute laryngitis, acute laryngotracheobronchitis (croup) (which could cause airway obstruction and **death)**, benign and malignant laryngeal neoplasms.

Infections of the lower respiratory tract are: Pneumonias, which can be classified based on onset (acute and chronic), on organisms (viruses, chlamydiae, rickettsiae, mycoplasmas, bacteria, fungi, parasites), on morphology (lobar, broncho, interstitial, granulomatous), on setting of origin (community-acquired typical and atypical, hospital-acquired, chronic, in immunodeficient people).

Obstructive lung diseases are:

1. Asthma.
2. Emphysema.
3. Chronic bronchitis.
4. Bronchiectasis.
5. Bronchiolitis.
6. Cystic fibrosis.

Restrictive lung diseases are due to:

A. *Pulmonary disorders:*

1. Acute interstitial lung disease–Acute respiratory distress syndrome (ARDS).
2. Chronic respiratory distress syndrome: Idiopathic pulmonary fibrosis, sarcoidosis, pneumoconiosis and

B. *Extrapulmonary disorders:*

1. Musculoskeletal (obesity, kyphoscoliosis).
2. Neurogenic, e.g. **Guillain-Barre syndrome**.

Vascular lung diseases are:

1. Pulmonary embolism.
2. Pulmonary hypertension, which could lead to right heart failure–cor pulmonale.
3. Pulmonary edema.

Neoplasms of the lung are: No benign, all malignant: Squamous cell carcinoma, adenocarcinoma, branchioloalveolar carcinoma, small cell carcinoma, large cell carcinoma, carcinoid.

Diseases of the pleura are:

1. Those with various substances within the pleural cavity, e.g. air, fluid, blood, lymph.
2. Pleuritis.
3. Neoplasms (mesothelioma).

Atelectasis is collapse of the part or whole lung. *Its types are:*

1. Resorption.
2. Compression.
3. Micro.
4. Contraction.

Diseases of the Upper Respiratory Tract (URT)

1. What are the acute infections of the URT?

Ans. 1. Common cold.
2. Acute pharyngitis.
3. Bacterial epiglottitis.
4. Acute laryngitis.
5. Acute laryngo-tracheo-bronchitis (croup).

2. What is common cold (infectious rhinitis)?

Ans. It is our commonest illness. *ETIO:* Rhinoviruses, viral infections such as most common coronaviruses, respiratory syncytial viruses, influenza and parainfluenza viruses, adenoviruses. *C/Fs:* Nasal congestion, sneezing, scratchy sore throat, mild fever. Heals spontaneously in ~1 week. Can cause complications, e.g. otitis media, sinusitis, pneumonia.

3. What is acute pharyngitis?

Ans. *ETIO:* Viruses: EBV **(infectious mononucleosis)**; coxsackievirus **(herpangina)**; adeno virus. Bacteria: Group A beta hemolytic streptococci: pharyngitis, tonsillitis. *COMPLI:* Peritonsillar abscess **(quincy)**, acute rheumatic fever, post-streptococcal glomerulonephritis.

4. What is bacterial epiglottitis?

Ans. *ETIO: H. influenzae. C/Fs:* Age—young children. Can occur in adults also. Acute onset with pain and airway obstruction—if this is not understood, it will cause **immediate death**.

5. What is acute laryngitis?

Ans. *ETIO:* Environmental irritants, allergens, organisms which cause common cold, *mycobacterium tuberculosis, Corynebacterium diphtheriae. M. tuberculosis:* Seen in people with chronic tuberculosis with exposure of larynx to sputum with tubercle bacilli for a long time. *C. diphtheriae:* Gram pos. bacillus, contracted by aerosols or fomites and produces an **exotoxin**, which causes necrosis of the pharyngeal and laryngeal mucosa with formation of thick fibrinopurulent exudate **(pseudomembrane)**, which causes the obstruction of airway and **death** Cervical l. nodes are swollen **(bull neck)**. Absorption of exotoxin can lead to **myocarditis**, **peripheral neuropathy, paralysis**.

6. What is acute laryngo-tracheo-bronchitis (croup)?

Ans. *ETIO:* Parainfluenza virus, respiratory syncytial virus. *C/Fs:* Age: Children. Dyspnea with inspiratory stridor and harsh, persistent cough. Inflammation with swelling of the larynx can lead to obstruction, respiratory failure and **death**.

7. What are nonmalignant (reactive) nodules/tumors?

Ans. 1. Vocal cord nodules (polyps).
2. Laryngeal papilloma.

8. What are vocal cord nodules (polyps)?

Ans. These are small growths commonly on the true vocal cords, made of fibrous tissue with overlying stratified squamous mucosa that can ulcerate by contact trauma with the opposite vocal cord. These occur mainly in heavy smokers or singers **(singer's nodes)**, due to chronic irritation.

9. What is laryngeal papilloma?

Ans. It is a benign neoplasm, consisting of a few mm size of soft growth commonly on the true vocal cords. Microscopically, it shows many finger-like projections covered by typical stratified squamous epithelium. Trauma may cause ulceration and bleeding. These are commonly single in adults; but, multiple in children, termed: **Juvenile laryngeal papillomatosis**. These tend to recur after excision, do **not** become malignant and usually regress spontaneously at puberty.

10. What is carcinoma of the larynx?

Ans. *Age:* > 40 yrs. *Sex:* Male: Female = 7:1. *ETIO:* **Nearly all occur in smokers**. Alcohol and asbestos are also risk factors.

MORPHO: 95% are squamous cell carcinoma, mostly beginning as CIS, appearing grossly as mucosal surface plaques eventually ulcerating and fungating and developing secondary infection. Tumor usually develops on the vocal cords; but, it may arise above or below the cords, on the epiglottis or aryepiglottic folds, or in the pyriform sinuses. Those limited to the larynx proper are called **intrinsic**, and those that arise outside or extend outside are called **extrinsic**. *C/Fs:* Main presenting feature is hoarseness of voice. Later: pain, dysphagia, hemoptysis. *TRT* and *PROG*: When initially seen ~2/3 are limited to larynx, with better prognosis than those that have spread into surrounding structures. Common cause of death is pneumonia or generalized metastases. With surgery, radiation, or combined therapeutic regimen **many patients can be cured, especially when diagnosed early**.

Diseases of the Lower Respiratory Tract

11. What is acute bronchitis?

Ans. *DEF:* Rapid-onset inflammation of the large- and medium-sized bronchi.
ETIO: Viral infection in healthy non-smokers. Smokers and people with COPD develop super added bacterial infection, commonly *Streptococcus pneumoniae, Hemophilus influenza.*

MORPHO: Bronchial wall BVs are hyperemic, glands are hyperactive with increased mucus and serous secretion and neutrophilic infiltration is present.

C/Fs: Cough, initially non-productive, later productive, mild tightness in chest, shortness of breath, wheezing, mild fever, mild lencocytosis spontaneous recovery within a week in healthy people. In children and debilitated people bronchiolitis and bronchopneumonia may develop.

12. What are the pneumonia?

Ans. *DEF:* Infection of the lungs.

13. What are the classifications of pneumonia/lung infections?

Ans. 1. *Based on onset:*

A. Acute.

B. Chronic.

2. *Based on organisms:*

a. Viruses.

b. Chlamydiae.

c. Rickettsiae.

d. Mycoplasma.

e. Bacteria.

f. Fungi.

g. Parasites.

3. *Based on morphology:*

a. *Lobar pneumonia:* Consolidation involves large continuous areas of the lung.

b. *Bronchopneumonia:* Consolidation involves small areas of the lung around inflamed bronchioles.

c. *Interstitial pneumonia* (pneumonitis): Inflammation of the alveolar septae with edema, hyperemia, and inflammatory cell infiltrate. Seen in infections with viruses, chlamydiae, (psittacosis/ornithosis) rickettsia, (Q fever), *Mycoplasma pneumoniae.*

d. *Chronic/granulomatous:* Inflammation of alveoli and interstitial tissue with granuloma formation, suppuration, fibrosis. Seen in infections with *Mycobacterium tuberculosis* and fungi.

4. *Based on settings of origin (narrows the list of organisms for giving early empirical antibiotic treatment):*

a. Community-acquired typical pneumonia.

b. Community-acquired atypical pneumonia.

c. Hospital-acquired (nosocomial) pneumonia.

d. Chronic pneumonia.

e. Pneumonia by opportunistic microorganisms in immunodeficient people.

14. What are the community-acquired typical pneumonias?

Ans. Bacterial in origin. Common bacteria: *Streptococcus pneumoniae, Haemophilus influenzae, Moraxella catarrhalis, Staphylococcus aureus, Legionella pneumophilia,* Enterobacteriaceae (*Klebsiella pneumoniae*) and Pseudomonas species. Preceding event usually is a viral infection. Onset is acute with fever, chills, mucopurulent productive cough. Commonest organism is *Streptococcus pneumoniae* (Pneumococcus).

15. What are some of the conditions which lead to susceptibility for development of pneumonia?

Ans.
1. Diminished or absent splenic function (splenectomy, sickle cell disease with autosplenectomy).
2. Immunodeficiency.
3. Chronic debilitating illnesses, CCF, COPD, DM.
4. Extremes of age.
5. Malnutrition.

16. What is lobar pneumonia?

Ans. *DEF:* Alveolar inflammation with consolidation involving large continuous areas of lung. *ETIO: Streptococcus pneumoniae* 90% of cases. Klabsiella, Pseudomonas, *Haemophilus influenzae, Staphylococcus aureus, Legionella pneumophilia. PATHOG:* Organisms are inhaled or aspirated into the alveoli, commonly involving the lower lobes or right middle lobe.

Stages:
1. **Acute congestion:** Hyperemia and fluid in alveoli. *S/S*: Fever, productive cough, chest pain with pleural involvement.
2. **Red hepatization:** RBCs and neutrophils in alveoli with consolidation with red liver-like appearance of involved lobe of the lung. *S/S*: High fever, cough and signs of consolidation.
3. **Gray hepatization:** Beginning of recovery with decreased exudates and no RBC in alveoli.
4. **Resolution:** Alveoli are clear.

C/Fs: As above. Dx: By sputum gram stain and culture. *COMPLI:* Respiratory failure, pleural effusion with pus in pleura (empyema), bacteremia, with meningitis, endocarditis, lung abscess. *DIAG:* Sputum gram stain and culture.

17. What is bronchopneumonia?

Ans. *DEF:* Focal consolidation of lung near inflamed bronchioles. *ETIO:* Aspiration of pharyngeal secretions. *Causative organisms:* Mostly *Streptococcus pneumoniae.* Also, gram-negative bacilli, *H. influenzae, S. aureus* super added infection over viral pneumonitis. *C/Fs:* Commonly in children and elderly with *S/S* of fever, cough, dyspnea, rales. There are no *S/S* of consolidation.

MORPHO: GROSS: 3–4 cm of slightly raised red patches in one or more lobes with large areas of normal lung in between these patches. *MICRO:* Suppurative exudates filling the bronchi, bronchioles and adjacent alveolar spaces.

18. What are community-acquired atypical pneumonias?

Ans. Called "atypical" because of absence of *S/S* of consolidation, not much sputum production, WBC not much elevated, no bacteria are found. Common organisms: *Mycoplasma pneumoniae*, Chlamydia species (*C. pneumoniae*, psittaci, trachomatis), *Coxiella burnetti* (Q. fever). *Viruses:* Influenza A and B (adults), parainfluenza (children), respiratory syncytial virus, adenovirus, measles, chicken pox, cytomegalo virus. Microscopically, mononuclear leucocytic infiltration of alveolar septa is seen. Occasionally, hyaline membranes linining alveoli may also be seen.

19. What is acute interstitial pneumonitis?

Ans. *DEF:* Inflammation of the alveolar septae. Alveolar spaces are clear. *C/Fs:* Fever, cough, dyspnea. *Signs:* Typical signs of pneumonia are absent because alveolar spaces are clear. Hence called atypical pneumonia. *MORPHO:* Alveolar septae are hyperemic and have inflammatory infiltrate of plasma cells, lymphocytes and macrophages. In cytomegalovirus, herpes simplex, chicken pox, adenovirus, measles, influenza, psittacosis **inclusion bodies** may be present. In measles, respiratory syncytial virus infection **multinucleated giant cells** may be present. In severe cases alveolar damage causes formation of **hyaline membranes**. *TRT:* Erythromycin, which is effective against both *Mycoplasma* and *Chlamydia pneumoniae*.

20. What is hospital-acquired (nosocomial) pneumonia?

Ans. Pneumonia in a hospitalized patient. Commonly seen in patients with some severe disease, immune deficiency, prolonged antibiotic treatment. *Common organisms:* Enterobacteriaceae, Pseudomonas, *S. aureus*.

21. What is chronic pneumonia (mainly granulomatous)?

Ans. *DEF:* Chronic inflammation of the lung parenchyma with granuloma formation. *ETIO: Mycobacterium tuberculosis*, fungi (Histoplasma, *Coccidioides immitis*, *Cryptocococcus neoformans*, Blastomyces, Nocardia).

22. What is lung abscess?

Ans. Abscess within lungs commonly due to anaerobic and saprophytic organisms, source usually is aspiration of vomitus or hematologic septic emboli. Pulmonary emboli and carcinomas may also develop secondary infection and develop abscess. *C/Fs* are fever, malaise and foul smelling purulent sputum. Complications can be empyema, pneumothorax, bronchopleural fistula, bronchiectosis, brain abscess, reactive amyloidosis. X-ray shows cavity with fluid level.

23. What is tuberculosis?

Ans. *DEF:* Chronic granulomatous infection of the lung caused by *Mycobacterium tuberculosis. ETIO: Mycobacterium tuberculosis. PATHOG:* In an immuno-competent host who has not been previously exposed to tuberculosis pathogenesis consists of: development of cell-mediated immunity, which gives immunity to the host and also causes delayed type of hypersensitivity (type IV) to the tuberculin antigens. The formation of caseating granulomas and cavitation are due to this hypersensitivity, because the effector cells which cause immunity also cause hypersensitivity with tissue destruction. Thus development of hypersensitivity to mycobacterium tuberculosis antigen also indicates development of immunity to *Mycobacterium tuberculosis*. This hypersensitivity can be detected by tuberculin **(Mantoux)** test.

24. What is Mantoux test (MT)?

Ans. It is a delayed-type hypersensitivity (type IV) response to the intradermal injection of tuberculin purified protein derivative (PPD). It is a cutaneous T-cell-mediated memory immune response with proliferation and differentiation of memory T-cells at the site of injection of PPD. Positive reaction is seen in people exposed to *Mycobacterium tuberculosis*, those immunized with the bacillus of Calmette and Guerin (BCG) vaccine. It does not mean that the person has TB infection (but, person could have TB infection). Negative PPD test means person does not have hypersensitivity to PPD or TB infection. However, **false negative test** can be due to sarcoidosis, Hodgkin's disease, immunosuppression.

25. What are the steps of pathogenesis in tuberculosis?

Ans. The pathogenesis of *M. tuberculosis* consists of the interaction between the cells and chemicals of the immune system of our body designated to fight the *M. tuberculosis* and the ability of the *M. tuberculosis* to withstand this as follows: Upon entry into our body the *M. tuberculosis* is engulfed by macrophage into phagosome where *M. tuberculosis* resists being killed by preventing fusion of phagosome with lysosome and multiplies there for approximately 3 weeks during which time macrophage processes the *M. tuberculosis* antigen and presents to CD_4T_HO cell and by IL-12 activate them into CD_4T_HI which secrete IFN-gamma which activate macrophage inducing them to secrete TNF become epithelioid cells and **Langhans giant cell**. Epithelioid cells group together and make a granuloma to prevent spread of *M. tuberculosis.* Also IFN-gamma and TNF stimulate production from epithelioid cells of nitric oxide and free radicals which cause destruction of *M. tuberculosis* and the tissue in the center of granuloma **(caseous necrosis)**. Also, in the center of the granuloma there is hypoxia which further kills *M. tuberculosis*. Also CD_4T_HI cells activate CD_8+ cytotoxic T-cells which kill macrophages containing *M. tuberculosis*. Inspite of all this killing of *M. tuberculosis* by the immune system of our body (that too at the expense of self injury by this type IV hypersensitivity reaction of tissue necrosis) some *M. tuberculosis* manage to **stay dormant** inside the granuloma and upon getting an opportunity get activated and cause secondary tuberculosis.

26. What is primary tuberculosis? What is Ghon focus? What is Ghon complex?

Ans. Non-immune host (usually child). Organism is inhaled and enters alveoli. Here it forms primary focus known as Ghon focus. (This is the initial focus of primary pulmonary tuberculosis).

Ghon focus is a small subpleural granuloma usually in the mid lobe, but could be large and present anywhere in the lung. In 95% cases this heals. In 5% cases it can progress and cause bacteremia, miliary tuberculosis, death. In many cases after healing TB bacilli remain dormant and can become reactivated many years later.

Ghon complex is Ghon focus + enlarged hilar lymph nodes.

27. What is secondary tuberculosis?

Ans. It is the tuberculosis usually seen in adults due to reactivation of primary tuberculosis or reinfection. Initial lesion is near the apex consisting of small area of consolidation, which in favorable conditions heals with fibrosis. In unfavorable conditions it cavitates and progresses called **progressive tuberculosis** consisting of spread of tubercle bacilli within the lungs continuously or passages such as bronchial tree or lymphatics. Furthermore, tubercle bacilli may enter bloodstream causing tuberculous bacteremia and approximately 1 mm millet-sized caseous lesions in all over lungs, liver, spleen, kidneys. This is called **miliary tuberculosis**. Also, spread beyond lungs causes tuberculous meningitis, vertebral TB **(Pott's disease)**, lymphadenitis, renal TB, intestinal TB, adrenal TB causing chronic adrenocortical insufficiency **(Addison's disease)**. In **Pott's disease** in paravertebral region abscess can be formed which does not have the warmth of acute pyogenic abscess and hence is called **cold abscess**. It may spread distally in the paravertebral region along the sheath of psoas muscle to the inguinal region and appear there as **cold abscess** called **psoas abscess**.

28. What microbial agents cause pneumonias in the immunocompromised host?

Ans.
1. Nontuberculous mycobacteria (*Mycobacterium avium*—intracellulare, *M. kansasii*).
2. *Viruses:* Cytomegalovirus, HIV.
3. Fungi (*Pneumocystis carinii*, Candida, Cryptococcus, Aspergillus, *Histoplasma capsulatum*, *Coccidioides immitis*, *Blastomyces dermatitidis*).

29. What are pulmonary vascular diseases?

Ans.
1. Pulmonary embolism.
2. Pulmonary hypertension.
3. Pulmonary edema.

30. What is pulmonary embolism?

Ans. *Sources:*

a. Venous thrombi, mostly from veins of the lower extremities or pelvis. Cause could be venous stasis due to CHF, prolonged bed rest, or immobilization due to prolonged sitting during air travel. Visceral cancer **(Trousseaus's syndrome)** due to use of oral contraceptives.

b. Fat, amniotic fluid.

MORPHO: GROSS: Hemorrhagic infarct *C/Fs:* Asymptomatic to s/o acute onset of: shortness of breath, chest pain, hemptysis, **respiratory arrest, death**.

31. What is pulmonary hypertension?

Ans. a. *Primary:* No known cause. Prognosis poor.

b. *Secondary:* More common than primary.

ETIO:

1. COPD.
2. Congenital heart diseases with L to R shunt with increased blood flow to the lungs.
3. Embolism causing increased pulmonary vascular resistance.
4. Hypoxia causing increased pulmonary vascular resistance.
5. Polycythemia causing increased viscosity of blood.
6. Restrictive lung diseases.

C/Fs: Leads to right ventricular hypertrophy, failure **(cor pulmonale)**.

32. What is pulmonary edema?

Ans. *DEF:* Collection of fluid within alveolar spaces.

ETIO: 1. *Increased hydrostatic pressure:* From left ventricular failure or mitral stenosis.

2. *Decreased oncotic pressure:* Hypoalbuminemia due to decreased intake, increased loss, decreased synthesis.
3. *Increased permeability of the alveolar capillaries:* Caused by alveolar inflammations from inhalation of irritant gases, pneumonia, shock, sepsis, pancreatitis, uremia, some drugs, ARDS (adult respiratory distress syndrome).

MICRO: Alveolar spaces have light-pink fluid. Alveolar septae vessels are congested. In long-standing cases alveoli have hemosiderin-laden macrophages, which give brownish color. Alveolar septae develop fibrosis which make lungs firm. This is called **brown induration**.

33. What are the obstructive lung diseases?

Ans. Here there is reduction in the flow of air in and out of lungs due to: Either narrowing of the airway or from reduced elasticity of the alveolar septae, which keep the terminal airways open during expiration, terminal airways collapse early during expiration resulting in obstruction to outflow of air. Main feature of obstructive lung diseases is that there is decreased expiratory flow rate. This is measured as forced expiratory volume at 1 second (FEV1). But, the total lung capacity and forced vital capacity (FVC) are normal or increased. So, the **ratio of FEV1/FVC is reduced**.

Types:

1. Asthma.

2. Emphysema.
3. Chronic bronchitis.
4. Bronchiectasis.
5. Bronchiolitis.
6. Cystic fibrosis.

34. What is bronchial asthma?

Ans. *DEF:* Episodic reversible bronchospasm and airway narrowing due to body's increased bronchial smooth muscle spasmodic and inflammatory response to various stimuli.

Types: 2:

1. Ig**E**-mediated (**E**xtrinsic) (in 1/5 cases).
2. **I**ndependent of IgE (**I**ntrinsic) (in remainder of the 4/5 cases).

ETIO:

1. *Extrinsic:* Reaction to external antigens/allergens.
2. *Intrinsic:* Reaction to several stimuli, that have no effect in normal people, causing bronchospasm, e.g. changes in environmental temperature, cold, viruses, aspirin, pulmonary infection, exercise, stress, etc.

PATHOG: Not well-understood about both above types. A little is understood about IgE-mediated asthma, the common type of which is atopic, i.e. due to familial predisposition to local type I hypersensitivity. In such a person an allergen stimulates TH_2 CD_4+ T-cells which secrete IL_{4+5}, cause B-cells to produce IgE, growth of mast cells and eosinophils. IgE-Ag-IgE bind to mast cells, cause mast cells to release several chemical mediators which cause bronchoconstriction increase vascular permeability and mucin secretion and narrowing of air passages and attract eosinophils which by peroxidase cause tissue destruction.

PATHOPHY: In an attack of asthma the patient has shortness of breath with wheezing. The chief difficulty is of expiration. Patient gets air into lungs, but cannot get it out due to spasm, thickening of the airway walls and increased thick secretion in the airway lumen resulting in hyperinflation of the lungs. This leads to **hypoxia**. With passage of time respiratory muscles get tired with diminished respiration, **decrease in arterial oxygen** and **increase in carbon-dioxide leading to respiratory acidosis resulting in respiratory failure** which could progress to **coma** and **death** if not appropriately treated. *GROSS:* Lungs are overdistended, bronchi and bronchioles are occluded with thick sticky mucus plugs. *MICRO:* Mucus plugs contain whorls of shed epithelium **(Curschman's spirals)**, many eosinophils and **Charcot-Leyden crystals** (collections of diamond-shaped crystals made of eosinophil granules/ proteins). Edema, hyperemia, and inflammatory infiltrate in bronchial walls with eosinophils, mast cells, macrophages, lymphocytes, plasma cells is seen. *C/Fs:* Severe dyspnea with wheezing—mainly expiratory, trapping air in the lung with hyperinflation of lungs. Usually resolves spontaneously or with treatment. However, it can progress into **acute severe asthma** (old term **status asthmaticus**) and thereafter into life-threatening asthma and if not treated very vigorously causes **death**.

35. What are the chronic obstructive pulmonary diseases (COPD)?

Ans. This includes 2 conditions:

1. Emphysema
2. Chronic bronchitis.

36. What is emphysema?

Ans. *DEF:* **Morphologic:** Permanent enlargement of airspaces distal to the terminal bronchioles with destruction of their walls.

TERMS: Acinus = Part of lung distal to terminal bronchiole: (Respiratory bronchiole + Alveolar duct + Alveolus). Lobule = Cluster of 3–5 acini.

Types of emphysema:

1. *Centriacinar (centrilobular):* Only respiratory bronchioles are dilated. More common in upper lobes.
2. *Panacinar (panlobular):* Respiratory bronchioles to alveoli are uniformly dilated. More common in lower lung fields. **Occurs in alpha 1-antitrypsin deficiency**.
3. *Distal acinar (Paraseptal):* Distal part of acinus is affected and proximal portion is normal.

ETIO:

1. Smoking.
2. Alpha 1-antitrypsin deficiency.

PATHOG:

1. Increased oxidants and decreased antioxidants.
2. Increased protease and decreased antiprotease.

With loss of elastic tissue in alveolar septa, resulting in reduced radial traction on the small airways. Therefore, they collapse during expiration causing chronic airflow obstruction in severe emphysema. *GROSS:* In panacinar lungs are large and pale. In centriacinar lungs are less large and pink. *MICRO:* There is thinning and destruction of alveolar walls. With progression neighbouring alveoli join making large airspaces. Alveolar capillaries are reduced in number and respiratory bronchioles become fibrotic. *C/Fs:* Progressive dyspnea. Later hypoxia develops leading to pulmonary vascular spasm, pulmonary hypertension and cor pulmonale. **Respiratory failure with hypoxia, acidosis and coma or cor pulmonale cause death**.

37. What is chronic bronchitis?

Ans. *DEF:* **Clinical:** Persistent productive cough for at least 3 consecutive months in at least 2 consecutive years.

PATHOG: Irritants, mainly cigarette cause bronchial mucus glands hyperplasia, bronchial epithelial metaplasia with formation of mucin-secreting goblet cells. Superadded infection is also present. *C/Fs:* Patients have cough with mucoid sputum. Some patients also have outflow obstruction with hypercapnia, hypoxemia and cyanosis. *MICRO:* Submucosal gland layer is thickened. This is estimated by the ratio of width of bronchial submucosal gland to the thickness of the bronchial wall and is called **Reid index**. (Increased to 0.41 to 0.80. Normally, it is <0.40).

Goblet cells are increased. There is loss of ciliated epithelial cells. Also there is squamous metaplasia followed by dysplasia and if this progresses it **can progress to neoplasia (bronchogenic carcinoma)**.

38. What is bronchiectasis?

Ans. *DEF:* Permanent dilation of bronchi and bronchioles due to destruction of the muscle and elastic supporting tissue, due to or with chronic necrotizing infections. This is due to:

1. Infection.
2. Obstruction.
3. Congenital or hereditary conditions.

Predisposing conditions:

1. *Infection:*
   a. Chronic bronchitis.
   b. Necrotizing or suppurative pneumonia.
   c. Pertussis.
2. *Bronchial obstruction:* Due to:
   a. Tumors.
   b. Foreign bodies.
3. *Congenital or hereditary conditions:*
   a. **Cystic fibrosis:** An autosomal recessive disorder-generalized severe bronchiectasis resulting from obstruction and infection due to secretion of abnormally thick-sticky mucus.
   b. **Immunodeficiency states:** By causing repeated bacterial infections.
   c. **Kartagener's syndrome:** An autosomal recessive disorder having structural abnormality of cilia with decreased motility causing impaired mucus clearance from the airways causing continuous infections.

PATHOG: This is due to:

1. *Obstruction:* Obstruction interferes with clearance of secretions thereby facilitating superimposed infection, which damages the bronchial wall resulting in irreversible dilatation.
2. *Chronic persistent infection:* Staphylococci, streptococci, *H. influenzae* cause increased secretion which obstruct the airways, cause inflammation with scarring and traction with dilatation of the bronchial wall.

GROSS: Airways are dilated and can be visualized as reaching upto pleural surface, which is not the case in normal lungs. *MICRO:* Acute and chronic inflammation with ulceration and fibrosis of the walls of the airways is seen. *C/Fs:* Productive cough, occasional hemoptysis. Later hypoxia, hypercapnia, and pulmonary hypertension develop, which can lead to cor pulmonale. *COMPLI:* Lung abscess, brain abscess, amyloidosis.

39. What are the restrictive lung diseases?

Ans. *DEF:* Reduced expandibility of lungs (stiff lungs) with increased pressure required to expand the lungs with less amount of air in the lungs. Total lung capacity and FVC are reduced. But, the expiratory flow rate is normal or only reduced proportionately. So, **the ratio of FEV1/FVC is normal**.

Types:

A. *Pulmonary diseases:* Here the lungs are affected.

Types:

1. Acute interstitial lung diseases: Acute respiratory distress syndrome **(ARDS)** and neonatal respiratory distress syndrome (hyaline membrane disease).
2. Chronic respiratory distress syndrome:

   a. Idiopathic pulmonary fibrosis b. Sarcoidosis c. Pneumoconiosis.

B. *Extrapulmonary diseases:* Here the chest wall is affected.

Types:

1. *Musculoskeletal:*

   a. Obesity b. Kyphoscoliosis.

2. *Neurogenic:* **Guillain-Barre syndrome**.

40. What is acute lung injury and acute respiratory distress syndrome (ARDS)? What is neonatal respiratory distress syndrome (hyaline membrane disease)?

Ans. *DEF:* Acute generalized damage of alveolar epithelium and capillary endothelium.

ETIO: 1. *Infections:* Sepsis, diffuse pulmonary infections, e.g. viral, mycoplasma, miliary tuberculosis, pneumocystic pneumonia.

2. *Injuries:* Pulmonary contusions, near drowning, head injuries, oxygen toxicity, inhalation of smoke and other irritant gases, heroin , methadone or barbiturate overdose.

3. *Miscellaneous:* DIC, pancreatitis, uremia.

PATHOG: Activated neutrophils and macrophages release chemical mediators, e.g. oxygen-free radicals, proteases, leukotrienes, prostaglandins which cause damage to the capillary endothelium and increase in vascular permeability. Endothelial injury starts the coagulation cascade leading to generalized intravascular coagulation culminating in DIC. *C/Fs:* Patient has severe dyspnea, hypoxia and respiratory distress. Hypoxia can also cause failure of the cardiac, renal and hepatic systems. Prognosis is poor with high mortality rate. *GROSS:* In the beginning lungs are dark red and edematous. Later, fibrosis occurs making them gray. *MICRO:* **Edema fluid and necrotic alveolar cells make hyaline membranes which line the alveolar ducts**. Hyperemia of capillaries and edema and hemorrhage of interstitial tissue is present. Later type II pneumocytes and fibroblasts proliferate, which cause fibrosis of alveoli and interstitial tissue with scarring and distortion of the normal pulmonary architecture.

Neonatal respiratory distress syndrome presents as severe tachypnea, dyspnea, cyanosis in the newborn soon after birth due to deficiency of surfactant, which is secreted by type II pneumocytes and helps in expansion of lungs during inspiration and prevents collapse during expiration by reducing surface tension. It is seen in premature babies, babies born by cesarean section, or babies of diabetic mothers. Blood vessels are congested and leakage from them cause formation of hyaline membranes formed by fibrin and cellular debris. Prognosis is poor with high death rate due to intraventricular brain hemorrhage and necrotizing enterocolitis.

41. What are chronic restrictive (interstitial) lung diseases?

Ans. Many conditions having common features, e.g.:

1. **Reduced FVC**. Equally reduced FEV1. So, **FEV1 to FVC ratio not reduced**.
2. Pathophysiologic changes: Stiff lungs which cannot expand normally.
3. *S/S*.
4. X-Ray findings.

These conditions are:

1. Idiopathic pulmonary fibrosis (IPF).
2. *Pneumoconiosis:*
   a. Asbestosis b. Silicosis c. Coal worker's pneumoconiosis.
3. Sarcoidosis.
4. Hypersensitivity pneumonitis.
5. Diffuse alveolar hemorrhage syndrome.
   a. **Goodpasture's syndrome**.
   b. Idiopathic pulmonary hemosiderosis.
6. Pulmonary angiitis and granulomatosis **(Wegener granulomatosis)**.
7. Collagen vascular diseases:
   a. SLE b. RA c. Scleroderma d. Dermatomyositis.
8. *Drugs:* Busulfan, bleomycin, methotraxate.

42. What is idiopathic pulmonary fibrosis (cryptogenic fibrosing alveolitis)?

Ans. *ETIO:* Unknown. *PATHOG:* Alveolar wall injury due to unknown cause — Interstitial edema + inflammation (alveolitis). If injury is limited there is resolution. If injury is continuous there is interstitial fibrosis. *MORPHO:* Pulmonary parenchyma with fibrosis and irregularly dilated airspaces make lung look like honey comb **(honeycomb lung)**. *C/Fs:* Gradual onset with cough, dyspnea. Later cyanosis and edema develop causing **pulmonary hypertension leading to cor pulmonale**.

43. What is sarcoidosis?

Ans. *See* chapter 2.

44. What is hypersensitivity pneumonitis?

Ans. *ETIO:* Alveolitis due to type III/IV hypersensitivity due to different antigens such as: Moldy hay **(Farmer's lung)**; Pigeons **(Pigeon breeder's lung)**; Bagasse

(Bagassosis), etc. *MORPHO:* Mononuclear infiltrate in interstitial tissue. Also, noncaseating granulomas. Diffuse interstitial fibrosis in advanced stage.

45. What is diffuse alveolar hemorrhage syndrome?

Ans. Triad:

1. **D**iffuse pulmonary infiltrates.
2. **A**nemia.
3. **H**emoptysis.

Types: Goodpasture's syndrome. Idiopathic pulmonary hemosiderosis.

46. What is Goodpasture's syndrome?

Ans. *ETIO:* Unknown. *PATHOG:* Type II alveolar wall hypersensitivity consisting of Ab against basement membrane antigen of pulmonary alveolar wall and renal glomerular capillaries. *MICRO:* Focal necrosis of alveolar walls + intra-alveolar hemorrhage + fibrous thickening of alveolar septae. Hemosidern-laden macrophages. *C/Fs:* Hemoptysis, hematuria, proteinuria. *TRT:* Plasma exchange—removes antibodies. Immunosuppressive treatment—inhibits antibody production.

47. What is Wegener granulomatosis (pulmonary angiitis granulomatosis)?

Ans. Necrotizing vasculitis.

Triad:

1. Necrotizing or granulomatous vasculitis of small-medium-sized BVs of upper respiratory tract and lungs.
2. Ac. necrotizing granulomas of up. resp. tract (nose, throat, sinuses, ears) and lungs.
3. Renal–glomerulonephritis.

S/S: Epistaxis, cough, hemoptysis.

48. What are the collagen vascular lung diseases?

Ans. Seen in SLE, RA, scleroderma, dermato-polymyositis. Interstitial pneumonitis + diffuse interstitial fibrosis. **End-stage** = **Honeycomb lung**.

49. What is pneumoconiosis?

Ans. *DEF:* Disorders caused by inhalation of physiochemical agents, e.g. aerosol, fumes, vapors, inorganic mineral dusts or organic dusts.

Responsible factors are:

1. *Amount of dust:* Affected by—amount of dust, duration of exposure, effectiveness of clearance.
2. *Size, shape and buoyancy of particles:* >5 mm particles are filtered in upper airways; <1 mm particles remain suspended and are exhaled; ***1–5 mm*** *particles stay in the alveoli and cause damage.*
3. *Physiochemical reactivity and solubility of particles:* Soluble particles cause rapid toxicity. Insoluble particles cause chronic fibrotic reaction.

Types:

1. Carbon dust-coal worker's pneumoconiosis.
2. Silicosis.
3. Asbestosis.

50. What is carbon dust—coal worker's pneumoconiosis?

Ans. Three types:

a. *Anthracosis:* Harmless inhalation of carbon dust. Endemic in urban areas.

   GROSS: Irregular black patches on the lung. *MICRO*: Carbon-laden macrophages, responsible for above stated gross appearance.

b. *Simple coal worker's pneumoconiosis (CWP):* Due to more coal dust-laden macrophages forming coal macules. Person might have cough and black sputum. **Harmless**—there is no significant dysfunction. *GROSS:* Coal macules around bronchioles. Micro: Macrophages containing coal dust particles.

c. *Complicated CWP with progressive massive fibrosis:* **Harmful**. Due to increased amount of dust leading to severe fibrosis and scarring in areas of dust accumulation with respiratory insufficiency. Can cause bronchiectasis, pulmonary hypertension leading to right-sided heart failure **(cor pulmonale)**, respiratory failure and **death**. *GROSS:* Fibrotic nodules filled with black fluid.

51. What is silicosis?

Ans. Pneumoconiosis due to silica dust. Seen in miners, glass makers, stone cutters. Pathogenesis: Alveolar macrophages engulf silica dust particles, and get damaged releasing lysosomal enzymes and other chemical mediators with inflammatory response leading to lung damage with formation of silicotic nodules, which enlarge causing obstruction of airways and blood vessels. Patients become susceptible to develop pulmonary tuberculosis called **silicotuberculosis**.

52. What is asbestosis?

Ans. Pneumoconiosis due to inhalation of asbestos fibres. Pathogenesis: Alveolar macrophages engulf asbestos fibres with release of fibroblast-stimulating growth factors leading to diffuse interstitial fibrosis.

Mainly 2 types of fibres:

a. Amphiboles brittle, straight-stiff fibres, reach deep in the lung and thus cause **more damage**.

b. Serpentines curled, flexible. Cause less damage. Some fibres are coated by hemosiderin to form beaded, dumbbell-shaped bodies called **Asbestos bodies** (ferruginous bodies). *GROSS:* Diffuse interstitial fibrosis. Calcified fibrotic plaques of the pleura. *MICRO:* Fibrosis, calcification, asbestos bodies. *COMPLI:* Asbestosis increases **risk of developing bronchogenic carcinoma**, which is further increased by cigarette smoking; and **risk of developing malignant mesothelioma of the pleura**.

53. What is Caplan syndrome?

Ans. *DEF:* Rheumatoid arthritis with pneumoconiosis due to **s**ilica, **a**sbestos, **c**oal **(sac)**. Miners of these who have or develop rheumatoid arthritis, may develop round nodules in the lung soon which are similar to rheumatoid nodules by LM.

54. What are some of the occupational pulmonary diseases (pneumoconiosis) due to organic materials?

Ans. Pneumoconiosis from organic materials is of 2 types:

1. Organic material itself causes pathology, e.g. cotton **(byssinosis)** which causes inflammatory chronic bronchitis.
2. Organic material is contaminated by moulds and fungi causing hypersensitivity reaction resulting in bronchiolitis and alveolitis **(extrinsic allergic alveolitis)**. Such recurrent attacks destroy alveoli and bronchi resulting in fibrosis. Few unaffected bronchioles develop compensatory dilatation giving the lungs a **honeycomb** appearance. Over many years pulmonary hypertension develops leading to right-sided heart failure **(cor pulmonale)**.

55. What are pulmonary neoplasms?

Ans. Predisposing factors:

1. Cigarette smoking—proportional to how many cigarettes smoked per day and for how many years.
2. Asbestos exposure.
3. Asbestos + cigarettes—worse.
4. Air pollution.
5. Radiation—radium and uranium.

Types: Benign: Almost none.

Malignant:

a. *Secondary cancers to the lung:* These are mostly from breast, GIT, kidneys, melanoma.

b. Primary lung cancers:

1. Squamous cell carcinoma (from metaplastic squamous cells).
2. Adenocarcinoma (from bronchiolar epithelium).
3. Bronchioloalveolar carcinoma (from bronchiolar epithelium).
4. Small cell carcinoma (from neuroendocrine cells).
5. Large cell carcinoma.
6. Carcinoid (from neuroendocrine cells—differentiation of **Kultchitsky cells**).
7. Mesothelioma (from pleura).
8. Miscellaneous.

Lung cancer is the most common cancer and cancer death in the world.
This is mainly due to cigarette smoking. *PATHOG:* Squamous cell carcinoma occurs in: Serial changes of metaplasia-dysplasia-CIS and invasive carcinoma. Adenocarcinoma develops as: Atypical adenomatous hyperplasia and invasive

carcinoma. Small cell carcinoma and carcinoid develop as diffuse idiopathic pulmonary neuroendocrine cell hyperplasia and invasive small cell carcinoma/carcinoid. *C/Fs: S/S:* Cough, hemoptysis, bronchial obstruction with shortness of breath, atelactasis, pneumonitis., extension to pleura, pericardium, ribs, superior vena cava **(superior vena cava syndrome)**. Tumors in the apex of the lung can compress brachial plexus with pain in the distribution of ulner nerve, cervical sympathetic plexus with **Horner's syndrome**. These apical tumors are called **Pancoast's tumor** and the clinical findings **Pancoast's syndrome**. They also spread to mediastinal, scelene, and supraclavicular **(virchow)** l. nodes. Also, they metastasize to opposite lung, liver, adrenal glands, bones, CNS. Also, associated with paraneoplastic syndromes (see below). *PROG:* Poor. Worse for small cell carcinoma, relatively better for bronchioloalveolar carcinoma.

56. What is squamous cell carcinoma of the lung?

Ans. *MICRO:* Anaplastic cells with intercellular bridges and keratin in individual cells with eosinophilic dense cytoplasm. **Keratin pearls**.

57. What are the adenocarcinomas of the lungs?

Ans. *MICRO:* Gland formation with mucin production. Patterns can be acinar, papillary, bronchioloalveolar. More common in nonsmokers and women. Usually more peripherally located and smaller in size.

58. What is bronchioloalveolar carcinoma of the lungs?

Ans. *MICRO:* Arises from terminal bronchioles. Grows along preexisting lung structures without destruction of alveolar architecture. This pattern is called **lepidic** (resemble the appearance of butterflies sitting on a fence). It is thought that some of these arise from the **Clara cells** (present in the lining of bronchioles before the alveolar acinus).

59. What is small cell carcinoma?

Ans. Very highly malignant tumor. *MICRO:* The tumor grows in group of epithelial cells having small, round to oval to spindle-shaped with nuclear molding with little cytoplasm. The nuclear chromatin is finely granular **(salt-pepper pattern)**.

60. What is superior sulcus tumor (Pancoast's tumor) and Pancoast's syndrome?

Ans. Neoplasms at the apex of the lung is called pancoast's tumor and the clinical findings due to them Pancoast's syndrome. These consist of erosion of adjacent ribs and involvement of lower part of brachial plexus (C8, T1, T2) causing severe pain in the shoulder and down the inner surface of the arm.

61. What is Horner's syndrome?

Ans. When lung cancer compresses cervical sympathetic chain it causes a condition called Horner's syndrome consisting of ipsilateral:

1. Enophthalmos

2. Ptosis.
3. Meiosis
4. Anhidrosis

62. What is superior vena cava syndrome (SVC syndrome)?

Ans. When lung cancer compresses superior vena cava (SVC) it causes a condition called superior vena cava syndrome which causes ipsilateral edema of the face and the upper limb.

63. What is the cause of hoarseness of voice with lung cancer?

Ans. Due to paralysis of recurrent laryngeal nerve.

64. What are paraneoplastic syndromes?

Ans. *DEF* of paraneoplastic syndrome: *See* chapter 4. Following hormone or hormone-like substances are secreted from lung cancers causing this syndrome:

1. *ADH:* Causes hyponatremia. Mainly by small cell carcinoma—**SIADH** (syndrome of inappropriate ADH secretion).
2. *ACTH:* Causes Cushing's syndrome. Mainly by small cell carcinoma.
3. *PTHrP (Parathyroid hormone-related polypeptide):* Causes hypercalcemia—mainly by squamous cell carcinoma.
4. *Calcitonin:* Causes hypercalcemia.
5. *Gonadotrophin:* Causes gynecomastia.

65. What is carcinoid?

Ans. *Histogenesis:* Kulchitsky cells (neuroendocrine cells present in bronchial mucosa). *C/Fs:* Age—40 yrs. Sometimes as part of MEN. Cure by surgical removal. Carcinoid syndrome: **VANISH**

1. ***V**asomotor:* Flushes and apparent cyanosis.
2. ***A**sthma:* Cough, dyspnea, wheezing.
3. ***N**iacin deficiency:* Due to niacin being used up in serotonin synthesis.
4. ***I**ntestinal:* Diarrhea, cramps, nausea, vomiting.
5. ***S**ystemic fibrosis:* Heart: Right ventricle endocardium; tricuspid and pulmonic valve thickening and stenosis.
6. **H**epatomegaly with nodular metastases.

66. What are mediastinal tumors masses?

Ans. *Superior:* Lymphoma, thymoma, thyroid, parathyroid, secondary.
Anterior: Lymphoma, thymoma, thyroid, parathyroid, teratoma.
Middle: Lymphoma, bronchogenic or pericardial cyst.
Posterior: Lymphoma, GIT hernia, Nr. tumors (neurofibroma, schwannoma).

67. What is atelectasis?

Ans. *DEF:* **Collapse**. Loss of lung volume due to **inadequate expansion of air spaces**. Results in shunting of inadequately oxygenated blood from pulmonary arteries into veins with ventilation-perfusion imbalance and hypoxia.

Types: Based on cause or part of lung involved: 4 types:

1. Resorption atelactasis
2. Compression.
3. Micro
4. Contraction.

68. What is resorption atelactasis?

Ans. Due to obstruction in the airway preventing air from reaching distal airway, with absorption of already present air in alveoli and alveolar collapse. Depending on level of obstruction collapse can occur of the entire lung, lobe or a segment of lobe.

Causes:

1. Mucous or mucopurulent plug—due to asthma, bronchiectasis, chronic bronchitis.
2. Foreign body aspiration, especially in kids.
3. Blood clots during oral surgery or anesthesia.
4. Tumors, e.g. bronchogenic carcinoma.
5. Enlarged lymph nodes, e.g. TB.
6. Vascular aneurysms.

69. What is compression atelactasis?

Ans. Also known as passive or relaxation atelactasis due to collection of fluid, blood or air in pleural cavity with mechanical collapse of the adjacent lung.

Causes:

1. CCF with pleural effusion.
2. Pneumothorax (air into pleural cavity).
3. Elevated diaphragm causing basal atelactasis during prolonged bed rest, long postoperative period.

70. What is microatelactasis?

Ans. Non-obstructive due to loss of surfactant with generalized loss of lung expansion.

Causes:

1. Neonatal respiratory distress syndrome.
2. Adult respiratory distress syndrome.
3. Several interstitial inflammatory pulmonary diseases.
4. Postsurgical.

71. What is contraction (cicatrization) atelactasis?

Ans. Due to local or generalized fibrotic changes in the lung or pleura thereby precluding expansion and increasing elastic recoil during expiration. Atelactasis, except due to contraction (cicatrization, fibrosis) is potentially reversible and should be treated promptly to prevent hypoxia and superimposed infection of the collapsed lung.

72. What are common disorders of the pleura?

Ans. 1. Substances within potential pleural cavities (air, fluid-transudate/exudates, blood, lymph).
2. Pleuritis.
3. Neoplasms.

73. What are the substances which can collect within the potential pleural cavity?

Ans. 1. *Air:* Pneumothorax.
2. *Fluid:*
   a. Transudate (hydrothorax).
   b. Exudate (pus = pyothorax or empyema).
   c. *Blood:* Hemothorax.
   d. *Chylothorax:* Milky lymphatic fluid.

74. What is pneumothorax?

Ans. A. *Spontaneous:* In apparently healthy young adults due to unknown etiology.
B. *Secondary:* Due to rupture of pulmonary lesion near the pleural surface, e.g. emphysema, abscess, tuberculosis. Also mechanical ventilation. Trauma.

75. What is tension pneumothorax? What is its significance?

Ans. Ball-valve phenomenon where air can enter the pleural cavity but cannot exit. **Surgical emergency**.

76. What is hydrothorax?

Ans. A. *Transudate:*
ETIO:
   a. CCF.
   b. **Meigs syndrome** = Thecoma-fibroma of ovary with ascites.

B. *Exudate:*
   a. Infections.
   b. Neoplasia: Primary of lung or pleura or secondary.
   c. Pulmonary infarction.

77. What is hemothorax?

Ans. a. *Internal:* Ruptured intrathoracic aneurysm.
b. *External:* Trauma.

78. What is chylothorax?

Ans. Due to obstruction of lymphatic duct usually from primary or secondary neoplasm.

79. What is mesothelioma?

Ans. *DEF:* Neoplasm of pleura—Less commonly of peritoneum and pericardium.
Types:
a. Benign.
b. Malignant.

a. *Benign*: Common in peritoneal cavity. Rare in pleural cavity. *GROSS:* Well-circumscribed, single, pinkish mass. *MICRO:* Papillary processes lined by single to many layers of cuboidal mesothelial cells without cellular atypia or mitotic figures.

b. *Malignant: ETIO*: Approximately 2/3 of cases have atleast 20 years exposure to asbestos (amphibole group). *GROSS:* Many grayish nodules and continuous plaques. *MICRO:* Spindle cell and cuboidal cell tumor with cellular atypia and mitotic figures. *C/Fs:* Chest pain and pleural effusion. *TRT:* Surgery, chemotherapy, radiation. *PROG:* Poor with death of almost all patients in 5 years.

11 Diseases of the Gastrointestinal System (GIS)

OVERVIEW

A. *Oral cavity:*
   1. Infectious.
   2. Premalignant.
   3. Malignant.

B. *Pharynx:* Acute pharyngitis/tonsillitis.

C. *Salivary glands:*
   1. Sialoadenitis.
   2. Neoplasms.

D. *Esophagus:*
   1. Congenital anomalies.
   2. Motor dysfunctions.
   3. Inflammation.
   4. Varices.
   5. Neoplasms.

E. *Stomach:*
   1. Congenital anomalies.
   2. Gastritis.
   3. Ulcers.
   4. Neoplasms.

F. *Intestines:*
   1. Congenital anomalies.
   2. Vascular diseases.
   3. Gastroenteritis.
   4. Malabsorption.
   5. IBDs.
   6. Diverticulosis.
   7. Obstruction.
   8. Neoplasms.

G. *Appendix:*
1. Appendicitis.
2. Neoplasms.

H. *Peritoneum:*
1. Peritonitis.
2. Neoplasms.

I. *Liver:*
1. Jaundice/cholestasis.
2. Cirrhosis.
3. Liver failure/LFTs.
4. Portal hypertension.
5. Infections.
6. Drug-toxic injuries.
7. Congenital anomalies.
8. Intrahepatic biliary tract diseases.
9. Vascular diseases.
10. Pre-eclampsia/eclampsia.
11. Reye's syndrome.
12. Neoplasms.

J. *Gallbladder:*
1. Stones.
2. Cholecystitis.
3. Neoplasms.

K. *Exocrine pancreas:*
1. Congenital anomalies.
2. Pancreatitis.
3. Neoplasms.

Oral cavity

Major diseases of the oral cavity are:
1. Inflammatory.
2. Premalignant.
3. Malignant.

Examples of inflammatory diseases are: Herpes labialis and oral candidiasis (moniliasis, thrush).

Premalignant diseases are: Leukoplakia and **erythroplasia, both of these are precancerous**—~10% leukoplakia and ~50% erythroplasia. Therefore, **biopsy is necessary in these diseases**.

Commonest malignant neoplasm of the oral cavity is squamous cell carcinoma. Its risk factors are leukoplakia, erythroplasia, tobacco, alcohol and betel nut use, human papilloma virus (HPV) infection, **Plummer-Vinson (Kelly-Peterson) syndrome**.

Pharynx

Common diseases of the pharynx are: Infections by viruses (EBV, coxsackie, adeno), bacteria (group A beta hemolytic streptococci) can result in rheumatic fever and poststreptococcal glomerulonephritis).

Salivary glands

Major diseases of the salivary glands are:

1. Inflammatory diseases (sialadenitis).
2. Neoplasms.

Inflammatory diseases of the salivary glands are:

1. Infectious.
2. Autoimmune.

Some of the infectious diseases of the salivary glands are due to viruses (e.g. mumps), bacteria, etc.

Some of the autoimmune sialadenitis are:

1. Sjogren syndrome-**Keratoconjunctivitis sicca** and **xerostomia** (isolated primary form of Sjogren syndrome-**Sicca syndrome**) and
2. Secondary form of Sjogren syndrome with RA, SLE, SS.
3. Mikulicz syndrome.
4. Mikulicz disease.

Some of the salivary gland neoplasms are:

1. Pleomorphic adenoma (mixed tumor).
2. Warthin tumor.
3. Mucoepidermoid carcinoma.

Esophagus

One of the **congenital anomalies** of the esophagus is tracheo-esophageal fistula.

Motor dysfunction of the esophagus is achalasia which is incomplete relaxation of the lower esophageal sphincter while swallowing.

Esophageal varices are varicose veins at the distal esophagus at portocaval anastomosis due to portal hypertension which when rupture cause death in ~ 50% patients.

Barrett's esophagus is metaplasia of distal esophageal mucosa from stratified squamous epithelium to columnar epithelium containing goblet cells in response to chronic reflux esophagitis.

Squamous cell carcinoma is the commonest esophageal neoplasm. Some of the risk factors are chronic esophagitis, **Plummer-Vinson syndrome**, alcohol, tobacco, etc.

Stomach

Gastritis is inflammation of the gastric mucosa. It is of two types:

1. Acute.
2. Chronic.

Acute gastritis is temporary acute mucosal inflammation usually due to NSAIDs, alcohol, *H. pyloi*, etc.

Chronic gastritis is chronic gastric mucosal inflammation which progresses to mucosal atrophy and metaplasia due to duodenogastric reflux, autoimmune disorder which leads to **pernicious anemia**, hypochlorhydria/achlorhydria, *H. pylori* infection, etc.

Ulcer of GIT is a mucosal breach extending to submucosa or deeper.

Acute gastric ulcer (stress ulcer) is due to severe stress, e.g. extensive burn **(Curling's ulcer)**, CNS injury **(Cushing's ulcer)**, NSAID, steroids.

Peptic ulcer is an ulcer in any part of the GIT having exposure to acid-peptic juices. 99 % are seen in duodenum and stomach out of which 75% are in the duodenum and 25% are in the stomach. Pathogenesis consists of decreased defensive factors and increased offensive factors. Decrease in defensive factors are ischemia, delayed gastric emptying, duodenogastric reflux. Increased offensive factors are NSAIDs, steroids, alcohol, cigarettes, COPD, hypercalcemia, *H. pylori*. Microscopically, from superficial to deep there are four layers: **DIGS**

1. Necrotic (**D**ead) tissue.
2. **I**nflammatory tissue.
3. **G**ranulation tissue.
4. **S**car.

Complications are: **HOP**

1. **H**emorrhage.
2. **O**bstruction.
3. **P**erforation (not CHOP, because cancer is very rare).

Neoplasms of the stomach are:

1. Benign (polyps).
2. Malignant.

Polyps are:

1. Hyperplastic.
2. Fundic (both harmless).
3. Adenomatous **(has risk of cancer development)**.

Malignant neoplasms are:

1. Adenocarcinoma.
2. Lymphomas.
3. Carcinoids.
4. Mesenchymal.

Adenocarcinomas are of two types:

1. Diffuse.
2. Intestinal.

Diffuse type arises in normal epithelium. Its risk factors are unknown.

Intestinal type arises in intestinal metaplastic epithelium. *Its risk factors are: H. pylori* infection, pernicious anemia, nitrites, smoked foods. Outcome is dependent on the depth of invasion. Adenocarcinomas have tendency for unknown reason to spread to supraclavicular lymph node **(Virchow's node)** and both ovaries **(Krukenberg tumor)**.

Intestines

Some of the developmental anomalies of the small intestine are:

1. Atresia or stenosis.
2. Meckel's diverticulum.

Some of the developmental anomalies of the large intestine are:

1. Malrotation.
2. Hirschprung disease.

Vascular diseases of the intestine are:

1. Ischemia.
2. Hemorrhoids.

Gastroenteritis is acute gastrointestinal infection causing diarrhea or dysentery with or without vomiting.

Dysentery is low volume bloody stools with abdominal pain. Some of the causative bacteria are Shigella species, Campylobacter species, enteroinvasive *E. coli* (EIEC) (mechanism of these is by mucosal invasion), Salmonella species, Campylobacter species, enterohemorrhagic *E. coli* (EHEC) (mechanism of these is by cytotoxin production). Causative protozoa is *Entamoeba histolytica* (mechanism is by mucosal invasion).

Diarrhea is loose watery stools with increased amount and frequency. Its cause can be noninfectious or infectious.

Examples of noninfectious causes of diarrhea are: IBDs, malabsorption, carcinoid, **Zollinger-Ellison syndrome**, thyrotoxicosis, carcinoma of the colon with change in bowel habits.

Examples of infectious causes of diarrhea are:

1. *Viruses:* Rotavirus, enteric adenovirus, noravirus.
2. *Bacteria:* Enteropathogenic *E. coli* (EPEC) (mechanism is by mucosal adherence), *Vibrio cholera*, Salmonella species, Campylobacter species, enterotoxigenic *E. coli* (ETEC), *Staphylococcus aureus, Clostridium perfringens* (mechanism of action is by enterotoxin production).
3. *Protozoa: Giardia lamblia* (mechanism is by attachment to the intestinal mucosa without invading it).

Malabsorption is deficient absorption of nutrients from GIT. Some of the causes are:

a. Defective digestion due to:
   1. Pancreatic insufficiency.
   2. **Zollinger-Ellison syndrome**.
   3. Decreased bile salts due to cirrhosis, cholestasis with decreased fat solubility.
   4. Lactose intolerance.
b. Defective transport from intestinal lumen into blood due to:
   1. **Celiac sprue**.
   2. **Tropical sprue**.
   3. **Whipple's disease**.
   4. Abetalipoproteinemia.
   5. Giardiasis.

Some of the manifestations of malabsorption are diarrhea, steatorrhea, dehydration, malnutrition causing anemia of iron, B_{12}, and folic acid deficiency, weight loss due to lack of calories, vitamin deficiencies (A, D, E, K) with their clinical manifestations.

Idiopathic inflammatory bowel diseases (IIBD) are:

1. Crohn's disease (CD).
2. Ulcerative colitis (UC).

CD is granulomatous, affects any part of the GIT from esophagus to anus, causes full-thickness inflammation with fissuring and fistula formation, has skip lesions with normal intestine between inflamed segments, is systemic disease and has less predisposition to development of cancer than UC.

UC is non-granulomatous, affects colon causing inflammation of mucosa and submucosa continuously without skip lesions, is systemic disease, can cause toxic megacolon and has predisposition to cancer development more than CD.

Colonic diverticulum is a blind pouch protruding out of the GIT.

Bowel obstruction can be due to:

1. *Mechanical causes*, e.g. hernia, adhesion, intussusception, volvulus, tumors, strictures, etc. or
2. *Non-mechanical causes*, e.g. paralytic ileus, bowel infarction, myo-neuropathies such as **Hirschprung disease**.

Peutz-Jegher syndrome is autosomal dominant condition consisting of hamartomatous polyps, melanotic mucosal and cutaneous pigmentation and risk of intestinal and extraintestinal malignancies.

Neoplasms of the small and large intestine are:

a. *Epithelial* such as adenoma, familial adenomatous polyposis syndromes **(FAP)**, adenocarcinoma, carcinoid, anal zone carcinoma and

b. Mesenchymal such as lipoma, leiomyoma, angioma, liposarcoma, leiomyosarcoma, **Kaposis's sarcoma**, lymphoma, **GIST** (gastrointestinal stromal tumor).

Appendix

Acute appendicitis has three stages:

1. Early.
2. Suppurative.
3. Gangrenous.

Neoplasms of the appendix are carcinoid, mucinous cystadenoma and adenocarcinoma.

Liver

Liver function tests (LFTs): AST, ALT, LDH, serum bilirubin (total and direct), urine bilirubin, serum bile acids, serum alkaline phosphatase, serum gamma glutamyl transpeptidase (GGTP), serum albumin, serum ammonia, prothrombin time.

Jaundice/Icterus/Cholestasis: **Jaundice** is yellow color of skin, **icterus** is yellow color of sclera due to elevated serum bilirubin at 2 to 2.5 mg/dl. **Cholestasis** is jaundice + pruritus (due to increased bile salts) + increased cholesterol (may cause **xanthomas**) (i.e. increased serum bilirubin, bile salts and cholesterol).

Pathophysiologic types of jaundice:

1. *Unconjugated hyperbilirubinemia due to:* Increased bilirubin production, e.g. hemolysis, decreased hepatic cellular uptake, e.g. **Gilbert's disease**, decreased conjugation, e.g. **Crigler-Najjar syndrome**.
2. *Conjugated hyperbilirubinemia due to:* Hepatic causes: Alcoholic hepatitis, viral hepatitis, cirrhosis, drugs (e.g. methyl dopa, isoniazid), neoplasms primary and secondary. Extrahepatic causes (obstructive): Biliary stricture and stones, pancreatic pseudocyst and carcinoma.

Hepatic failure

Types:

1. Massive hepatic necrosis.
2. Cirrhosis.
3. Without overt necrosis.

C/Fs:

1. Jaundice.
2. Cholestasis.
3. Hypoalbuminemia.
4. Hyperammonemia.
5. Fetor hepaticus.
6. Palmar erythema and spider angioma.
7. Male hypogonadism and gynecomastia.
8. Coagulopathy.
9. Encephalopathy.
10. Hepatorenal syndrome.

Cirrhosis

End stage of liver diseases.

Characteristics:

1. Fibrosis.
2. Regenerating nodules.
3. Entire liver architecture is disrupted.

ETIO:

1. Alcoholic liver diseases.
2. Viral hepatitis.
3. Biliary diseases.
4. Genetic hemochromatosis.
5. Wilson's diseases.
6. Alpha 1-antitrypsin deficiency.
7. Miscellaneous, e.g. schistosomiasis.

Portal hypertension

Increased pressure in the portal circulation.

ETIO:

1. Prehepatic, e.g. portal vein thrombosis.
2. Hepatic, e.g. cirrhosis.
3. Posthepatic, e.g. right heart failure.

Consequences:

1. Ascites.
2. Portosystemic venous shunts.
3. Congestive splenomegaly.
4. Hepatic encephalopathy.

Hepatomegaly

Liver larger than the normal (~1500 gm).

ETIO:

1. Inflammatory, e.g. hepatitis.
2. Congestive, e.g. right-sided heart failure.
3. Neoplastic, e.g. hepatocellular carcinoma, lymphoma/leukemia.
4. Infiltrative, e.g. amyloidosis.

Hepatotropic viral hepatitis

Types: A, B, C, D, E.

Hepatitis A: Transmission by fecal-oral. No chronic hepatitis or carrier state. Rarely fatal.

Hepatitis B: Transmission by body fluids (serum, semen, etc.). Can cause chronic disease, carrier state, death. Presence in the serum of HBeAg means person is infective and the disease might progress to chronic hepatitis, of anti-HBe means the infection is declining, of IgG-anti-HBs means the person has recovered from the disease and has protection for life and person is not infective.

Hepatitis C: Transmission by IV route. *C/Fs:* Similar to hepatitis B.

Hepatitis D: Transmission by IV route. Cannot cause hepatitis without the help of hepatitis B virus: When coinfection with HBV complete recovery; when superinfection of a chronic carrier of HBV severe chronic hepatitis develops.

Hepatitis E: Transmission by drinking water. Endemic in India. Self-limited without chronic liver disease.

Hepatic amebiasis

From chronic intestinal amebiasis due to amebic trophozoites entering portal venous radicals in colonic mucosa and forming amebic abscesses.

Drugs/toxins hepatic injuries

Due to alcohol abuse and exposure to various drugs, e.g. acetaminophen, OCs, isoniazid, etc.

Alcoholic liver disease

Types:

1. Fatty liver.

2. Hepatitis.
3. Cirrhosis.

Hemochromatosis

Excess iron collection in liver with injury leading to hepatomegaly and eventually cirrhosis.
Types:

1. Hereditary (autosomal recessive).
2. Acquired.

Wilson's disease

Autosomal recessive with increased copper deposition in liver, brain, eyes and injury to liver and brain.

Alpha 1-antitrypsin deficiency

Autosomal recessive with deficiency of protease inhibitor and increased protease activity causing lung injury (emphysema) and liver injury (cirrhosis and occasionally hepatocellular carcinoma).

Circulatory liver disorders (impaired blood flow)

Types:

1. Into liver via hepatic artery, portal vein **(Banti's syndrome)**.
2. Through liver due to cirrhosis, congestion.
3. Out of liver due to hepatic vein thrombosis **(Budd-Chiari syndrome)**.

Neoplasms

Benign: Adenoma.

Malignant: Primary – Hepatocellular carcinoma (HCC), cholangiocarcinoma.
Secondary – More common than primary. From common site GIT, breasts, lungs.

Gallbladder

Cholelithiasis

80% cholesterol–More common in Europe and N. America, **female, fat, fertile, forties, flatulent**.
20% pigment–More common in Asia, with chronic hemolysis, biliary infection.

Cholecystitis

Acute, chronic, acute on chronic. Majority associated with stones.

Carcinoma

Majority are adenocarcinoma, discovered late, therefore, prognosis poor. Predisposition in West is stone and in East is infections of biliary tree.

Exocrine pancreas

Fibrocystic Disease of Pancreas (Cystic Fibrosis) (Mucoviscidosis)

Autosomal recessive with defect in transport of chloride ions across epithelia with decreased chloride in pancreatic ducts followed by compensatory sodium and water outflow causing plugging of pancreatic ducts with thick, viscid secretion resulting in atrophy of exocrine glands and islets of Langerhans, fibrosis and cyst formation leading to exocrine pancreatic insufficiency and diabetes mellitus.

Acute pancreatitis

Inflammation of pancreas with leakage of enzymes causing injury, mostly due to alcoholism and gallstones. Diagnosis by elevated serum amylase and lipase. Presents as acute abdominal pain, shock and cause death in 25 to 50% cases.

Carcinoma of pancreas

Adenocarcinoma of the exocrine pancreas. Poor prognosis due to late discovery. Recognition of migratory phlebothrombosis **(Trousseau's sign)** might help in early diagnosis. **Courvoiser's law/ sign:** Painless, non-tender, dilated gallbladder is usually due to obstruction from carcinoma of the pancreas.

Diseases of the Oral Cavity

1. What are the main categories of oral cavity diseases?

Ans. 1. Inflammatory diseases.
2. Premalignant diseases.
3. Malignant diseases.

2. What are common inflammatory diseases of the oral cavity?

Ans. 1. Herpes labialis.
2. Oral candidiasis (moniliasis, thrush).

3. What is herpes labialis?

Ans. *ETIO:* Herpes simplex virus type 1 (HSV-1). Sometimes HSV-2, which usually causes genital herpes (which can be sometimes caused by HSV-1). All herpes viruses establish lifelong latent infections in our body, e.g. varicella zoster virus (cause of chickenpox and herpes zoster-shingles), cytomegalovirus (CMV), Epstein-Barr virus (EBV), human herpes virus type 8 (associated with Kaposi's sarcoma). *MORPHO:* Small, vesicles containing clear fluid. Microscopically, intranuclear acidophilic viral inclusions are seen. Some giant cells are also seen. *PATHOG:* Transmitted between people by kissing. Virus stays inactive within ganglia, e.g. trigeminal ganglia of the V cranial nerve. Stimuli such as fever, sun or cold exposure, etc. reactivate the virus and small vesicles appear. Vesicles are formed from filling of edema fluid in spaces created by death of viral-infected epithelial cells. Vesicles rupture soon with formation of shallow, painful ulcers which heal within a few weeks. *DIAG:* By **Tzanck test:** Smear of fluid blisters is made, with observation of giant cells or cells containing intranuclear inclusions.

4. What is candidiasis (moniliasis, thrush)?

Ans. *DEF/DES:* Disease caused by *Candida albicans* in vulnerable people. *ETIO:* Infection by *Candida albicans* in susceptible people due to diabetes mellitus, steroid treatment, AIDS, widespread malignancy. *MORPHO:* Gross examination shows adherent, white, membrane-like area in the oral cavity. Microscopic examination of membrane shows sheet of candida in chains with budding yeasts. There is no epithelium present. Therefore, these membranes are called **pseudomembranes**. *C/Fs:* In general, it is not a serious condition and easily treatable. However, in severely vulnerable people, it can cause life-threatening generalized infection requiring very aggressive treatment.

5. What are premalignant diseases of the oral cavity?

Ans. 1. Leukoplakia.
2. Erythroplasia.

6. What is leukoplakia of the oral cavity?

Ans. *DEF:* A whitish, mucosal patch due to epidermal thickening or hyperkeratosis. *ETIO:* Unknown. Associated with: Use of tobacco, (pouches, snuff, chewing) alcohol, chronic friction, e.g. Ill-fitting dentures. Human papillomavirus (HPV). *MORPHO: GROSS:* One or more diffuse, white, areas of mucosal thickening. *MICRO:* Microscopic appearance varies from hyperkeratosis without dysplasia to mild to severe dysplasia [carcinoma *in situ* (CIS)]. **These can be determined only by histologic examination** and **not** by gross/clinical examination. **Hence, biopsy is mandatory**. *C/Fs:* More common in older men. Most often sites are vermilion border of lower lip, buccal mucosa, hard and soft palates. Approximately 10% develop squamous cell carcinoma.

7. What is erythroplasia of the oral cavity?

Ans. *DEF:* Red, circumscribed areas, with irregular border. Microscopically, severe epithelial dysplasia is usually present. **Malignant transformation is >50%.**

8. What is the common neoplasm of the oral cavity?

Ans. Squamous cell carcinomas. *Risk factors:* Erythroplasia, leukoplakia, tobacco use, alcohol abuse, betel nut chewing, human papilloma virus (HPV), **Plummer-Vinson syndrome**. Common sites of occurrence:

1. Vermillion border of the lip.
2. Lateral border of the tongue.
3. Floor of the mouth.

MORPHO: GROSS: White gray thickenings of the mucosa. Fungating or ulcerating lesion. *MICRO:* Well differentiated keratinizing squamous cell carcinomas. *C/Fs:* Usually asymptomatic, therefore, present in late stage with poor prognosis.

Diseases of Pharynx

9. What is acute pharyngitis?

Ans. *ETIO:* Viruses: EBV (infectious mononucleosis); coxsackievirus (herpangina); pharyngitis, tonsillitis, peritonsillar abscess (quincy). Can cause acute rheumatic fever and poststreptococcal glomerulonephritis.

Diseases of the Salivary Glands

10. What are the common diseases of the salivary glands?

Ans. 1. Inflammatory diseases.

2. Neoplasms.

11. What are the common inflammatory diseases (sialadenitis) of the salivary gland?

Ans. 1. Infectious 2. Autoimmune.

12. What are the common infectious sialadenitis?

Ans. *ETIO:* Viruses (mumps), bacteria.
Viruses: Several viruses can cause mumps. Commonest virus to cause mumps is a paramyxovirus. *MORPHO:* Generalized mononuclear inflammatory cell infiltration with edema. *C/Fs:* Mumps in childhood is usually benign and self-limited. Mumps in adults can cause pancreatitis, orchitis which occasionally causes sterility.
Bacteria: Predisposing factors: Stone (sialolithiasis) with obstruction of the salivary duct, dehydration, immune deficiency diseases. *MORPHO*: Polymorphonuclear inflammatory cell infiltrate is seen.

13. What is autoimmune sialadenitis?

Ans. This is usually seen in:
Sjogren's syndrome consisting of involvement of salivary and lacrimal glands leading to dry mouth **(xerostomia)** and dry eyes with inflammation of conjunctiva and cornea **(keratoconjunctivitis)**. In approximately 1/2 the cases there are other associated autoimmune diseases, e.g. RA, SLE, etc. Approximate other 1/2 of the cases consist of the **sicca syndrome** having only **xerostomia** and **keratoconjunctivitis** (known as **primary form of Sjogren syndrome**). Also *see* chapter 3.

14. What are Mikulicz syndrome and Mikulicz disease?

Ans. **Mikulicz syndrome:** Here there is salivary and lacrimal gland involvement with xerostomia and keratoconjunctivitis of unknown etiology, however, it can be seen with Sjogren's syndrome.
Mikulicz disease: Same like Mikulicz syndrome with known etiologic conditions, e.g. lymphoma, leukemia, sarcoidosis, etc. Some authors describe these 2 terms the other way around. **Due to this confusion some authors recommend to stop altogether the use of these 2 terms.**

15. What are the common salivary gland neoplasms?

Ans.
1. Pleomorphic adenoma (mixed tumor of the salivary gland).
2. Warthin tumor (cystadenoma lymphomatosum).
3. Mucoepidermoid carcinoma.

16. What is pleomorphic adenoma (mixed tumor) of salivary glands?

Ans. Most common benign tumor of salivary glands which grows very slowly over many years. *GROSS:* Firm in consistency. *MICRO:* Epithelial elements consisting of ducts and acini together with myxoid cartilage-like elements are seen. Capsule shows penetration by tumor cells requiring resection with clear margins to prevent recurrence. Tumors of very long duration of approximately 20 years may develop malignant transformation.

17. What is Warthin tumor (cystadenolymphoma, cystadenoma lymphomatosum)?

Ans. *DES:* Benign tumor. Common site is parotid gland. Small, round mass. Cut section shows small cysts with mucin. *MICRO:* Cysts are seen which are lined by two layers of epithelial cells. Lymphoid tissue with occasional germ center is present in adjacent area. *C/Fs:* Excision is curative.

18. What is mucoepidermoid carcinoma of the salivary glands?

Ans. It is the commonest malignant neoplasm of the salivary glands. *MICRO:* 4 cell types are seen:

1. Mucin producing
2. Squamous
3. Intermediate
4. Clear.

It can be of low to high grade, where only 1/2 the patients survive for 5 years.

Diseases of the Esophagus

19. What is hiatal hernia?

Ans. *DEF/DES:* A part of the stomach projects into the thoracic cavity.

Types:

1. Sliding.
2. Paraesophageal.

C/Fs: From reflux of gastric acid consisting of heart burn. *COMPLI:* Ulcer, bleeding, perforation.

20. What is achalasia of the esophagus?

Ans. *DEF/DES:* Incomplete relaxation of lower esophageal sphincter upon swallowing. *ETIO/PATHOG:* Primary unknown. Secondary, e.g. **Chagas disease** by *Typanosoma cruzi* cause destruction of the myenteric plexus of the esophagus. *S/S:* Dysphagia. *COMPLI:* Development of squamous cell carcinoma.

21. What is Mallory-Weiss syndrome?

Ans. *DEF/DES:* Longitudinal tears in the esophagus at the esophagogastric junction. *ETIO/PATHOG:* During severe vomiting, due to inadequate relaxation of the lower esophageal sphincter resulting in bleeding. Severe vomiting for any reason can cause this; however, commonly it is seen with alcoholics.

22. What are the esophageal varices?

Ans. *DEF/DES:* Varicose veins within the submucosa of the distal esophagus and proximal stomach at the site of porto-caval anastomosis due to portal hypertension, which when rupture cause **severe bleeding with death in approximately half the patients** and recurrent episode of hemorrhage in the others with death in certain percentage of patients with each episode.

23. What is Barrett's esophagus?

Ans. *DEF/DES:* In distal esophagus instead of normal stratified squamous epithelium abnormal metaplastic columnar epithelium containing goblet cells is produced. *ETIO:* Due to reflux esophagitis of long duration. *COMPLI:* Development of adenocarcinoma.

24. What is the commonest esophageal neoplasm?

Ans. Carcinoma. *DEF/DES:* Malignant neoplasms of the esophageal mucosa. Squamous cell carcinoma is the commonest. Adenocarcinoma develops in Barrett's esophagus. Risk factors for squamous cell carcinoma are chronic esophagitis, **Plummer-Vinson or Kelly-Peterson syndrome (esophageal web, microcytic hypochromic anemia, atrophic glossitis)**, alcohol and tobacco, deficiency of vitamin A, C, B (1, 2, 6), food contaminated by fungus. Also there is geographic prevalence in region of Asia extending from Northern China to Northern Iran. *C/Fs:* Slowly developing dysphagia more for solids than liquids.

Diseases of the Stomach

25. What is gastritis?

Ans. *DEF:* Inflammation of the gastric mucosa.

26. What are the types of gastritis?

Ans. 1. Acute gastritis.
2. Chronic gastritis.

27. What is acute gastritis?

Ans. *DEF/DES:* Temporary acute mucosal inflammation generally due to **(HUG IS ANS²)** NSAIDs, **A**lcohol, **S**moking, **U**remia, **S**evere stress, **S**hock, **G**astric intubation, *H. pylori* infection where patient may be asymptomatic or have nausea, vomiting, epigastric pain, and may develop hematemesis, melena, severe hemorrhage with death.

28. What is chronic gastritis?

Ans. *DEF/DES:* Chronic gastric mucosal inflammation which progresses to mucosal atrophy and intestinal metaplasia.

ETIO/PATHOG: **(HA^{2}DS)**

1. ***H**elicobacter pylori.*
2. **A**utoimmune destruction of parietal cells which leads to pernicious anemia, hypochlorhydria and achlorhydria.

   COMPLI: Peptic ulcer, **gastric cancer**. *H. pylori* infection predisposes to development of **MALToma**.
3. **A**lcohol.
4. **D**uodenogastric reflux.
5. **S**moking.

29. What are acute gastric ulcers?

Ans. Acute gastric ulceration (stress ulcers). *DEF/DES:* Ulcers due to severe stress such as extensive burn **(Curling's ulcer)**, CNS injury **(Cushing's ulcer)**, severe trauma, or NSAID/steroids. *MORPHO:* Small with normal adjacent mucosa, without any gastritis.

30. What are chronic peptic ulcers?

Ans. *DEF/DES:* Ulcers in any part of the GIT exposed to increased acid-peptic juices. *PATHOG:* Decreased defenses due to ischemia, delayed gastric emptying, duodenal gastric reflux and aggravating factors consisting of *H. pylori* infection, NSAID, alcohol, cigarettes, steroids, COPD, hypercalcemia. *GROSS:* 1 to 4 cm, punched out with straight margins without any irregularity of edges (unlike cancer) commonly seen in the first part of duodenum or the lesser curvature of the stomach. *MICRO*: Ulcers extend into submucosa, muscularis propria and sometimes, even deeper, and have 4 zones: **DIGS**

1. Necrotic tissue (**D**ebris) at base
2. **I**nflammatory tissue
3. **G**ranulation tissue
4. **S**car.

S/S: Epigastric pain, 1–3 hours after meals, worse at night, relieved with alkali or food ingestion. *COMPLI:* **H**emorrhage, **P**erforation, **O**bstruction, **C**ancer (rare). **HOP not CHOP** as cancer is rare.

31. What are neoplasms of the stomach?

Ans. 1. Benign (polyps).
2. Malignant.

32. What are the polyps of the stomach?

Ans. *DEF/DES:* Mass due to proliferation of the mucosa with protrusion.

Types:

1. Hyperplastic.
2. Fundic gland, both harmless.
3. Adenomatous: Risk of cancer development.

ETIO/PATHOG: Chronic gastritis is the precursor.

MORPH: HISTO:

1. *Hyperplastic:* Not true neoplasms but reparative response to chronic mucosal damage. Made of hyperplastic epithelium.
2. *Fundic gland polyp:* Collection of dilated glands, possibly hamartoma.
3. Adenomatous polyps are true adenomas.

33. What are the malignant neoplasms of the stomach?

Ans. a. Adenocarcinoma.

b. Lymphomas.

c. Carcinoids.

d. Mesenchymal.

34. What is the adenocarcinoma of the stomach?

Ans. These are of 2 types:

1. Intestinal. 2. Diffuse

Intestinal type: PATHOG: Arises in intestinal metaplastic epithelium.

Risk factors: H. pylori infection, pernicious anemia, nitrites, smoked foods.

Diffuse: Arises in normal epithelium. Risk factors unknown.

C/Fs: Could be asymptomatic. May have abdominal discomfort, dysphagia when in cardia, obstruction when in pylorus. Depth of invasion determines the outcome. Peculiar spread to supraclavicular lymph node **(Virchow's node)** and to both ovaries **(Krukenberg tumor)**. *MORPHO*: Location: Cardia—1/4; Body, fundus—1/4, Pylorus, antrum 1/2. Gastric carcinoma is classified on the basis of:

1. Depth of invasion.
2. Macroscopic growth type.
3. Histologic type.

1. *Depth of invasion:* Early confined to mucosa and submucosa. Advanced deeper than submucosa into muscular wall.
2. *Macroscopic growth types:*
   a. Exophytic.
   b. Flat or depressed.
   c. Excavated (linitis plastica).
3. *Histologic type:*
   a. Intestinal type (neoplasm appears like adenocarcinoma of colon, with presence of neoplastic cells in gland formation).
   b. Signet ring type (neoplasm consists of single cells which appears as signet-ring which infiltrate the mucosa and wall of the stomach).

Diseases of the Intestine and Anal Canal

35. What are some of the developmental anomalies of the small intestine?

Ans. 1. Atresia or stenosis.

2. Meckel's diverticulum.

36. What is atresia or stenosis of the small intestine?

Ans. Involves only a segment of bowel. Complete failure of development of intestinal lumen is atresia. Only narrowing is **stenosis**.

37. What is Meckel's diverticulum?

Ans. It is a blind-ended protrusion which is present in 2% of the population, located on ileum within 2 feet from the cecum and is 2 inches long. *C/Fs:* Generally asymptomatic. Symptoms when:

a. Bacterial overgrowth uses up vitamin B_{12} causing megaloblastic anemia.

b. Heterotopic gastric mucosa causing peptic ulceration, bleeding and pain **mimicking acute appendicitis**.

c. Perforation secondary to peptic ulceration.

d. Volvulus, especially when it is attached to the umbilicus by the obliterated omphalomesenteric duct.

e. Intussusception due to inversion of the diverticulum.

38. What are the common developmental anomalies of the large intestine?

Ans. 1. Malrotation.

2. Congenital megacolon (Hirschprung disease).

39. What is malrotation of large intestine?

Ans. Intestines not in their normal positions, e.g. cecum may be in any location in abdomen, such as left upper quadrant and if a person has acute appendicitis causing pain in left upper quadrant could be quite confusing to make the correct diagnosis.

40. What is Hirschprung disease (congenital megacolon)?

Ans. Megacolon can be congenital or acquired. *In Congenital megacolon* parasympathetic ganglion cells of the submucosal Meissner's and muscular Auerbach's plexuses are absent in a segment of colon causing functional obstruction at this segment resulting in **distention of the bowel proximal to it**. *S/S*: Initial passage of meconium is delayed followed by vomiting in 48–72 hours. Complications are enterocolitis, perforation. *DIAG*: Demonstration of absence of ganglion cells **in non-distended segment**. *Acquired megacolon* may occur from **Chaga's disease** , where trypanosomas invade the colon wall and destroy the plexuses. Also, seen in **ulcerative colitis**.

41. What are the common vascular diseases of the intestine?

Ans. 1. Ischemic bowel diseases 2. Hemorrhoids.

42. What is ischemic bowel disease?

Ans. *ETIO:*

1. Arterial thrombosis of one of the three major arteries:
   a. Celiac.
   b. Superior mesenteric.
   c. Inferior mesenteric
2. Arterial embolism.
3. Venous thrombosis.
4. *Nonocclusive ischemia:* CHF, dehydration, shock.
5. *Miscellaneous:* Radiation injury, volvulus, stricture, internal or external herniation.

C/Fs:

a. *Transmural:* Sudden onset of pain, sometimes with bloody diarrhea. **Within a few hours can cause shock, vascular collapse, gangrene, and/or perforation**. Therefore, high index of suspicion and prompt diagnosis is necessary.

b. *Mural and mucosal:* Gradual onset of abd. pain, discomfort, distension, GI bleeding. If cause of hypoperfusion corrected, heals.

43. What are hemorrhoids?

Ans. Varices of anal and perianal submucosal venous plexuses. Due to elevated venous pressure.

Causes:

1. Straining at stool due to constipation.
2. Venous stasis of pregnancy.
3. Portal hypertension due to cirrhosis of liver.
4. Pressure due to tumors.

Types:

1. Internal.
2. External.

1. *Internal:* Vericosities in the superior and middle hemorrhoidal veins appear above the anorectal line and are covered by rectal mucosa. May prolapse during straining at stool, get trapped by anal sphincter and get strangulated. May also get thrombosed.
2. *External:* Vericosities in the inferior hemorrhoidal veins and are covered by anal mucosa.

Both are thin-walled, dilated vessels that commonly bleed. **Sometimes, these can mask the bleeding from more serious conditions such as a cancer.**

44. What is gastroenteritis?

Ans: *DEF:* It is acute gastrointestinal infection presenting with diarrhea (loose watery stools with increased amount and frequency) or dysentery (low-volume bloody stools with abdominal pain) and sometimes, with vomiting.

ETIO:

1. Viruses (commonly in children).
2. Bacteria (commonly in adults).
3. Protozoa.
4. Helminths.

PATHOG:

1. Mucosal adherence causing **diarrhea**, e.g. enteropathogenic *E. coli* (EPEC), *Giardia lamblia*.
2. Mucosal invasion causing **dysentery**, e.g. Shigella spp., Campylobacter spp., enteroinvasive *E. coli* (EIEC), *Entamoeba histolytica*.
3. Toxin production:
   a. Enterotoxin causing severe watery **diarrhea**, e.g. *Vibrio cholera*, Salmonella spp., Campylobacter spp., enterotoxigenic *E. coli* (ETEC), *Staphylococcus aureus*, *Clostridium perfringens*.
   b. Cytoxin causing **dysentery**, e.g. Salmonella spp., Campylobacter spp., enterohemorrhagic *E. coli* (EHEC).

45. What is dysentery? What are some of its causes?

Ans. *DEF:* Dysentery is defined as low-volume bloody stools with abdominal pain.

ETIO: E. coli (EIEC, EHEC), *S. typhi*, Shigella, Campylobacter, *Claustridium difficille*, *Yersinia pseudotuberculosis*, *Mycobacterium tuberculosis*, *Entamoeba histolytica*. *Some detailed description of some of these is as follows:*

Salmonella: By *S. typhi*. Spread by fecal-oral route. *S. typhi* invades small intestinal lymphoid tissue, multiplies there and enters the bloodstream causing systemic infection (typhoid fever). *First week*, there is bacteremia. *Second week*, there is reticuloendothelial system involvement with splenomegaly. *Third week*, there is ulceration of mucosa overlying Peyer's patches parallel to long axis of the intestine. Gallbladder colonization produces a chronic carrier state. Chronic infection may affect joints **(arthritis)**, bones **(osteomyelitis)**, meninges **(meningitis)**.

Shigella: Affects mainly the distal colon, causing acute mucosal inflammation and erosion.

Mycobacterium tuberculosis: From ingested or swallowed from the sputum bacteria, there is chronic inflammation and granuloma formation with ulceration of the epithelium in transverse axis to the intestine in the terminal ileum.

Entamoeba histolytica: It spreads by fecal-oral route. Amebas invade crypts of colonic glands and burrow into submucosa making a flask-shaped ulcer. In many cases amebas penetrate the portal veins and reach the liver causing liver abscess.

46. What is diarrhea? What are some of its causes?

Ans: *DEF:* Diarrhea is defined as loose, watery stools with increase in amount and frequency.

ETIO:

a. *Infectious causes:* Viruses (rotavirus, enteric adenovirus, noravirus), *E. coli* (EPEC, ETEC), *Vibrio cholera*, Salmonella spp., Campylobacter spp., Staphylococcus, *Clostridium perfringens* spp., *Giardia lamblia*.

b. *Non-infectious causes:* Inflammatory bowel diseases, carcinoma of the colon with change in bowel habits, malabsorption, Zollinger-Ellison syndrome, carcinoid syndrome, thyrotoxicosis.

47. What are some of the causes of malabsorption?

Ans. A. *Defective digestion*:

1. *Pancreatic insufficiency:* Mainly due to chronic pancreatitis or cystic fibrosis.
2. *Zollinger-Ellison syndrome:* Increased gastric acid inactivates pancreatic enzymes.
3. *Cirrhosis, cholestasis:* Decreased bile salts with decreased fat solubility.
4. *Lactose intolerance:* Due to inherited deficiency *of* disaccharidase, milk intolerance leading to diarrhea and malabsorption.

B. *Defective transport from the intestinal lumen to blood:*

1. *Celiac sprue (Gluten-sensitive enteropathy):* Sensitivity to the gluten-part of wheat, oat, barley, rye. Sensitized B lymphocytes and plasma cells damage the intestinal mucosal cells resulting in flattening of mucosal villi thereby decreasing the surface area resulting in diarrhea and malabsorption.
2. *Tropical sprue:* Occurs in tropics. Its cause is unknown; however, infection is suspected because it responds to treatment by tetracycline. Intestinal villi are flattened resulting in reduced absorptive surface area leading to malabsorption.
3. *Whipple's disease:* This is a systemic infection by Tropheryma whippelii mainly affecting small intestine, joints and CNS. In the lamina propria of the small intestine many macrophages containing above rod-shaped bacilli are present which can be identified by EM. This also responds to treatment by tetracycline.
4. *Abetalipoproteinemia:* This is an autosomal recessive disorder consisting of lack of formation of apoprotein necessary for transport of lipoprotein through intestinal mucosal cells.
5. Giardiasis.

48. What are some of the manifestations of malabsorption?

Ans. 1. Diarrhea, dehydration, steatorrhea, electrolyte imbalance.

2. Malnutrition resulting in anemia (iron deficiency, folic acid deficiency, vitamin B_{12} deficiency), weight loss (calorie deficiency), bleeding (vitamin K deficiency), also various manifestations of vitamin A, B, C, D deficiencies (e.g. B_1—beriberi, B_6—pellagra, C—scurvy, D—rickets/osteomalacia).

49. What are the idiopathic inflammatory bowel diseases (IIBD)?

Ans. *ETIO:* Unknown. These cause inflammation of the bowel mucosa with loss of absorptive space resulting in dysentery and malabsorption. Actually, these are not confined to GIT; but, are systemic diseases causing in many patients such as enteropathic arthritis, ankylosing spondylitis, uveitis, in liver causing cholangitis and skin lesions. These are of two types:

1. Ulcerative colitis (UC) and 2. Crohn's disease (CD). Brief further description of these consists of:

Ulcerative colitis (UC): It is **non-granulomatous** chronic inflammatory disease of the mucosa and submucosa of the colon. Usually, it begins distally in the rectum and progresses continuously up to cecum.

GROSS: Mucosa is edematous, hyperemic with ulcers which may extend to muscularis propria affecting the function of the neural plexus with dilatation of the colon leading to gangrene **(toxic megacolon)**. In between inflamed areas, regenerating mucosa bulge into lumen appearing like polyps **(pseudopolyps)**. *MICRO:* Mononuclear and neutrophilic infiltration of the mucosa is present. Neutrophil collection can cause crypt abscesses. Inflammation can progress to ulceration which extend only up to submucosa. During remission the ulcers heal by formation of granulation tissue and regeneration of epithelium. *COMPLI:* Development of **adenocarcinoma** of the colon.

Crohn's disease: It is a **granulomatous** chronic inflammatory disease of the GIT, which can affect any part of the GIT from esophagus to anus; but, usually it involves the colon and small intestine, mainly the terminal ileum. *GROSS:* There is full-thickness involvement of the wall of the intestine. Normal **skip areas** are present in between inflamed areas. *MICRO:* Inflammation involves the full thickness of the intestinal wall. In approximately 1/2 the cases non-caseating granulomas are present. Fissures and fistulas are seen, mucosa is ulcerated, mucosal cells may show gastric metaplasia, dysplasia, which might eventually progress to neoplasia **(adenocarcinoma)**, mainly in the colon. Differences of *CD* and *UC* are: In *CD* the presence of:

1. "Skip areas".
2. Granulomas.
3. Full-thickness involvement.
4. Fissures and fistula; whereas in *UC* these are absent. Also, the risk of development of cancer in *CD* is less than *UC*.

50. What is colonic diverticulosis?

Ans. A diverticulum is a blind pouch from the GIT. Increased intraluminal pressure predisposes. Almost all are in sigmoid colon.

COMPLI: a. Diverticulitis.

b. Bleeding.

c. Perforation.

d. Abscess formation.
e. Fistula formation.

51. What are the causes of bowel obstruction?

Ans. *Causes:*

1. *Mechanical:*
   a. Hernias.
   b. Adhesions.
   c. Intussusception.
   d. Volvulus.
   e. Tumors.
   f. Strictures.
2. *Non-mechanical:*
   a. Paralytic ileus.
   b. Myo-neuropathies, e.g. Hirschprung disease.

52. What are the potentially neoplastic and neoplastic lesions of the small and large intestine?

Ans. 1. Potentially neoplastic:
   A. Hyperplastic polyps.
   B. Hamartomatous polyps.
2. Neoplastic epithelial lesions:
   A. Adenoma.
   B. Familial polyposis syndromes.
      a. Familial adenomatous polyposis (FAP).
      b. Gardner's syndrome.
      c. Adenocarcinoma.
      d. Carcinoid.
      e. Anal zone carcinoma.
3. Neoplastic mesenchymal lesions.
   A. *Benign:*
      a. Lipoma.
      b. Leiomyoma.
      c. Angioma.
   B. *Malignant:*
      a. Liposarcoma.
      b. Leiomyosarcoma.
      c. Kaposi's sarcoma.
      d. Lymphoma.

53. What are the hyperplastic polyps of the intestine?

Ans. Small, mucosal protrusions mostly in rectosigmoid area. *MICRO:* Crypts lined by well-differentiated goblet or absorptive epithelial cells. No malignant potential in most of the cases; however, a few might develop into adenocarcinoma of the colon.

54. What are the hamartomatous polyps?

Ans. a. Juvenile polyps b. Peutz-Jeghers polyps.

55. What are the Juvenile polyps of the intestine?

Ans. Usually, in children<5 years of age. *GROSS*: Small, round pedunculated. *MICRO*: Hamartomatous proliferation, mainly of lamina propria with dilated cystic glands. No malignant potential.

56. What is Peutz-Jeghers syndrome?

Ans. Hamartomatous polyps occur as part of rare autosomal dominant **Peutz-Jeghers syndrome. Has increased risk of both intestinal and extraintestinal malignancies.** Melanotic mucosal and cutaneous pigmentation.

57. What is adenoma of the intestine?

Ans. Mainly in colon. Has familial predisposition. Strong malignant potential. Sessile to pedunculated. *MICRO:* Three subtypes:

1. Tubular adenomas—with glands mostly tubular.
2. Villous adenomas—with mostly villous projections.
3. Tubulovillous adenomas—mixture of above two. **Size of the above is the main risk factor for these to have adenocarcinoma.**

58. What is the familial adenomatous polyposis (FAP) syndrome?

Ans. Multiple adenomas are present in colon and in other parts of GIT. All patients will develop colonic cancer by approximately 40 years of age. **Therefore, prophylactic colectomy is recommended.**

59. What is the Gardner's syndrome?

Ans. Adenoma of colon and extraintestinal tumors, e.g. osteomas, gliomas, soft tissue tumors, etc.

60. What is the adenocarcinoma of the large intestine?

Ans. Almost all cancers of large intestine are adenocarcinoma.

PATHOG:

1. Adenoma-carcinoma sequence due to loss of tumor suppressor genes (APC and TP53) and mutation of oncogene (K-RAS). Knudson's hypothesis of "Two Hits"=

Loss of one allele of APC, inherited or acquired, (first hit), followed by loss of second, (second hit).

2. *Hereditary non-polyposis colon cancer (HNPCC):* Due to loss of DNA mismatch repair gene, e.g. MSH2.

GROSS: In proximal colon (~30%): Polypoid, fungating mass. In distal colon (~60%): Circular lesions producing narrowing. *MICRO:* All above microscopically similar. Well differentiated to undifferentiated anaplastic. Many secrete mucin, which dissects through gut wall, facilitating extension, thereby worsening prognosis. *C/Fs:* Initially asymptomatic, lesions in proximal colon usually present as anemia; distal as change in bowel habits. In West, all old people with anemia should be suspected to have carcinoma of the GIT. Carcinoembryonic antigen **(CEA)** is elevated, it is non-specific, so not useful for diagnosis, but is useful for follow-up.

Staging:

A. Limited to mucosa. Survival 100%.
B1. Extending into m. propria, but not penetrating it. Survival 70%.
B2. Penetrating through m. propria. Survival 50%.
C1. B1 + Nodes involved. Survival 40%.
C2. B2 + Nodes involved. Survival 20%.
D. Distant metastases. Survival very low.

PROG: Main criterion is extent of tumor at diagnosis as above.

61. What are the carcinoids?

Ans. Tumors of cells which secrete hormones. In GIT mostly arise in small intestine. *GROSS:* Solid yellowish. *MICRO:* Islands and strands of uniform round cells with little cytoplasm and stippled nuclei. *C/Fs:* Some cause carcinoid syndrome: with flushing, diarrhea, cramps, coughing, wheezing. pulmonic, tricuspid valve thickening, endocardial fibrosis mainly in right side (bronchial carcinoid affects left side of the heart). 5-HT and 5HIAA (5-hydroxy tryptamine and 5-hydroxy indole acetic acid) present in blood and urine. *PROG:* Rectal and appendiceal carcinoids very rarely or never metastasize. (Also *see* chapter 10).

62. What are the anal zone carcinoma?

Ans. Usually squamous cell carcinoma.

63. What are the neoplastic mesenchymal lesions?

Ans. 1. Benign:

a. Lipoma b. Leiomyoma c. Angioma.

2. Malignant:

a. Liposarcoma b. Leiomyosarcoma.
c. Kaposi's sarcoma d. Lymphoma.

Diseases of the Appendix

64. What is acute appendicitis?

Ans. *DEF:* Acute inflammation of the appendix. *ETIO:* Exact etiology is not known. Obstruction of the lumen is seen in some cases by fecalith, gallstone, tumor or ball of worms, (*oxyuriasis vermicularis*). Ischemia and edema predispose to bacterial growth. *Stages:*

1. *Early acute appendicitis:* Consisting of small amount of polymorphonuclear inflammatory cell infiltrate. Subserosal vessels are congested. The serosa looks dull in color.
2. *Acute suppurative appendicitis:* With progression of inflammation the mucosa develops focal necrosis. Also increased neutrophilic infiltrate involving all the layers of the appendix with focal necrosis and abscess formation. The serosa develops fibrinopurulent exudates.
3. *Acute gangrenous appendicitis:* Further progression causes hemorrhagic ulceration of the mucosa. Gangrenous necrosis with greenish-blackish discoloration involves the full thickness of the appendix wall including the serosa. *C/Fs:* Acute onset with mild fever, mild periumbilical discomfort followed by anorexia, nausea, vomiting, followed by right lower quadrant pain with tenderness usually at the McBurney's point. Test shows increased white cell count with neutrophilia. If not promptly diagnosed and surgically removed the appendix ruptures and has an approximate mortality of 2%. *D/D:* Viral mesenteric lymphadenitis, Meckel diverticulitis. In females: **Mittelschmerz (ovulation)**, ectopic pregnancy.

65. What are the tumors of the appendix?

Ans.
1. Carcinoid.
2. Mucinous cyst adenoma.
3. Mucinous cyst adenocarcinoma.

66. What is the carcinoid of the appendix?

Ans. Commonest neoplasm of appendix. Metastasize rarely. Prognosis is good.

67. What is the mucocele of the appendix?

Ans. *DEF/DES:* Dilation of appendix due to filling of its lumen by its mucinous secretion. *ETIO:* Usually due to obstruction of the lumen due to fecalith. *C/Fs:* Usually asymptomatic because of spontaneous stoppage of mucous secretion due to pressure atrophy of the mucus-secreting cells. Sometimes, the mucocele ruptures with spread of mucin in the peritoneal cavity.

68. What is mucinous cyst adenoma of the appendix?

Ans. Benign tumor made of cystic glands lined by benign columnar mucin-secreting cells.

69. What is mucinous cyst adenocarcinoma of the appendix?

Ans. Tumor made of cystic glands lined by mucin-secreting cells with anaplastic features. It invades the appendix wall resulting in generalized peritoneal involvement with cancer **(pseudomyxoma peritonei)**.

Diseases of the Liver

70. What are the liver function tests?

Ans. a. *Functions of hepatocyte integrity:*

1. AST.
2. ALT.
3. LDH.

b. *Biliary functions-serum bilirubin:* Total (unconjugated and conjugated), direct (conjugated only). Urine bilirubin. Serum bile acids, plasma membrane enzymes (from damage to bile canaliculus): Serum gamma glutamyl transpeptidase, serum alkaline phosphatase.

c. *Hepatocyte function:*

1. Serum albumin.
2. Prothrombin time: Factors V, VII, X, fibrinogen, prothrombin.
3. Serum ammonia.

71. What is jaundice? What is icterus?

Ans. *DEF:* Jaundice is yellow color of skin and icterus is yellow color of sclera due to elevated serum bilirubin at 2 to 2.5 mg/dl (normal is approximately half of this). Increased serum carotene also makes skin color yellow but not of sclera.

72. What are the pathophysiologic types of jaundice?

Ans. These are of 2 types as follows:

1. Unconjugated hyperbilirubinemia.
   a. Due to increased bilirubin production, e.g. hemolysis.
   b. Due to decreased hepatic cellular uptake, e.g. Gilbert's disease.
   c. Due to decreased conjugation, e.g. Crigler-Najjar syndrome.
2. *Conjugated hyperbilirubinemia:* Due to interference with secretion of bilirubin into bile canaliculi or excretion through intra/extrahepatic biliary passages. Seen in:
   a. Alcoholic hepatitis.
   b. Hepatotropic viral hepatitis.
   c. Other infectious hepatitis, e.g. infectious mononucleosis, CMV, yellow fever, herpes, etc.
   d. Cirrhosis.

e. Drugs, e.g. acetaminophen, isoniazid, nitrofurantoin, methyl dopa.
f. Dubin-Johnson syndrome.
g. Rotor syndrome.
h. Hepatic neoplasms—primary and secondary.
i. Common bile duct stones.
j. Biliary stricture.
k. Pancreatic pseudocyst.
l. Neoplasms of head of pancreas and bile duct.

73. What is the *D/D* of jaundice?

Ans. *Hemolytic:* Hyperbilirubinemia—unconjugated. Urine bilirubin—absent. Urobilinogen—increased. Other findings—degree of urobilinogen increase directly related to increased hemoglobin catabolism.

Hepatocellular: Hyperbilirubinemia—conjugated + unconjugated. Urine bilirubin—increased; urobilinogen—normal to decreased. Other findings-intrahepatic cholestasis may result in retention of conjugated bilirubin; hepatocellular damage may result in impaired conjugation of bilirubin; ALT and AST increased; increased alkaline phosphatase indicates intrahepatic obstruction, viral markers for HAV, HBV, HCV.

Obstructive: Hyperbilirubinemia—conjugated; urine bilirubin—increased; urobilinogen—decreased; other findings—alkaline phosphatase and cholesterol increased.

74. What is hepatic failure?

Ans. It is the most severe consequence of liver disease. It indicates loss of 90% of liver function. Three types:

1. *Massive hepatic necrosis:* Due to:
   a. Fulminant viral hepatitis.
   b. Drugs and chemicals, e.g. acetaminophen, halothane, anti-TB drugs (rifampin, isoniazid), CCl_4, mushroom poisoning (*Amanita phalloides*).
2. *Chronic liver disease:* Most common end-point of cirrhosis.
3. *Without overt necrosis:* Hepatocytes may be viable but unable to perform normal metabolic function, e.g. Reye's syndrome; tetracycline toxicity; and acute fatty liver of pregnancy.

C/Fs:

1. Jaundice.
2. Hypoalbuminemia.
3. Hyperammonemia—Due to defective hepatic urea cycle function.
4. *Fetor hepaticus:* "Musty", "sweet-sour" odor due to formation of mercaptans by GIT bacteria.
5. *Palmer erythema and spider angioma* (due to local vasodilation): Due to impaired estrogen metabolism.

6. Male hypogonadism + gynecomastia due to impaired estrogen metabolism.
7. *Coagulopathy:* Due to lack of clotting factors I, II, VII, IX, X.
8. *Hepatic encephalopathy:* CNS symptoms:
   a. Subtle behavioral abnormalities—marked confusion-stupor-coma-death.
   b. Signs: Rigidity, hyperreflexia, asterixis. *Pathophysiology:* Elevated blood ammonia impairing neuronal function and causing generalized brain edema.
9. *Hepatorenal syndrome:* Renal failure in patients with liver disease without any intrinsic renal cause. Renal failure reverses if liver failure reverses. *Cause:* Exact cause unknown. *Manifestations:* Drop in urine output, increase in BUN and creatinine. Ability to concentrate urine is retained. Urine is hyperosmolar, is devoid of protein and is low in sodium.
10. Cholestasis: Jaundice, pruritus, hypercholesterolemia with xanthomas.

75. What is cirrhosis?

Ans. End stage of liver disease.

Three characteristics:

1. Scarring with replacement of normal liver architecture with fibrosis forming fibrous septae.
2. Parenchymal nodules formed by regeneration of encircled hepatocytes (<3 mm = micronodular cirrhosis; >3 mm = macronodular cirrhosis).
3. Entire liver architecture is disrupted.

ETIO:

1. Alcoholic liver disease 3/4 cases.
2. Viral hepatitis 1/10 cases.
3. Biliary diseases.
4. Genetic hemochromatosis.
5. Wilson's disease and miscellaneous, e.g. schistosomiasis.
6. Alpha-1 antitrypsin deficiency.

C/Fs: Anorexia, weight loss, weakness, jaundice, portal hypertension with all its *S/S* (see below), hepatic failure with all its manifestations (see above). *Causes of death:*

1. Liver failure.
2. Portal hypertension complications.
3. Hepatocellular carcinoma (in macronodular).

76. What is portal hypertension?

Ans. *DEF:* Increased pressure in portal circulation.

ETIO/CLASSI:

1. *Prehepatic:* Thrombosis of portal vein.
2. *Hepatic:* Cirrhosis.
3. *Posthepatic:* Right heart failure, constrictive pericarditis hepatic vein thrombosis **(Budd-Chiari syndrome)**.

Consequences:

1. *Ascites:* Due to:
   a. Increased portal capillary pressure.
   b. Decreased colloid osmotic pressure (due to low albumin).
   c. Low functional volume causing increase in aldosterone and Na with water retention.
2. *Porto-systemic venous shunt:* Esophageal varices (lower end of esophagus); (these are esophageal tributaries of the azygos vein (systemic vein) which connect with portal vein); caput-medusae around umbilicus; hemorrhoids.
3. Congestive splenomegaly.
4. Hepatic encephalopathy.

77. What are some of the causes of hepatomegaly?

Ans. 1. *Inflammatory:* Hepatitis, tuberculosis, sarcoidosis, early stage of cirrhosis.

2. *Congestive:* Right-sided heart failure, **Budd-Chiari syndrome**.
3. *Infiltrative:* Amyloidosis, fatty liver, hemochromatosis, extramedullary hematopoiesis, glycogen storage disease.
4. *Neoplastic:* Lymphoma, leukemia, adenoma, hepatocellular carcinoma, metastatic neoplasms.

78. What are the inflammatory disorders of the liver?

Ans. 1. Infectious.

2. Non-infectious.

1. Infectious:
   A. *Viral:*
      a. Hepatotropic viruses (A, B, C, D, E).
      b. Non-hepatotropic viruses: EBV, CMV, herpes simplex, yellow fever.
   B. *Bacterial:* Syphilis (secondary and tertiary stages), *E. coli*, *Staphylococcus aureus*, Borrelia, *Leptospira icterohaemorrhagica*, etc.
   C. *Protozoal:* Amebic, *Pneumocystis carinii* (in AIDs), *Toxoplasma gondii*.
   D. *Helminthic: Schistosoma mansoni* and *japonicum* (not hematobium), *Echinococcus granulosus*.
2. Non-infectious.
   A. Alcohol
   B. Hypothyroidism.
   C. Cholelithiasis
   D. Drugs.
   E. Autoimmune.

79. What is viral hepatitis?

Ans. Five types according to the viruses:

a. Hepatitis A (infectious hepatitis).
b. Hepatitis B (serum hepatitis).
c. Hepatitis C.
d. Hepatitis D (delta hepatitis).
e. Hepatitis E.

Hepatitis A (Infectious Hepatitis)

DEF: Hepatitis caused by virus, is infectious and transmitted via fecal oral route *ETIO:* RNA, entero virus, *C/Fs:* Incubation period 2–6 weeks. Worldwide distribution. Poor hygienic condition favor it. Epidemics can occur. Mild disease with spontaneous recovery in a few weeks. No chronic hepatitis, no carrier state. Rarely fatal. In early stage IgM antibodies followed by IgG antibodies.

Hepatitis B (Serum Hepatitis)

DEF: Hepatitis caused by a virus, transmitted by exposure to body fluids (serum, blood, blood products by IV routes, drug abusers with contaminated needles, semen, renal dialysis). *ETIO:* DNA virus called Dane particle. Core of the virus causes infection, not the surface envelope or surface antigen (HbsAg) *C/Fs:* Incubation period 6 weeks to 6 months. Causes chronic disease, carrier state, and even death. During acute stage HbsAg appears followed by HbeAg. Both disappear when recovery begins. Anti-HBc appear during acute illness, then anti-Hbe and anti-HBs appear. Presence of HbeAg and hepatitis B-DNA means person is infective. Presence of anti-Hbe means Dane particle is absent and person is not infective. Hepatocytes have a ground glass appearance. In summary, anti-HBc in serum is early indication of infection; HBeAg indicates high degree of infectivity, HBsAg indicates active infection; Anti-HBe indicates resolution of infection. Anti-HBs indicates recovery and immunity.

Hepatitis C

DEF: Hepatitis caused by virus, which was in the past called non-A, non-B and is transmitted by IV route. *C/Fs:* Incubation period 2 weeks to 6 months. *C/Fs* similar to hepatitis B.

80. What is hepatitis D (delta hepatitis)?

Ans. *DEF:* Hepatitis by an RNA virus, which has the envelope of hepatitis B, but core of delta antigen. It cannot cause hepatitis by itself without the help of hepatitis B virus. *C/Fs:* Transmission by IV route. Delta hepatitis happens in 2 ways:

1. Coinfection by exposure to serum with both HBV and HDV where patients recover completely and only rarely develop chronic hepatitis.
2. Super infection of a chronic carrier of HBV with new exposure to HDV where in majority of patients there is acceleration of hepatitis to severe chronic hepatitis. Diagnosis is made by finding delta antigen in blood or liver cells.

81. What is hepatitis E?

Ans. Hepatitis E virus is an RNA virus which is endemic in India which causes an enterically transmitted water-borne infection which is self-limited without chronic liver disease.

82. What are the clinical syndromes after exposure to hepatitis virus?

Ans. 1. Carrier state without apparent disease.

2. *Acute viral hepatitis:* Diffuse hepatic swelling, focal or centrizonal necrosis, plasma cell and lymphocytic infiltrate in the portal tracts. *C/Fs:* Sudden onset of fever, loss of appetite, vomiting, jaundice and tender hepatomegaly. Jaundice is hepatocellular and cholestatic. Urine has bile and increased urobilinogen. Liver enzymes are elevated. Recovery in 2–3 weeks.
3. *Fulminant viral hepatitis:* Acute liver failure with massive or submassive liver cell necrosis. Seen in 1% cases of hepatitis B and C. Mortality rate is very high. Survivors recover completely with normal regeneration of liver when the liver framework is intact. Regeneration is nodular when liver framework is not intact.
4. *Chronic active viral hepatitis:* Caused by hepatitis B, C and delta agent. *C/Fs:* Chronic illness with severe elevation of liver enzymes. May develop portal hypertension. Progresses to cirrhosis and liver failure with bad prognosis. Histologically focal necrosis of hepatocytes, portal tracts have fibrosis and chronic inflammation extending into liver lobule with piecemeal necrosis of liver cells.
5. *Chronic persistent hepatitis:* Common condition due to hepatitis B and C. *C/Fs:* Symptoms mild, liver function tests are mildy elevated, lasting 6 months. Benign self-limited, may last years, but does not progress to cirrhosis. It is a chronic carrier state patient being infective. *MICRO:* Increased plasma cells and lymphocytes are present in portal tract. Limiting plate of hepatocytes is intact and there is no hepatocytic necrosis.

83. What is hepatic amebiasis?

Ans. Due to entry of amebic trophozoites into portal venous radicals in the colonic submucosa. Usually in patients with chronic intestinal amebiasis. In the liver amebas cause focal enzymatic necrosis forming many micro abscesses which fuse to form large abscesses. *C/Fs:* High fever, RUQ pain, tender hepatomegaly. Diagnosis is by chest X-ray, US, CT scan. *COMPLI:* High mortality rate without treatment. Death due to rupture into peritoneal cavity, pleural cavity, lung, pericardial sac, systemic spread into brain. *GROSS:* Abscess lined by irregular wall with reddish brown pus **(anchovy sauce)**.

84. What is hydatid disease?

Ans. It is caused by tapeworm *Echinococcus granulosis*, which infects sheep, cattle, pigs. When dogs eat their tissue adult worms develop in dogs' GIT from where ova are excreted which are ingested by animals and men in whose GIT embryos are liberated and via portal vein reach liver or via systemic vein reach brain, spleen, kidneys and muscles where they form multilocular cysts.

85. What is hepatic *Leptospira icterohaemorrhagiae* infection?

Ans. *Leptospira icterohemorrhagiae* is a spirochaete whose reservoir is rat and it is present in the rat excreta and via skin abrasion infect people who work in sewers. It causes focal necrosis and inflammation in the liver manifesting as fever, jaundice. It also causes hemorrhage into lungs, kidneys which may be severe and cause death.

86. What is schistosomal disease of the liver?

Ans. *S. mansoni* (Egypt and Africa) and *S. japonicum* (Japan, China, Philippines) infect liver. These colonise intestine and via portal blood reach liver causing granulomatous inflammation, which may progress to portal fibrosis, cirrhosis and portal hypertension.

87. What is clonorchiasis?

Ans. It is infection by Chinese fish fluke due to eating under-cooked fish, which causes ascending cholangitis which may develop into cholangio carcinoma.

88. What are hepatic injuries from drugs and toxins?

Ans.
1. *Fatty change:* Ethanol, tetracycline, salicylates.
2. *Centrilobular necrosis:* Acetaminophen, halothane, carbon tetrachloride, rifampin.
3. *Diffuse necrosis:* Acetaminophen, halothane, isoniazid.
4. *Hepatitis and cirrhosis:* Ethanol, isoniazid, nitrofurantoin, phenytoin
5. *Cholestasis:* Oral contraceptives, erythromycin estolate, chlorpromazine, anabolic steroids.
6. *Hepatic or portal vein thrombosis:* Oral contraceptives.
7. *Adenoma:* Oral contraceptives.
8. *Hepatocellular carcinoma:* Thorotrast, vinyl chloride.
9. *Cholagiosarcoma:* Thorotrast.

89. What is alcoholic liver disease?

Ans. Three types:
1. Fatty liver (hepatic steatosis).
2. Alcoholic hepatitis.
3. Alcoholic cirrhosis.

1. *Fatty liver: C/Fs:* Reversible, if alcohol intake is stopped. *MORPHO: GROSS:* The liver is large, soft, yellow, greasy. *MICRO:* In early stage small lipid droplets (microvesicular) collect within the hepatocytes. Later, increased collection of lipids in hepatocytes makes these droplets larger, which push the nucleus to the periphery (macrovesicular). If alcohol intake continues, irreversible fibrosis develops around the central veins extending into adjacent sinusoids.
2. *Alcoholic hepatitis: C/Fs:* Usually acute after a bout of heavy drinking. If patient does not die after a few bouts of hepatitis within a few years cirrhosis develops.

MORPHO:

a. *Hepatocyte swelling and necrosis:* **(ballooning)** due to collection of water and fat.

b. *Mallory's bodies:* Pinkish intracytoplasmic bodies made of intermediate cytokeratin filaments.

c. *Neutrophilic reaction:* Neutrophils seen around degenerating hepatocytes containing **Mallory's bodies**.

d. *Fibrosis:* Fibrosis is seen in sinusoids, around central veins and portal tracts.

3. *Alcoholic cirrhosis:* This is the last irreversible phase of alcoholic liver disease. *C/Fs:* These are related to portal hypertension which occurs with cirrhosis consisting of distended abdomen with ascites, caput medusae, bleeding varicose veins, hepatic encephalopathy. *PROG:* Poor. Patients who continue to drink die of liver failure, severe GIT hemorrhage, hepatocellular carcinoma.

90. What is hemochromatosis?

Ans. *DEF:* Excessive iron accumulation commonly in liver and pancreas.

Types:

1. Congenital 2. Acquired.

1. *Congenital:* Autosomal recessive. Homozygotes suffer from the disease. *PATHOG:* Increased iron absorption from the GIT. When iron accumulates to approximately 20 gm of storage iron in several years disease manifests itself with hepatomegaly, abdominal pain, pigmentation of the skin, diabetes due to injury to the islets of Langerhans, cardiomyopathy with arrhythmia, arthritis. *PROG:* With early treatment good. *MORPHO:* Hemosiderin deposition is seen in liver, pancreas, myocardium, pituitary, adrenal, thyroid, parathyroid glands, joints, skin (with bronze color); cirrhosis, pancreatic fibrosis with diabetes **(bronzed diabetes)**.

2. *Acquired:* Due to:

a. *Increased oral iron intake:* **Bantu siderosis**.

b. *Due to increased parenteral iron:* Transfusions for sickle cell disease, leukemias, aplastic anemia.

c. *Ineffective erythropoiesis:* Beta thalassemia, sideroblastic anemia.

91. What is Wilson's disease (hepatolenticular degeneration)?

Ans. *DEF:* Autosomal recessive disorder of copper metabolism with increased collection of copper in the body with injury, mainly, to liver, brain and eyes. *C/Fs:* Liver disease, Parkinson's-like disease, psychosis, **Keyser-Fleischer ring** around the cornea due to copper deposition. *DIAG*: Serum ceruloplasmin is decreased, urinary copper is increased.

92. What is alpha 1-antitrypsin deficiency?

Ans. *DEF:* Autosomal recessive disorder with diminished serum protease inhibitor, with increased activity of proteases with destruction of pulmonary alveoli and development of emphysema. Due to deficiency of alpha-1 antitrypsin, liver cannot make the normal antitrypsin but makes a mutant protein which collects in the liver where it is seen as PAS (periodic acid-Schiff) positive pinkish round intracytoplasmic inclusion. Some patients develop cirrhosis and some hepatocellular carcinoma.

93. What is Reye's syndrome?

Ans. *DEF:* A disease of the liver with fatty change of the liver and encephalopathy. *ETIO:* Unknown. Usually seen after approximately 4 days of a viral illness in children under 4 years of age, mostly when treatment with salicylate is given. *PATHOG:* Derangement of mitochondria. *C/Fs:* Acute onset with severe vomiting, irritability or lethargy and hepatomegaly followed by liver failure, coma and death in 25% cases. *MORPHO:* Liver, heart, kidney cells have fatty change. Brain has edema. By EM astrocytes, liver, heart, kidney cells have mitochondrial enlargement.

94. What are the circulatory disorders of the liver?

Ans. a. Impaired blood flow into the liver:

1. Hepatic artery obstruction.
2. Portal vein obstruction, e.g. **Banti's syndrome**.

b. Impaired blood flow through the liver:

1. Cirrhosis.
2. Passive congestion and centrilobular necrosis.

c. Impaired blood flow out of the liver (hepatic vein outflow obstruction)

1. Hepatic vein thrombosis **(Budd-Chiari syndrome)**.
2. Veno-occlusive disease.

95. Describe some conditions with impaired blood flow into the liver.

Ans. A. Hepatic artery obstruction:

ETIO:

1. Hepatic artery thrombosis in transplanted liver.
2. Thrombosis or compression of an intrahepatic branch due to polyarteritis nodosa, embolism, neoplasia, sepsis.

B. Portal vein obstruction:

Blockage of portal vein due to thrombosis. Could be acute or gradual.

ETIO:

1. **Banti's syndrome:** Subclinical thrombosis of portal vein, e.g. from neonatal omphalitis which does not cause complete obstruction and many years later manifests with *S/S* of portal hypertension such as splenomegaly and esophageal varices.
2. Pancreatitis with splenic vein thrombosis followed by extension into portal vein.
3. Enlarged lymph nodes due to metastatic cancers.

Manifestations: Ascites, esophageal varices, splenomegaly, intestinal congestion.

96. Describe some conditions with impaired blood flow through the liver.

Ans. 1. *Cirrhosis: Manifestations:* Ascites, esophageal varices.

2. *Passive congestion and centrilobular necrosis: ETIO:* Right side heart failure. *MORPHO: GROSS:* Liver slightly enlarged. *MICRO:* Hemorrhage and necrosis of liver cells around central veins. (Area depressed and dark in color) periportal liver cells are viable. (Area slightly elevated and pale) = Gross **nutmeg** appearance. *LAB:* Mild jaundice, mild elevation of serum aminotransferase. *COMPLI:* Fibrosis. **Cardiac cirrhosis.**

97. Describe some conditions with impaired blood flow out of the liver.

Ans. A. Hepatic vein thrombosis **(Budd-Chiari syndrome)**, inferior vena cava thrombosis: *ETIO:*

1. Polycythemia vera or other myeloproliferative disorders.
2. Pregnancy and postpartum state.
3. Oral contraceptives.
4. Paroxysmal nocturnal hemoglobinuria.
5. Intra-abdominal cancers mainly HCC. (Due to stasis or hypercoagulability).
6. Idiopathic.

MORPHO: GROSS: Liver swollen, with tense capsule and red in color. *MICRO:* Severe centrilobular congestion and necrosis. *Course:* Mortality from acute Budd-Chiari syndrome is high. Prompt surgical creation of portosystemic venous shunts allows reverse flow through portal vein and improves the prognosis.

B. Veno-occlusive disease:

Originally it was seen in Jamaican people who drank bush tea. Now it is seen in people who receive bone marrow transplantation due to toxic endothelial injury of the hepatic vein radicals from chemotherapy/radiation given before the transplantation. *Course:* Incidence in approximately 1/3 cases out of which approximately 1/3 die. *Manifestation:* Ascites, hepatomegaly, abdominal pain, elevated transaminases, jaundice.

98. What are the neoplasms of the liver?

Ans. 1. *Benign:* Liver cell adenoma.

2. *Malignant—primary:*
   a. Hepatocellular carcinoma (HCC)–origin: Hepatocytes.
   b. Cholangiocarcinoma–origin: Bile ducts.
   c. Hepatoblastoma–origin: Immature hepatocytes.
   d. Angiosarcoma–origin: Endothelial cells of the blood vessels.
3. *Malignant—secondary*, e.g. from colon, breast, lung, etc.

99. What is adenoma of the liver?

Ans. Seen in women using oral contraceptives. Regresses when oral contraceptives stopped. *GROSS:* Pale nodule. Can become 30 cm in size. *MICRO:* Sheets and cords of hepatocytes which look like normal hepatocytes. Portal tracts are absent. *COMPLI:* Can rupture, particularly during pregnancy (due to stimulation by estrogen) with fatal intra-abdominal hemorrhage.

100. What is hepatocellular carcinoma (HCC)?

Ans. Etiologic associations:

1. Infection with HBV, HCV.
2. Chronic alcoholic liver disease.
3. Aflatoxins

GROSS: Unifocal or multifocal, diffuse. Strong tendency to invade vessels: Portal, hepatic vein, extending into inferior vena cava and into right heart. *MICRO:* Well-differentiated: Hepatocytes arranged in cords or small groups. Poorly differentiated: Large multinucleate anaplastic tumor giant cells. *C/Fs:* Alpha fetoprotein elevated. (Also, in several other conditions, e.g. cirrhosis, liver necrosis, chronic hepatitis, normal pregnancy, fetal distress, or death, fetal neural tube defects, gonadal germ cell tumors.) Very high levels >1000 ng/ml are usually not seen in other conditions. *PROG:* Poor. Median survival 1/2 year.

Diseases of the Gallbladder

101. What is cholelithiasis?

Ans. 4/5 of gallstones are cholesterol stones, 1/5 are pigment stones composed of bilirubin calcium salts.

Risk factors for cholesterol stones:

1. *Demography:* More incidence in Europe and North America.
2. *Age:* Advancing age.
3. *Female sex hormones:* Female gender, oral contraceptives, pregnancy.
4. Obesity.

(Forty, fat, flatulent, fertile, female).

Risk factors for pigment stones:

1. *Demography:* More incidence in Asia.
2. Chronic hemolysis.
3. Biliary infection.

C/Fs: Most patients are asymptomatic, a few have symptoms consisting of biliary pain, continuous or spasmodic. *COMPLI:* Empyema, perforation, fistulae, inflammation, obstructive cholestasis, pancreatitis. Larger the stone, less likely it can enter the ducts to cause obstruction and symptoms. Therefore, very small stones are worse.

102. What is cholecystitis?

Ans. It could be acute, chronic or acute on chronic. *Acute:* Gallbladder is enlarged. Almost all have stones with obstruction of neck of gallbladder or cystic duct. *GROSS:* In mild cases the wall is thick, edematous. In severe cases it is necrotic with gangrene. *MICRO:* Acute inflammation with neutrophilic infiltration, edema and hyperemia. *Chronic:* Size could be normal, small or large. *MICRO:* Sometimes, mucosa has ulcer. Most of the times submucosa and serosa are thick with fibrosis.

103. What is carcinoma of the gallbladder?

Ans. In West predisposing factors are stones. In the East these are pyogenic and parasitic diseases of the biliary tree. Usually, these are discovered late with poor prognosis. *GROSS:* Two patterns:

1. Exophytic.
2. Infiltrating.

MICRO: 9/10 are adenocarcinomas. 1/10 are squamous or mixed adenosquamous. *S/S:* Abdominal pain, jaundice, anorexia, nausea, vomiting.

Diseases of the Exocrine Pancreas

104. What is cystic fibrosis (CF): (fibrocystic disease of pancreas/mucoviscidosis)?

Ans. Autosomal recessive disorder with defect in the transport of chloride (Cl^-) ions across epithelia leading to high level of sodium chloride in the sweat and defect in the secretory process of all exocrine glands, including pancreas, where the ducts are filled with mucoid (thick), viscid (sticky) secretion, giving the name: "mucoviscidosis"; with dilatation of the ducts (cystic change) and atrophy of the exocrine glands with fibrosis giving the condition its name: "cystic fibrosis" and "fibrocystic disease of the pancreas".

PATHOG: Primary defect is the transport (passage) of chloride (Cl^-) ions across epithelia, leading to changes in the mucus. In normal epithelia Cl^- ion passes across cell membrane (go in and/or out) through channels (passages/doors/gates) formed by membrane proteins. In CF these channels are defective. Hence, they are also called cystic fibrosis transmembrane-conductance regulators (CFTCRs). These channels are under the control of a gene. This gene is called CFTR gene. Mutation in this gene makes the epithelial membrane relatively impermeable to Cl^- ions. The resultant effect of this is tissue-specific as follows:

1. *In the sweat glands:* Concentration of Na^+ and Cl^- is normal inside the gland lumen. But the epithelium of the sweat ducts is impermeable to Cl^-. So, normal reabsorption of NaCl into blood does not occur and NaCl concentration is high inside duct lumen.
2. *In the respiratory tract:* Transport of Cl^- into the lumen of the airways is impaired. So, Na^+ and water are re-absorbed in excess amount from the lumen of the airways into blood, causing dehydration inside the lumen of the airways leading to defective mucociliary action and accumulation of viscid secretions that obstruct the air passages and predispose to recurrent pulmonary infections. Same mechanism is for the pancreas, biliary tract and seminiferous tubules.

MORPHO:
Pancreas: Plugging and blockage of ducts with mucus causes atrophy of exocrine glands with replacement by fibrous tissue, dilatation of ducts, converting them to cysts and atrophy of islets of Langerhans. *Pulmonary:* Plugging and blockage of small airways with mucus with dilatation of bronchioles and bronchi. Secondary infection of bronchioles and bronchi leading to severe chronic bronchitis, bronchiectasis, and lung abscesses. Emphysema and atelectasis of pulmonary parenchyma. Cor pulmonale. *Biliary tract:* Plugging and dilatation of bile ducts. *Male reproductive system:* Plugging of vas deferens, epididymis and seminal vesicle. Atrophy of seminiferous tubules. Azoospermia and sterility in almost all cases.

C/Fs: **Meconium ileus at birth**. Later *S/S* of deficiency of fat soluble vitamins: A/D/E/K: Vitamin A: Night blindness, xerophthalmia, keratomalacia, metaplasia of columnar epithelium into squamous epithelium. Vitamin D: Rickets in children, osteomalacia in adults, hypocalcemic tetany. Vitamin E: Spinocerebellar syndrome. Vitamin K: Bleeding diathesis. Hypoproteinemia, edema, anemia. Sweat more salty. Excessive sweating which may lead to dehydration and circulatory failure. Chronic cough and wheezing, clubbing and cyanosis. Cor pulmonale. Insulin-dependent diabetes mellitus.

DIAG: Quantitative pilocarpine iontophoresis sweat test—Na or Cl concentration: >60 mEq/L is diagnostic. *PROG:* Depends on the extent of pulmonary involvement, which is usually extensive with poor prognosis.

105. What is acute pancreatitis?

Ans. Inflammation of pancreas with acinar injury and leakage of proteolytic and lipolytic enzymes with resultant injury to pancreas and adjacent tissues. *ETIO/PATHOG:* Most of the cases are due to alcoholism and gallstones. Other causes are infections, e.g. mumps, *Mycoplasma pneumonia*, shock, atheroembolism, hypercalcemia, hyperlipoproteinemia, etc. *C/Fs:* Abdominal pain localized in epigastric region with radiation to back, shock which can cause death in 25 to 50% of cases. Tests: Serum amylase and lipase are elevated which together are sensitive and specific. *MORPHO:* Four basic changes:

1. Proteolytic destruction of pancreatic tissue.
2. Lipolytic destruction of fat with fat necrosis and superadded calcification.
3. Necrosis of BVs with hemorrhage.
4. Acute inflammation. Liquefied areas of pancreatic tissue with surrounding fibrosis make cystic space without an epithelial lining. Therefore, called **pseudocysts**.

106. What is carcinoma of pancreas?

Ans. Adenocarcinoma of the exocrine pancreas. *C/Fs:* 3/5 are in the head, 1/5 in body, 1/5 in tail. Ones in the head invade the ampullary region with obstruction of the bile flow causing jaundice, which can help in relatively earlier detection. Carcinoma of the body and tail are silent until they spread posteriorly to the retroperitoneal spaces and adjacent nerves and cause pain. Spontaneous phlebothrombosis, migratory, **(Trousseau's sign)**. Fatal within first year in most of the cases. *MORPHO*: Adenocarcinoma made of atypical irregular small glands lined by anaplastic cuboidal to columnar cells.

107. What is Courvoiser's law/sign?

Ans. Painless, non-tender, dilated gallbladder is usually due to obstruction from carcinoma of the pancreas.

12 Diseases of the Urinary System (US)

OVERVIEW

1. Congenital disorders.
2. Obstructive diseases.
3. Glomerular diseases.
4. Tubular diseases.
5. Interstitial diseases.
6. Blood vessel diseases.
7. Neoplasms.
8. Renal failure.
9. Diseases of the ureters.
10. Urinary bladder diseases.

Some of the congenital disorders of the urinary system are: Ectopic kidney, **horse-shoe** kidney, adult and childhood polycystic diseases. Adult polycystic kidney disease (ADPK) is autosomal dominant and has better prognosis than childhood polycystic diseases which is autosomal recessive and where patients usually die in infancy due to renal failure.

Obstructive diseases may cause hydronephrosis consisting of dilation of the renal pelvis and calyces with atrophy of the renal parenchyma. *Causes of the obstruction can be* congenital or acquired. When the cause is not diagnosed early it can result in renal failure.

Renal calculi are made of calcium oxalate, uric acid, cystine, which are due to their increased amount in blood or urine and magnesium ammonium phosphate **(staghorn)**, which are due to urinary tract infection (UTI) causing urine alkaline with resultant stone formation. Calcium, cystine and staghorn calculi are radiopaque; uric acid stones are radiolucent.

Glomerulonephritis can be classified based upon clinical syndromes into:

1. Nephrotic syndrome.
2. Nephritic syndrome.

Nephrotic syndrome consists of:

1. Proteinuria >4 gm/day.
2. Hypoalbuminemia <3 gm/100 mls.
3. Generalized edema.
4. Hyperlipidemia.

It is mostly seen in:

1. Minimal change disease (lipoid nephrosis).
2. Focal and segmental glomerulosclerosis.
3. Membranous glomerulonephritis.
4. Membranoproliferative glomerulonephritis.
5. SLE.
6. Amyloidosis.
7. Diabetes mellitus.

Nephritic syndrome consists of:

1. Hematuria.
2. Oliguria.
3. Azotemia.
4. Hypertension.

It is mostly seen in:

1. Alport's syndrome.
2. Goodpasture's syndrome.
3. Rapidly progressive glomerulonephritis.
4. IgA nephropathy.
5. Poststreptococcal glomerulonephritis.
6. SLE.

Pyelonephritis is suppurative inflammation of the pelvis of the kidney and the kidney proper. Its types are:

1. Acute.
2. Chronic.

Acute pyelonephritis is commonly due to ascending infection from lower urinary tract. Less commonly, it is due to hematogenous. Some of the common organisms are *E. coli*, Proteus, Klebsiella, Enterobacter, etc.

Chronic pyelonephritis is due to chronic obstruction (commonly by enteric bacteria) or chronic reflux.

Acute tubular necrosis is a clinicopathological condition of destruction of tubular epithelial cells with acute suppression of renal function. Its types are:

1. Ischemic
2. Toxic.

Ischemic is due to any general causes of ischemia. Some of the toxic causes are due to mercuric chloride, carbon tetrachloride, ethylene glycol, gentamicin/tobramycin.

Nephrosclerosis is arteriolosclerosis of the renal arterioles. Its types are:

1. Benign.
2. Malignant.

Benign is seen in mild hypertension, diabetes mellitus and old age.

Malignant is seen in malignant hypertension, i.e. severe (diastolic pressure >120 mmHg) rapidly accelerated hypertension.

Renal failure is loss of kidney's ability to maintain the volume and composition of the body fluids under conditions of normal dietary intake. It is always associated with azotemia (increased serum creatinine and/or urea of renal origin) and in advanced stages results in uremia (patient has various symptoms and signs). Its types are:

1. Acute.
2. Chronic.

Renal neoplasms are:

1. Benign (adenoma).
2. Malignant (renal cell carcinoma—RCC, Wilms' tumor).

Diseases of the urinary bladder are:

1. Cystitis (acute and chronic).
2. Neoplasms (benign—transitional cell papilloma and malignant—transitional cell carcinoma).

Kidneys

Congenital Diseases

1. What is ectopic/pelvic kidney?

Ans. Kidney does not reach the normal adult position and stays in the pelvis. This can cause problems such as arterial supply, differential diagnosis of pelvic infections and neoplasms.

2. What is "horse-shoe" kidney?

Ans. Fusion of kidneys at the lower poles. This can cause problems such as ureteral obstruction resulting in stone formation, hydronephrosis and infection.

3. What is adult polycystic kidney disease (APKD)?

Ans. *DEF/DES:* Inheritance: Autosomal dominant. Multiple cysts of the kidney involving any structure from the Bowman's space to the collecting ducts. *C/Fs:* At birth cysts are small, which grow with age and at approximately 30 years of age present with symptoms of flank pain, hematuria, hypertension, urinary tract infection, aneurysms of the circle of Willis liver cysts, eventually renal failure requiring dialysis or renal transplant. *GROSS:* Kidneys very large in size up to 5000 gm (normal 150 gm). Multiple cysts up to 5 cm in diameter, having clear to hemorrhagic fluid. *MICRO:* Small amount of normal renal parenchyma. Cysts lined by atrophic lining.

4. What is childhood polycystic kidney?

Ans. *DEF/DES:* Inheritance is autosomal recessive. It is less common and more serious than APKD: *C/Fs:* Bilateral multiple cysts, and cysts of the liver are present making child sick since birth. Most of the patients die in infancy due to renal failure. *GROSS:* Kidneys have multiple small cysts in the cortex and medulla. *MICRO:* Cysts are lined by cuboidal cells.

Obstructive Diseases

5. What are renal calculi?

Ans. *Types:* Calcium oxalate, calcium oxalate plus calcium phosphate, magnesium ammonium phosphate (staghorn), uric acid cystine. *ETIO:* Increased concentration of calcium or uric acid in case of calcium and uric acid stones. In case of magnesium stones, urinary tract infection, which causes urine alkaline. *C/Fs:* Pelvic stones usually produce no symptoms. Ureteral stones produce renal colic and gross hematuria. Stones can cause obstruction, and hydronephrosis. Also, they predispose to infection. Calcium, cystine and staghorn stones are radiopaque, uric acid stones are radiolucent.

6. What is hydronephrosis?

Ans. *DEF:* Dilation of the renal pelvis and calyces, with atrophy of the parenchyma, caused by obstruction to the outflow of urine. *ETIO*: Obstruction could be due to congenital or acquired.

Causes:

A. *Congenital:*

1. Urethral atresia or valve.
2. Ureteral compression due to kinking or aberrant renal artery.

B. *Acquired:*

1. *Intraluminal:* Calculi; neoplasms of ureter, urinary bladder, prostate; urethritis; prostatic hyperplasia.
2. *Extraluminal:* Carcinoma of uterus, colon; normal pregnancy; aortic aneurysm.

Types:

1. *Bilateral:* When blockage is below the level of the ureters.
2. *Unilateral:* When blockage is at the level of ureter or above.

GROSS: Kidney is large consisting of distended pelvis and calyces with atrophied parenchyma. *MICRO*: Atrophy of renal parenchyma including tubules and glomeruli is present. *C/Fs:* Flank pain—dull or sharp, constant or intermittent. Malaise, fever, septicemia if super added infection present.

Early detection and treatment can reverse hydronephrosis prior to the development of the irreversible pressure atrophy of renal parenchyma.

Glomerular Diseases

7. What are the terms used to describe the distribution of glomerular diseases?

Ans. 1. *Focal:* Involvement of only some of the glomeruli.
2. *Generalized/diffuse:* Involvement of almost all the glomeruli.
3. *Segmental:* Involvement of only a segment of glomerulus.
4. *Global:* Involvement of the entire glomerulus.

8. What is glomerulonephritis?

Ans. Classification can be based upon the following clinical syndromes:

1. Nephrotic syndrome.
2. Nephritic syndrome.

9. What is nephrotic syndrome?

Ans. *DEF:* Consists of:

1. Massive proteinuria (> 4 gm per day) (due to increased basement membrane permeability).
2. Hypoalbuminemia, (serum albumin reduced to < 3 gm/ 100 mls) (due to massive proteinuria).

3. Generalized edema (due to hypoalbuminemia with decreased plasma oncotic pressure) and hypernatremia.
4. Hyperlipidemia (due to increased lipid synthesis by the liver).

The main pathologic feature is increased basement membrane permeability with increased loss of low-weight protein (albumin) without any inflammation (seen in nephritic syndrome). Commonly seen in the following conditions:

1. Minimal change disease (lipoid nephrosis).
2. Focal and segmental glomerulosclerosis.
3. Membranous glomerulonephritis.
4. Membranoproliferative glomerulonephritis.
5. SLE.
6. Amyloidosis.
7. Diabetic nephropathy.

10. What is minimal change disease?

Ans. By LM: Glomeruli appear normal. By EM: Epithelial foot processes are fused. Seen most often in young children. Responds well to steroid therapy.

11. What is focal and segmental glomerulosclerosis?

Ans. Sclerosis of some of the glomeruli (i.e. focal) and only of some portions of the affected glomeruli (i.e. segmental). *C/Fs:* Similar to lipoid nephrosis, but seen in older patients, does **not** respond to steroids and progresses to chronic glomerulonephritis.

12. What is membranous glomerulonephritis?

Ans. Immune complex disease. Most of the cases have SLE, hepatitis B, syphilis, malaria, or malignancy. *MICRO*: Severe thickening of the capillary basement membrane seen both by LM and EM. Also, by EM, electron dense deposits are seen in intramembranous and subepithelial areas. By special stain, **a spike and dome (tooth comb)** pattern is seen, where dome is due to immune complex deposits and spike due to deposition of new basement membrane around and over the domes. Immunofluorescence shows IgG and C3 as granular deposits. *C/Fs:* Slowly progressive. Response to steroids is poor. Approximately 50% cases develop renal failure approximately within 20 years.

13. What is membranoproliferative glomerulonephritis?

Ans. Both nephrotic and nephritic. Slowly progressive disease with chronic renal failure of unknown etiology. *MORPH:* Basement membrane thickening. Mesangial cellular proliferation with mesangial expansion into basement membrane with duplication of membrane into 2 layers: **tram-track** appearance by silver methenamine stain. Two types by EM and IM, (but LM same in both):

Type I: Immune complex-mediated injury. Ag unknown. Seen with SLE, hepatitis B and C. **Tram-track** appearance prominent, EM: Subendothelial deposits. IM: C3, C1q, C4 and IgG in granular pattern.

Type II: Dense deposit disease: Tram-track appearance not as prominent as Type I EM: dense deposit within lamina densa of BM giving it an irregular, extremely electron dense appearance. IM: C3 seen in irregular linear pattern in BM. Serum C3 is reduced. Pathogenesis: IgG autoantibody (called **C3 nephritic factor**), which reacts with C3 convertase of the alternate complement pathway with its activation resulting in complement-mediated injury.

14. What are renal disease from SLE (lupus nephritis)?

Ans. SLE is an autoimmune disease affecting many systems with many manifestations with a remitting, relapsing course. It mainly involves skin, kidneys, serosal membranes, joints and heart. Many autoantibodies are present, mainly antinuclear antibodies. Lesions are due to immune complexes (Type III hypersensitivity). DNA-anti-DNA complexes in glomeruli causing inflammatory reaction resulting in proliferation of the endothelial, mesangial, and epithelial cells and necrosis of the glomeruli resulting in *S/S* **of both syndromes: nephrotic and nephritic**. Six patterns are seen as per WHO morphologic classification:

1. *Type I:* No observable renal involvement by LM, IM and EM.
2. *Type II:* Mesangial form: Focal and segmental glomerular involvement with increase in number of mesangial cells and mesangial matrix. There is slight proteinuria and hematuria with mild illness.
3. *Type III:* Focal proliferative: Involves less than 50% of the glomeruli. In some patients may progress to severe renal illness.
4. *Type IV:* Diffuse proliferative: Involves glomeruli diffusely with proliferation of endothelial and mesangial cells. Proliferated epithelial cells may fill Bowman's space forming crescent shape (hence, called **crescents**). EM shows subendothelial immune complexes when immune complex severe they cause thickening of capillary wall which appears like rigid **wire loops** by LM. Glomeruli gradually become sclerosed. Patients have hematuria, proteinuria, hypertension and renal insufficiency.
5. *Type V:* Membranous: Appears similar to primary membranous with sub-epithelial immune complex deposits. These patients have severe proteinuria.
6. *Type VI:* Chronic glomerulonephritis: Glomeruli are fibrosed in generalized distribution and global pattern. Clinical features are of azotemia and uremia.

15. What is renal disease from amyloidosis?

Ans. Shows subendothelial and mesangial amyloid deposits—seen by special stains, e.g. congo red or birefringence under polarized light and also by EM. Renal amyloidosis causes nephrotic syndrome.

16. What is diabetic nephropathy?

Ans. a. Glomerular lesions:

i. Capillary basement membrane thickening.

ii. Mesangial global glomerulosclerosis.

iii. Mesangial nodular glomerulosclerosis-**KW kidney**. **(Kimmelstiel-Wilson kidney)**.

b. Hyaline arteriolosclerosis.

c. Pyelonephritis, necrotizing papillitis.

d. Collection of glycogen and fat in convoluted tubular epithelial cells.

17. What is nephritic syndrome?

Ans. *DEF:* Consists of:

1. Hematuria due to inflammatory injury of the glomerular capillaries with bleeding into Bowman's space. Grossly urine appears brownish in color. Microscopically-RBC casts can be seen due to RBCs mixed with proteinaceous material in renal tubules forming a cylindrical cast-like shape of renal tubule.
2. Oliguria.
3. Azotemia (increased BUN and creatinine).
4. Hypertension.

Main pathology is the inflammatory injury of the glomerular capillaries. Seen in conditions such as:

1. Alport's syndrome (hereditary nephritis).
2. Goodpasture's syndrome.
3. RPGN (Rapidly progressive glomerulonephritis).
4. IgA nephropathy (Berger's disease).
5. Poststreptococcal GN.
6. SLE.

18. What is Alport's syndrome?

Ans. Nerve deafness, eye problems (cataract, lens dislocation, corneal dystrophy). By EM: glomerular basement membrane. Splitting.

19. What is Goodpasture's syndrome?

Ans. Type II autoimmune diseases with antibodies against glomerular capillary basement membrane and alveolar basement membranes. IM: Linear IgG deposit. *C/Fs:* Glomerulonephritis, pneumonitis, hemoptysis. Can present with nephritic and nephrotic syndromes.

20. What is RPGN (rapidly progressive glomerulonephritis) (crescentic)?

Ans. Nephritic syndrome progresses rapidly to renal failure in weeks or months. *ETIO*: Poststreptococcal glomerulonephritis, Goodpasture's syndrome, SLE, IgA nephropathy, unknown (membranous and membranoproliferative can also progress to this form). It is of three types:

Type I: Anti-GBM disease with linear deposits of IgG and C3, e.g. Goodpasture's syndrome. Benefit by plasmapheresis.

Type II: Immune complex-mediated. Lumpy-bumpy granular staining.
Type III: Pauci-immune. No antibody by IM or EM. Many cases have ANCA (antineutrophilic cytoplasmic antibody) in serum, thus, seen with microscopic polyangiitis and WG (Wegener's granulomatosis). *PATHOG:* Proliferation of epithelial cells, deposition of fibrin in Bowman's space with formation of crescent between Bowman's capsule and glomerular tuft.

21. What is IgA nephropathy (Berger's disease)?

Ans. **Most common glomerular disease in the world**. IgA deposits in mesangium. Benign recurrent hematuria in children and young adults. **One of the most common causes of hematuria**. Definite cause unknown usually follows URI. *PROG:* In most children benign course. In adults slowly progresses—resulting in renal failure in approximately 1/2 cases in approximately 20 years.

22. What is poststreptococcal glomerulonephritis?

Ans. Type III hypersensitivity reaction to group A beta hemolytic streptococci due to **molecular mimicry**. Diffuse global bilateral glomerular inflammation causing **punctate hemorrhages on the kidney surfaces bilaterally**, enlarged, hypercellular glomeruli with PMNs. By EM: Electron dense subepithelial humps, also subendothelial **(Lumpy-bumpy deposits)**. By IF: Coarse granular IgG and C3, Immunofluorescence. Glomerular basement membrane of normal thickness and uniform. Lab: Hematuria with RBCs and RBC casts, azotemia, decreased serum C3, increased ASO titer. Prognosis is good. Mostly all children get completely well and also many adults. Very few patients develop rapidly progressive glomerulonephritis (RPGN).

Tubular and Interstitial Diseases

23. What is pyelonephritis?

Ans. *DEF:* Suppurative inflammation of the pelvis of the kidney and kidney proper.
Types: Two:
1. Acute
2. Chronic.

24. What is acute pyelonephritis?

Ans. *ETIO:* Bacterial infection:
1. *Escherichia coli* (most common)
2. Proteus
3. Klebsiella
4. Enterobacter
5. Pseudomonas
6. Staphylococci
7. *Streptococcus faecalis*

PATHOG: Two routes of infection:
1. Ascending (from lower urinary tract) (more common).
2. Hematogenous (through the bloodstream) (less common).

Predisposing factors:

1. Urethral instrumentation (catheterization, cystoscopy).
2. Outflow obstruction (prostatic hyperplasia, uterine prolapse).
3. VUR (vesicouretral reflux).
4. DM.
5. Pregnancy.
6. Immunosuppression and immunodeficiency.

Urinary tract infection (UTI) most commonly affects females due to short urethra with its external opening being close to external anal opening. Also, common with urinary tract obstruction, e.g. due to hyperplasia of prostate and prolapse of uterus. *MORPHO: GROSS:* Yellow-colored abscesses are present. *MICRO:* Suppurative infiltration is present, initially in the interstitial tissue which later extends into tubules with many WBCs, which are seen in urine as WBC casts. When severe obstruction develops pus cannot drain into urine and fills the renal pelvis (pyonephrosis).

25. What is chronic pyelonephritis?

Ans. *DEF:* Chronic recurrent infection with interstitial inflammation and scarring of renal parenchyma.

Types:

a. *Chronic obstructive.* b. *Chronic reflux-associated.*

MORPHO: GROSS: Scarring involving pelvis and calyces with severe papillary blunting and calyceal deformity. Scarring is always uneven leading to uneven contraction of the kidney as opposed to even contraction of kidney in chronic glomerulonephritis and benign nephrosclerosis.

MICRO: 1. Infiltration by lymphocytes and plasma cells.

2. Dilation of tubules, many of which have pinkish casts known as colloid casts and appear like thyroid **(thyroidization)**.

26. What is acute tubular necrosis?

Ans. *DEF:* Destruction of tubular epithelial cells with acute suppression of renal function.

Etiologically 2 types:

1. Ischemic.
2. Nephrotoxic.

1. Ischemic ATN: Causes:
   a. Severe trauma, burns.
   b. Acute pancreatitis.
   c. Septicemia.
   d. Mismatched blood transfusion.
   e. Myoglobinuria, crush syndrome.
   f. Heat stroke.

g. Hemolytic crises due to any other cause.

h. Shock due to any other cause.

PATHOG: Ischemic necrosis of the tubular basement membrane causes decreased renal function. *GROSS:* Kidneys are large and pale. *MICRO:* Necrosis of the epithelial cells of the tubule extending deep to the tubular basement membrane causing rupture of the basement membrane called **tubulorrhexis**. Proteinaceous casts in the tubules seen.

2. Toxic ATN: Causes:

a. Mercuric chloride.

b. Carbon tetrachloride.

c. Ethylene glycol.

d. Gentamicin/tobramycin.

e. Radiographic contrast agents.

PATHOG: Above agents cause direct injury to the structure of the cells of the tubules. *MORPHO: GROSS:* Kidneys are swollen, pale or red. *MICRO:* Necrosis of the tubular cells, but the necrosis does not damage the basement membrane of the tubules. *C/Fs* (common to both): ATN is the most common cause of acute renal failure. There is acute suppression of renal function with oliguria of less than 400 ml of urine in 24 hours to anuria in very severe cases. Clinical course has 4 stages:

1. *Initiating stage:* For about 24 hours. There is slight reduction of urine output and slight elevation of BUN.
2. *Maintenance stage:* Begins after 2nd day. Urine output is severely decreased. Lasts from a few days to 2–3 weeks. Patient is uremic and has fluid overload. **If not managed well in this stage patient will die**. If managed well during this stage patient will go to the third stage.
3. *Recovery stage:* There is gradual increase in urine output. But the tubules have not completely healed. So, patient can suffer from electrolyte imbalance and **needs intensive care, otherwise patient can die**. If treated well patient goes to the next stage.
4. *Final stage:* Patient recovers completely with normal renal function and urine output.

Vascular Diseases

27. What is nephrosclerosis?

Ans. *DEF:* Arteriolosclerosis of the renal arterioles.

Types:

1. Benign
2. Malignant.

1. *Benign: MORPHO: GROSS:* Kidneys are atrophic uniformly and have finely granular surfaces. *MICRO:* Arteriolar walls are thick with homogenous pink

glassy appearance **(hyaline arteriolosclerosis)**, causing narrowing of the arteriolar lumen with decreased blood flow leading to ischemic atrophy of glomeruli and tubules with interstitial fibrosis. Seen in mild hypertension, diabetes mellitus and old age.

2. *Malignant: PATHOG:* Endothelial injury with fibrinoid necrosis with reactive hyperplasia of smooth muscles. *GROSS:* Due to rupture of arterioles and glomerular capillaries there are small, pinpoint petechial hemorrhages on the cortical surface giving the kidney a **flea-bitten** appearance. *MICRO:* Arterioles have **fibrinoid neurosis** and superadded inflammation **(necrotizing arteriolitis)**. Large arterioles have proliferation of smooth muscle of intima as circular layers in an onion-skin configuration **(hyperplastic arteriolosclerosis)**. *C/Fs:* Diastolic pressure is more than 120 mmHg. Most patients die due to renal failure.

Renal Failure/Uremia

28. What is renal failure?

Ans. *DEF:* Loss of kidneys' ability to maintain the volume and composition of the body fluids under conditions of normal dietary intake. Is always associated with **azotemia** (increased serum creatinine and/or urea of renal origin). In advanced stages results in **uremia** [biochemical plus clinical features of symptomatic renal disease].

29. What are the types of renal failure?

Ans. *Two types:*

1. Acute.
2. Chronic.

30. What is acute renal failure?

Ans. Rapid, severe decrease in glomerular filtration rate (GFR) with increase in serum blood urea nitrogen (BUN) and creatinine and reduction in urine output.

ETIO:

1. *Prerenal:* Decreased blood supply due to diarrhea, vomiting, hemorrhage, sepsis, CCF.
2. *Renal:* Glomerulonephritis, interstitial nephritis, toxins, drugs.
3. *Postrenal:* Obstruction from calculi, neoplasms, fibrosis.

31. What is chronic renal failure?

Ans. Irreversible loss of renal function occurring in many months to years.

ETIO: Diabetes mellitus, hypertension, obstruction, interstitial nephritis, glomerulonephritis due to various causes.

C/Fs: As of uremia (described in next question).

32. What are features of uremia?

Ans. 1. Azotemia.
2. Acidosis—due to accumulation of sulphates, phosphates, and organic acids.
3. Hyperkalemia.
4. Abnormal control of fluid volume.
5. Hypocalcemia—due to failure to synthesize active form of vitamin D. Hypocalcemia can lead to renal osteodystrophy.
6. Anemia—due to decreased secretion of erythropoietin.
7. Hypertension—due to hyperproduction of renin.
8. Anorexia, nausea and vomiting.
9. Neurologic disorders—ranging from diminished mental function to convulsions and coma.
10. Bleeding—due to disordered platelet function.
11. Pruritus—due to accumulation of urochrome and other urinary pigments.
12. Fibrinous pericarditis.

Neoplasms

33. What are renal neoplasms?

Ans. *Benign:* Cortical adenoma. *Malignant:* Renal cell carcinoma, Wilms' tumor.

34. What is renal cell carcinoma?

Ans. *DEF:* Adenocarcinoma of the kidney. Histogenesis (cell of origin): Tubular epithelial cells. *ETIO:* No definite etiology known; but cigarette smoking is a contributory factor, also, in von Hippel-Lindau syndrome there is mutation of the tumor suppressor gene on chromosome 3. In von Hippel-Lindau syndrome many patients have multiple bilateral renal cell carcinomas, and hemangioblastomas of CNS and retina. *MORPHO: GROSS:* It can occur anywhere on the kidney, but often is located at the upper pole. It is large, yellow in color with extensive hemorrhage and necrosis seen on the cut surface. Often it extends into renal vein, to inferior vena cava and sometimes even into the right atrium. *MICRO:* Cells are in groups, they are large with clear cytoplasm, nuclei are located at the base of the cells. *C/Fs:* Most common symptom is hematuria. Patient can have a triad of symptoms:

1. Hematuria.
2. Palpable abdominal mass.
3. Flank pain.

Patient can also present with **paraneoplastic syndromes** such as: polycythemia, hypercalcemia, Cushing's syndrome, hypertension. Metastases are to bones, lungs, which are sometimes discrete round masses called **Cannon balls**. *DIAG:* US, CT scan, pyelography, renal angiography, biopsy, urine cytology may show neoplastic cells. *PROG:* 5 year survival is 50% with radical nephrectomy with regional node dissection.

35. What is Wilms' tumor?

Ans. *DEF:* Adenosarcoma. Congenital malignant neoplasm. Histogenesis: Originates from metanephrogenic blastema. *ETIO:* Many patients have deletion of short arm of chromosome 11 resulting in deletion or mutation of tumor suppressor gene. *MORPHO: GROSS:* Grayish, soft, smooth tumor.

MICRO: Three elements.

1. Epithelial tubular elements lined by cells with hyperchromatic nuclei.
2. Tightly packed blastemal elements composed of small round blue cells with hyperchromatic nuclei.
3. Spindle-shaped stromal cells.

C/Fs: **WAGR** syndrome (**W**ilms' tumor, **A**niridia, **G**enital abnormalities, **R**etardation mental). Also can have hemihypertrophy. Age of presentation: 2–3 years. Presenting symptoms: abdominal mass, pain, hematuria, fever, anorexia, nausea, vomiting, hypertension. *DIAG:* US, CT scan, IVP, Bx. *TRT:* Surgery, chemotherapy, radiotherapy. *PROG:* Excellent. 90% cure.

Urinary Bladder
Cystitis

36. What is cystitis?

Ans. *Types:* Two types:

1. Acute
2. Chronic.

ETIO: Escherichia coli, Proteus, Klebsiella, Enterobacter. *Schistosoma hamatobium* in Egypt. *MORPHO: GROSS:* Hyperemia of the mucosa, sometimes hemorrhage—(hemorrhagic cystitis) sometimes exudate: (Suppurative cystitis). Sometimes ulceration of the mucosa: (ulcerative cystitis). *MICRO:* In acute: PMN infiltrate. In Chronic: Lymphocytic infiltrate. *C/Fs:* Triad:

1. Frequency
2. Suprapubic pain
3. Dysuria.

Systemic: Fever, chills, malaise.

Neoplasms

37. What are urinary bladder neoplasms?

Ans. *Types:* Benign: Transitional cell papilloma cells, 7 layers thick, no dysplasia/atypia. Malignant: Transitional cell carcinoma:

1. CIS.

2. Grade I.
3. Grade II.
4. Grade III.

1. Papillary: Non-invasive.
2. Papillary: Invasive.
3. Flat: Non-invasive.
4. Flat: Invasive.

Squamous cell carcinoma. Mixed adenocarcinoma.

Factors implicated in causation:

1. Industrial exposure to 2-naphthylamine.
2. Smoking.
3. *Schistosoma haematobium*.
4. Long-term use of phenacetin.
5. Cyclophosphamide.
6. Coffee.
7. Saccharin.
8. Alcohol.

MORPH: GROSS: Papillary: Exophytic, polypoid, attached by a stalk to the mucosa. Flat: Plaque–like thickening of the mucosa. Non-invasive: Thickening of the mucosa without penetration of basement membrane by cancer cells. Invasive: Penetration of the mucosal basement membrane. *MICRO:* Grade I: No. of layers of cells >7, Some atypia, mitoses rare, slight loss of polarity. Grade II: No. of layers of cells > Gr. I. No. of mitoses >Gr. I. Loss of polarity >Gr. I. Variability in size, shape and chromaticity. Cells still recognizable as transitional cells. Grade III: Cells barely recognizable as transitional cells. All the changes seen in Gr. II are more pronounced. *C/Fs*: Painless hematuria. Sometimes frequency, urgency, dysuria. If ureteral orifice involved—pyelonephritis and hydronephrosis. *PROG:* Depends on depth of invasion and grade: More the extent of invasion and higher the grate, worse the prognosis. *DIAG:* Cytology of urine, cystoscopy, biopsy.

38. What are some of the causes of hematuria?

Ans. 1. *Urinary tract disorders:* Trauma, infection, polycystic kidney diseases, stones, renal infarction, renal vein thrombosis, glomerulonephritis, neoplasms, etc.

2. *Hematologic disorders:* Bleeding disorders, anticoagulation, sickle cell anemia, etc.

13 Diseases of the Nervous System (NS)

OVERVIEW

1. Some special features of the nervous system.
2. Congenital-perinatal diseases.
3. Trauma.
4. Vascular diseases.
5. Nutritional, metabolic, toxic diseases.
6. Degenerative diseases.
7. Demyelinating diseases.
8. Infections.
9. Neoplasms.
10. Peripheral nerves.

Nervous system has some structural and physiologic special/unique features which are of clinical importance:

1. Brain is placed inside the confined bony skull, which causes herniations (**cut** = **c**ingulated, **u**ncinate, **t**onsillar) upon increased intracranial pressure causing different deleterious effects, **even death**.
2. Nerve cells (neurons) do not regenerate and since brain controls the body, when brain is permanently injured the **person dies**.
3. Specific areas of the brain have specific functions and injury to such areas can cause loss of these functions, e.g. occipital lobe—loss of vision, Broca's area—loss of speech, etc.
4. Small area of brain controls function of large area of the body, consequently injury to such area results in major loss of function, e.g. injury to internal capsule causes contralateral hemiplegia.

Congenital disorders of the nervous system consist of:

1. Defects which cause outpouching of brain tissue, meninges and spinal cord.
2. Hydrocephalus (increased CSF), and
3. Various neurocutaneous syndromes.

Trauma to the skull with:

1. *Epidural hemorrhage* can present with **lucid interval, which can give false sense of security leading to death**.

2. Subdural hematomas can also cause serious morbidities and in due course even mortality.

Other traumatic injuries consist of:

3. Concussion.
4. Contusions and intracerebral hemorrhage.

Vascular disorders are very serious, which consist of generalized hypoxic-ischemic encephalopathy, infarcts due to thrombosis (commonest cause), embolism, non-traumatic hemorrhage (commonly as complication of hypertension) and from berry aneurysm of circle of Willis (which can sometimes present with leak before the full-blown hemorrhage **which can be prevented if timely recognized and treated**. Transient ischemic attacks also worth remembering because ~ 1/3 of patients develop infarcts within 5 years, **which may also be prevented if timely recognized and treated.**

Degenerating diseases consist of **Alzheimer's disease** and **Pick's disease** with dementia, **Parkinsonism** with loss of dopamine-producing cells in substantia nigra causing motor function disturbances (slow rigid with resting tremors), **Huntington disease** (hereditary, but not congenital-presenting at ~ 45 years of age) involving basal ganglia with reduced GABA and acetylcholine resulting in chorea and dementia; **amyotrophic lateral sclerosis** with upper and lower motor neuron degeneration with loss of motor functions resulting in death in ~ 5 years due to respiratory failure.

Demyelinating diseases consist of:

a. *Congenital:* Leukodystrophies.
b. *Acquired:*
   1. Multiple sclerosis.
   2. Acute disseminated encephalomyelitis.
   3. Central pontine myelinosis.
   4. Progressive multifocal leukoencephalopathy.

Some of the nutritional and toxic diseases of the nervous system are:

A. *Nutritional:*
   1. Vitamin B_1 deficiency—**Wernicke's encephalopathy, Korsakoff's psychosis**.
   2. Vitamin B_{12} deficiency—Subacute combined degeneration of the spinal cord and **megaloblastic madness.**
B. *With systemic diseases:*
   1. With hepatic failure.
   2. With renal failure
C. *With Industrial toxins:*
   1. Metals (lead, arsenic, mecury).
   2. Organophosphate.
   3. Methyl alcohol.
   4. Carbon monoxide.
D. *With therapeutic agents:*
   1. Metronidazole.
   2. Vinca alkaloids.
   3. Methotrexate.

Infectious diseases of the nervous system are:

A. *Meningitis:*

1. *Acute bacterial:* In neonates mostly by *E. coli* and group B streptococci; in children and adults mostly by pneumococcus and meningococcus. In elderly mostly by *Listeria monocytogenes*.
2. *Acute viral:* Mostly mumps, E-B virus, coxsackie virus.
3. Chronic mostly by *Mycobacterium tuberculosis*, Cryptococcus, *Treponema pallidum* (meningovascular syphilis).

B. *Syphilis consisting of:*

1. *Tabes dorsalis* causing degeneration of dorsal nerve roots and posterior columns of the spinal cord causing loss of vibration, position and pain sensation resulting in ataxia and joint injuries **(Charcot joints)**.
2. *General paralysis of insane (GPI)* causing cortical atrophy with neuronal loss, resulting in gradual weakness and dementia.
3. Meningovascular syphilis.

C. *Encephalitis* (infection of the brain parenchyma). Some of the types are:

1. Localized bacterial abscess.
2. Tuberculosis.
3. Toxoplasmosis.
4. Neurocysticercosis.
5. Viral encephalitis (herpes, polio, rabies, cytomegalo virus, HIV, etc.)

D. *Prion disease (spongiform encephalopathy):* Caused by prions which are proteins without any nucleic acids such as DNA or RNA. PrPc is normal cellular protein. PrPsc is its abnormal isoform.

Types:

1. Sporadic.
2. Familial.
3. Infectious.
4. Transmissible.

Examples:

1. CJD (Creutzfeldt-Jacob disease).
2. New-variant CJD.
3. Kuru.
4. Gerstmann-Straussler-Scheinker (GSS) syndrome.
5. Fatal familial insomnia.
6. Scrapie, "mad cow" disease.

Spongiform appearance with many small cysts are present in the gray matter. *C/Fs:* Generally, dementia, ataxia. Rapidly progressive, death in 1/2–1 year.

Neoplasms of the CNS are:

1. Meningioma.
2. Neurocytoma.

3. Glial tumors (Astrocytomas—fibrillary including well differentiated, anaplastic and glioblastoma multiforme; oligodendroglioma, ependymoma).
4. Primitive neuroectodermal tumors (medulloblastoma).
5. Miscellaneous (germ cell tumors, lymphomas).
6. Metastatic (carcinomas, e.g. from lungs, breast, melanoma).

Diseases of the peripheral nervous system (PNS) are:

A. Neuropathies.
B. Neoplasms.

Some neuropathies by causes are: **MINT**

1. **M**etabolic (DM).
2. **I**nfectious.
3. **N**utritional (B_1 deficiency).
4. **T**oxic.

Neoplasms are:

1. Schwannoma (neurilemmoma).
2. Neurofibroma—has the potential to become malignant. Can be seen as sporadic and also with hereditary condition—**Neurofibromatosis—types 1 and 2.**

Introduction

1. What are special anatomic and physiologic features of the CNS, which influence the outcome of the diseases of the CNS?

Ans. 1. Located in a confined space—vulnerable to pressure-related problems.
2. Specific area has specific function—vulnerable to focal lesions.
3. Controls whole body functions: Brain dead = Body dead.
4. Neurons (nerve cells) permanent cells—So, defect from injury is permanent.
5. Nervous system is more susceptible to relatively mild, transient injuries such as hypoxia, hypoglycemia, etc.
6. CSF circulation.

2. What are cells of the CNS which are different from the other cells of our body?

Ans. 1. Neurons (nerve cells).
2. Specialised support cells (glial cells):
   a. Astrocytes—These have delicate cytoplasmic processes, with which they provide a framework for nerve and other cells of the CNS. These proliferate after injury.
   b. Oligodendrocytes—Their cytoplasm provide wrap-up sheath (myelin) around axons of neurons of the CNS. In the PNS Schwann cells do this function.
   c. Microglia—Derived from circulating monocytes, protective function similar to histiocytes/macrophages in other tissues.
   d. Ependymal cells—These provide a lining to the cerebral ventricles and canal of spinal cord.

3. How blood vessels and connective tissue cells of CNS are different than at other sites in our body?

Ans. Blood vessels in the CNS have specialized structure to maintain blood-brain barrier which limits transport of substances from blood vessels to the brain. Connective tissue is present only in meninges, choroid plexus, and around BVs. There are only a few fibroblasts which limit fibrous scarring after injury.

4. What is the basic microscopic appearance of brain and PNS?

Ans. Brain parenchyma shows as neurons (nerve cells) supported by a framework of glial cells (astrocytes, oligodendrocytes and ependyma), microglia and blood vessels. Processes of these cells combine to form a delicate fibrillar background called the **neuropil**. Nerve cells (neurons) are present in the cortex of the brain and inner part of spinal cord. This area appears grey and is called **gray matter**. The areas which do not contain nerve cell bodies appear white due to white appearing fatty myelin sheaths of the axons in this area which is called **white matter**.

In the PNS, connective tissue and associated blood vessels are present with individual axons **(endoneurium)** bundles of axons **(perineurium)** and peripheral nerves **(epineurium)**.

Congenital Malformations

5. What are some of the common congenital malformations of the CNS?

Ans. Common congenital malformations of the CNS include:

1. Neural tube defects.
2. Malformations with hydrocephalus.
3. Neurocutaneous syndromes.

6. What are the neural tube defects?

Ans. *DEF/DES:* These are a group of disorders where there is a failure of closure of the neural tube. These can involve either:

A. Vertebrae or

B. Skull.

These can be with or without involvement of meninges, spinal cord or brain.

A. Involving skull/brain:

1. Encephaloceles.
2. Cranial meningoceles.

B. Involving vertebrae/spinal cord:

1. *Spina bifida:* Posterior vertebral arches not closed.
2. *Spina bifida occulta:* Spina bifida without any clinically apparent abnormalities.
3. *Spinal meningocele:* Herniation of meninges only through spina bifida.
4. *Meningomyeloceles:* Herniation of both meninges and spinal cord through the defect.

7. What are some of the congenital malformations of CNS associated with hydrocephalus?

Ans. Malformations causing hydrocephalus can be due to:

a. Developmental abnormalities, e.g.

1. Arnold-Chiari malformation,
2. Dandy-Walker malformation.

b. Acquired conditions, e.g.

1. Hemorrhage,
2. Inflammation, or
3. Neoplasms.

8. What are neurocutaneous syndromes?

Ans. Major neurocutaneous syndromes are following:

1. *Neurofibromatosis type I:* Autosomal dominant, gene located on chromosome 17. *C/Fs*: Hyperpigmented skin lesions **(café-au-lait spots)**, pigmented nodules on iris **(Lisch nodules)**, gliomas, meningiomas, neurofibromas, schwannomas, malignant neoplasm of peripheral nerves.
2. *Neurofibromatosis type II:* Autosomal dominant, gene located on chromosome 22. *C/Fs*: Meningioma, schwannoma of VIII cranial nerve (acoustic neuroma).
3. *Sturge-Weber syndrome:* Genetic defect unknown. *C/Fs*: Angiomas of skin in distribution of VII cranial nerve, seizures.
4. *Tuberous sclerosis:* Autosomal dominant, gene on chromosome 9. *C/Fs*: Renal angiomyolipomas. Cardiac rhabdomyoma, seizures.
5. *von Hippel-Lindau disease:* Autosomal dominant, gene on chromosome 3. *C/Fs*: Renal cell carcinoma, pheochromocytoma, cerebellar hemangioblastoma.

Edema, Herniation and Hydrocephalus

9. What is cerebral edema and it is of how many types?

Ans. *DEF:* Increased fluid within brain parenchyma.
Types:

1. *Intercellular:* Generalized-due to blood-brain barrier disruption fluid escapes from B.V. to interstitial space of brain.
2. *Intracellular:* Due to cellular injury, e.g. from hypoxia/ischemia causing sodium pump failure leading to increased water in the cell.
   Morphology: Gyri flattened, sulci narrowed, ventricular cavities compressed. Expansion of the brain may lead to **herniation**.

10. What is herniation of the brain? What are its common locations?

Ans. *DEF:* Displacement of a part of the brain due to increased intracranial pressure.
Common locations: These are three:

1. *Cingulate gyrus (subfalcine):* Due to unilateral or asymmetric expansion of cerebral hemisphere displaces the cingulate gyrus under the falx cerebri leading to compression of branches of the anterior cerebral artery.
2. *Uncinate (mesial temporal, transtentorial):* Due to medial aspect of temporal lobe being compressed against the free margin of tentorium cerebelli leading to compression of III cranial nerve (resulting in pupillary dilation and impairment of ocular movements on the side of the lesion) and posterior cerebral artery (causing ischemic injury to the territory of its supply, importantly primary visual cortex resulting in homonymous hemianopia). Brainstem herniation commonly causes hemorrhagic lesions in the midbrain and pons, called secondary brainstem

or **Duret's hemorrhages** which are linear hemorrhagic infarcts in midline and paramedian regions, due to kinking of branches of basilar artery during herniation. **Life threatening like tonsillar herniation**.

3. *Tonsillar:* Due to cerebellar tonsils being displaced through foramen magnum. This is **life-threatening** because it causes brainstem compression and compromises vital respiratory centers in medulla oblongata.

11. What is normal CSF circulation?

Ans. CSF is produced by the choroid plexus in the lateral and IV ventricles, exits the ventricular system, via the foramina luschka and magendie and flows over the superior cerebral convexities, where it is absorbed by the arachnoid granulations.

12. What is hydrocephalus?

Ans. *DEF:* Increased CSF in the cranial cavity.

Types:

1. Internal.
2. External.
3. Non-communicating.
4. Communicating.
5. Hydrocephalus ex vacuo.
6. Hydrocephalus before closure of cranial sutures.
7. Hydrocephalus after closure of cranial sutures.
8. Acquired.
9. Congenital.

1. *Internal:* Increased CSF is present only in the ventricles.
2. *External:* Increased CSF is present only in the subarachnoid space.
3. *Non-communicating:* Obstruction to CSF flow is within ventricular system without flow of CSF from the ventricles to the subarachnoid space.
4. *Communicating:* Obstruction to CSF flow is outside the ventricular system (e.g. in the subarachnoid space or at the arachnoid granulations) with flow of CSF from the ventricles to the subarachnoid space.
5. *Hydrocephalus ex vacuo:* Due to loss of brain parenchyma dilation of ventricles with compensatory increase of CSF within the ventricles. CSF production is not increased and its flow is normal.
6. *Hydrocephalus before closure of cranial sutures:* Head is enlarged with increase in head circumference. In neonates eyes are deviated downward **(setting-sun sign)**.
7. *Hydrocephalus after closure of cranial sutures:* Dilation of VS with increased intracranial pressure without change in head circumference.
8. *Acquired:* Due to tumors, hemorrhage, inflammations, etc.
9. *Congenital:* Involve the cerebellum, A-C malformation; DW syndrome (*see* next page).

13. What is Arnold-Chiari malformation (A-C malformation)?

Ans. Congenital downward displacement of cerebellar tonsils and medulla through foramen magnum causing obstruction of CSF outflow resulting in hydrocephalus.

14. What is Dandy Walker syndrome (DW syndrome)?

Ans. Aplasia/hypoplasia of cerebellar vermis, IV ventricle dilation, large post fossa, hydrocephalus.

Trauma

15. What is epidural hematoma? What is lucid interval?

Ans. *DEF:* Hematoma above the duramater. *Cause:* Rupture of meningeal artery, or commonly, its branch between squamous portion of temporal bone and duramater with fracture of the bone. Hematoma is formed beneath the bone above the dura. **If not drained immediately, it will compress the underlying brain and cause uncal and cerebellar tonsillar herniation, brainstem compression and death.** Immediately after the injury many patients have a brief period of unconsciousness due to concussion. Then, the patient recovers consciousness for a short interval of time. This short-recovery of consciousness is known as **lucid interval**. This recovery can give a false sense of security and well-being. After a few minutes or hours, due to continuous bleeding and increase in the size of hematoma there is progressively increased intracranial pressure **leading to progressive loss of consciousness, coma and death if not promptly diagnosed and treated**.

16. What is subdural hematoma?

Ans. *DEF:* Hematoma beneath the duramater. *Cause:* Rupture of bridging veins between dural sinuses and the surface of brain due to quick changes in head movement velocity, e.g. whiplash injury, blows to the head, violent shaking of head of infants.
Types:

1. *Acute:* Clotted blood mostly in hematoma. Known history of trauma. Unilateral usually, except in infants bilateral. Swelling of the underlying brain causing compression of the opposite side of the brain against the skull bone and herniation. Symptoms develop gradually and hematoma liquefies gradually.
2. *Chronic:* Due to mild trauma with no known history causing mild transient hemorrhage and the resultant hematoma. By osmosis increases slowly causing *S/S* of compression.

17. What are some of the traumatic parenchymal brain injuries?

Ans. 1. Concussion.

2. Contusions.

18. What is concussion?

Ans. Temporary loss of consciousness and generalized paralysis with recovery within a few to 24 hours, caused by blunt head trauma possibly due to mild reticular activating system injury without any structural lesion. Recovery is complete; however, patient has no memory of the event.

19. What are contusions of the brain?

Ans. Consist of injury to the superficial brain by blunt trauma. There are 2 types:

a. Coup b. Contrecoup.

a. *Coup contusion:* Injury at the point of contact when the head is immobile.

b. *Contrecoup contusion:* Injury at the **opposite end** of the point of contact when head is in motion which when abruptly stopped by impact against an immobile object causes the brain to hit against the skull opposite to the site of impact.

Vascular Diseases

20. What are the types of the vascular diseases of the brain?

Ans. a. Generalized hypoxic-ischemic encephalopathy: Due to generalized blood flow reduction.

b. Infarcts: Caused by local vascular obstruction. **80% of total cases** due to:
   1. Thrombosis **(more common)**.
   2. Embolism.

c. Hemorrhages:
   1. Within brain parenchyma; or
   2. Subarachnoid space.

21. What are the infarcts of the brain?

Ans. *DEF:* Local brain injury due to local circulatory disturbances. **80% of all CVA (cerebrovascular accidents) (strokes).**

ETIO:

Atherosclerosis—Most common cause of brain infarcts.

1. Thrombosis is most common cause of occlusion of an atherosclerotic artery. Other conditions which could cause occlusion of the cerebral arteries are:
2. Emboli.
3. Vasculitis.
4. Trauma.

Atherosclerosis: Common blood vessels involved are: internal carotid, proximal middle cerebral and basilar arteries. Since atherosclerosis is the most common cause of the cerebrovascular accident; and, since atherosclerosis takes many years to develop to cause ischemic brain injury leading to infarctions it can be very well anticipated and prevented by vigilant management. **So, it is a misnomer to call this disease an accident** because "accident" means "by chance—unexpected". Therefore, the correct term should be "brain infarction", similar to "myocardial infarction". (We do **not** call it "myocardial accident"), prevention of which by appropriate medical intervention has become a routine medical practice.

Thrombosis: Occurs most commonly near carotid bifurcation or in the basilar artery.

Emboli: Commonly occur in intracranial blood vessels and most commonly in branches of middle cerebral artery. Basilar artery emboli can occur in extracranial region. Emboli often originate from heart and proximal segment of carotid arteries. Common types of emboli are: Cardiac mural thrombi, vegetations from infected valves, air bubbles, fat droplets, clusters of tumor cells.

22. What are the *C/Fs* of brain infarcts?

Ans. *Middle cerebral artery:* Contralateral hemiparesis, spasticity, loss of sensation, aphasias (with dominant hemisphere involvement); visual field defects.

Internal carotid artery: Less common than occlusion of middle cerebral artery. Since arterial anastomosis at circle of Willis supplies blood to the area the deficit is less than expected. Severe cases develop large infarction of the ipsilateral cerebral hemisphere with monocular blindness.

Vertebrobasilar system: Could cause fatal infarcts (commonly thrombotic) due to brainstem injury or small silent infarcts. Neurologic deficits with infarction are dependent on location and extent of brain damage. Besides the infarction, edema of adjacent brain also causes additional neurologic deficits and leads to **brain herniation** and **death**.

23. What are the transient ischemic attacks (TIAs)?

Ans. *DEF:* Transient episodes of neurologic dysfunction lasting from several minutes to several hours (maximum 24 hours). *ETIO:* Due to temporary vascular obstruction by atheromatous emboli. **TIAs are important conditions because approximately 1/3 of these patients develop infarcts within approximately 5 years.**

24. What do you know about the types of intracranial hemorrhages?

Ans. Types:

1. Primary intraparenchymal
2. Primary subarachnoid.

25. What is primary intraparenchymal hemorrhage?

Ans. *DEF:* Acute nontraumatic intraparenchymal hemorrhage.

ETIO:

1. Hypertension.
2. Vascular malformations and aneurysms.
3. Vasculitis.
4. Coagulation disorders.

26. How does hypertension (HTN) cause primary intracranial hemorrhage?

Ans. HTN is the commonest cause of primary intracranial hemorrhage, usually due to rupture of an arteriole. Occasionally-vessels < 300 micrometer in diameter develop minute aneurysms called **Charcot-bouchard microaneurysms**, which may rupture, commonly within basal ganglia. *PATHOG:* HTN makes vessels prone to rupture by increasing atherosclerosis in larger arteries. Hyaline arteriolosclerosis in smaller vessels in mild HTN. Hyperplastic arteriolosclerosis in severe HTN. Frank necrosis of arterioles in malignant HTN.

MORPHO: Common sites: Basal ganglia, thalamus, cerebral white matter, pons, cerebellum. Hemorrhage can extend into ventricles and subarachnoid space and can also cause herniation of cerebellar tonsils and brainstem **(Duret's)** hemorrhage.

C/Fs: Acute onset with *S/S* of increased intracranial pressure such as severe headache, vomiting, loss of consciousness, irregular, intermittent respirations **(Cheyne-Stokes respiration)**; dilated non-responsive pupils, deep coma and death.

27. What is primary subarachnoid hemorrhage?

Ans. *DEF:* Commonly due to rupture of congenital berry aneurysms of vessels of circle of Willis. *C/Fs*: Onset is very sudden with severe headache **(worse headache of my life)**, vomiting, loss of consciousness and neck rigidity are usually present. CSF is grossly bloody. **Within a few days approximately 50% patients die**. Survivors usually develop hydrocephalus due to organization of blood in the leptomeninges resulting in obstruction of the CSF flow.

28. What are vascular malformations of the brain?

Ans. These are developmental abnormalities, e.g.

1. Arteriovenous malformations.
2. Cavernous angiomas.

These can rupture suddenly and spontaneously causing severe intracranial hemorrhage.

Degenerative Diseases

29. What are some of the degenerative diseases of the nervous system?

Ans. *DEF:* Diseases that cause degeneration of the neurons, such as:

1. Alzheimer's disease.
2. Pick's disease.
3. Parkinsonism.
4. Huntington's disease.
5. Diseases of motor neurons.
   a. ALS.
   b. Werding-Hoffman disease (Floppy infant syndrome).

30. What is Alzheimer's disease?

Ans. *DEF:* Brain disorder causing dementia. *C/Fs:* Onset is after 50 years of age, progressive, with average life 10 years after the onset. Symptoms are of loss of memory, understanding, and other higher mental functions, resulting in confusion and disorientation and inability to take care of oneself and one's daily needs. This results in susceptibility to various infections such as UTI, bronchopneumonia, which cause death of the patient. *MORPH*: *GROSS:* Generalized atrophy of the brain. *MICRO:* (*see* mnemonic in appendix I)

1. Neurofibrillary tangles.
2. Senile plaques.
3. Amyloid angiopathy.
4. Hirano bodies.
5. Granulovacuolar degeneration.
6. Lewis bodies.
7. Loss of neurons.

31. What is Pick's disease?

Ans. *DEF:* It is a neurodegenerative atrophic disease of the brain involving frontal and temporal lobes causing dementia. *MICRO:* Large nerve cells **(Pick's cells)** and inclusions **(Pick's bodies)**.

32. What is parkinsonism?

Ans. *DEF:* Group of degenerative brain disorder where there is progressive loss of dopamine-producing cells in substantia nigra resulting in disturbance in motor functions with rigidity, difficulty in initiating movements (akinesia) with slowing of voluntary movements, expressionless face, stooped posture, gait disturbance, and "pill-rolling" tremor at rest. *ETIO:* Trauma, toxins, chronic ischemia, infections (encephalitis).

33. What is Parkinson's disease (idiopathic parkinsonism) (paralysis agitans)?

Ans. *DEF:* Parkinsonism where the cause is unknown. *C/Fs:* Gradual onset usually at 60 years. Slowly progress over ~10 years with death due to infection or trauma due to unsteady gait. *S/S*: Disturbances of motor functions with rigidity, expressionless face, stooped gait, slow voluntary movements, and a "pin-rolling" tremor of the hands/fingers. *MORPHO: GROSS:* Brain might be slightly atrophic or normal appearing. Substantia nigra and locus ceruleus appear very pale due to loss of nerve cells containing melanin pigment. *MICRO:* The neurofibrillary area (neuropil) is fibrotic (gliotic) due to loss of nerve cells (neurons). Some of the remaining nerve cells (neurons) have collection of circular layered eosinophilic material called **Lewy bodies**.

34. What is Huntington's disease?

Ans. *DEF:* Autosomal dominant hereditary (but not congenital) brain disease involving extrapyramidal motor system with involuntary movements (chorea) and dementia. *C/Fs*: Age of onset is approximately 50 years. Slow onset and progression with a life of ~20 years from the onset. *S/S* are involuntary twisting movements called choreiform movements. Mental problems, consisting of failure of understanding, depression are also present. *MORPHO: GROSS:* Brain is small with atrophy of caudate nucleus, putamen, and globus pallidus with compensatory dilation of adjacent ventricles. *MICRO:* Severe loss of neurons in caudate and putamen and some in cortical areas.

35. What is amyotrophic lateral sclerosis (ALS) (Lou Gehrig's disease)?

Ans. *DEF/DES:* Degenerative, progressive disorder of the both upper and lower neurons of the pyramidal system with loss of motor nerve cells in the anterior horns of spinal cord, brainstem and cerebral motor cortex causing muscle weakness, atrophy, and spasticity. *ETIO:* Unknown. *C/Fs:* Onset is gradual with slow progression with average life expectancy of 5 years. Death usually occurs from respiratory insufficiency or infection. Initially, there is weakness of muscles which later become atrophied and there is fine tremors called fasciculations. Since, upper motor nerve cells are involved there is spasticity, hyperactive tendon reflexes, and positive Babinski reflex. *MORPHO: GROSS:* Mild atrophy of the anterior spinal nerve roots may be present, otherwise brain and spinal cord usually appear normal on gross examination. *MICRO:* There is loss of nerve cells with compensatory gliosis in the motor areas of the spinal cord, brainstem and cerebral cortex. There is a resultant loss of corticospinal fibres in the cerebral peduncles, basal pons, medullary pyramids and lateral anterior columns of the spinal cord. Peripheral nerves carrying motor fibers are also atrophied and also the affected skeletal muscles.

Demyelinating Diseases

36. What are the demyelinating diseases?

Ans. *DEF:* Diseases characterized by loss of myelin.

CLASSI:

A. Congenital: Leukodystrophies

B. Acquired demyelinating diseases:

1. Multiple sclerosis (multiphasic, multicentric, multi onset—acute or gradual).
2. Acute disseminated encephalomyelitis (monophasic) (hypersensitivity reaction).
3. Central pontine myelinolysis.
4. Viral encephalitis-related demyelination (infection).

37. What is multiple sclerosis?

Ans. Multiple sclerosis (MS) is the most common demyelinating disease of the CNS. It is more common in people of temperate climates and of European origin.

ETIO: Unknown. Most likely it is an autoimmune disease mediated by T lymphocytes.

MORPHO: GROSS: Multiple areas of demyelination are present. These are called **plaques**. Plaques are present in multiple areas of the brain and spinal cord giving rise to multiple signs and symptoms. Common sites of plaques are: Periventricular white matter, the optic nerves, and the white matter of the spinal cord.

MICRO: Perivascular lymphocytic infiltrate is present. In active lesions: lipid-filled macrophages are present due to break down of myelin.

C/Fs: The onset of MS may be suddenly or slowly. Common symptoms are visual disturbances (blurred vision, diplopia, scotomata), paresthesias, spasticity of one or more extremities, speech disturbances, and gait abnormalities.

Tests: In the CSF, a few lymphocytes are present. Protein is slightly increased with relative increase of the gamma globulin portion with increase in the oligoclonal bands of immunoglobulins as seen by electrophoresis. But, these immunoglobulin antibodies are thought to be in response to myelin break down and not the cause of it, which is thought to be T lymphocyte-mediated.

38. What is acute disseminated encephalomyelitis?

Ans. *ETIO:* Unknown. It is immune-mediated which occurs after some infections, e.g. **measles, chickenpox, rubella** and **vaccinations**, possibly **due to hypersensitivity reaction** to some foreign antigen.

MICRO: Areas of perivascular demyelination and mononuclear infiltration.

C/Fs: It is a monophasic illness of acute onset. *S/S:* Fever, seizures, coma, spinal cord dysfunction. Death occurs in approximately 1 in 5 cases.

39. What is central pontine myelinolysis?

Ans. Demyelination in the base of pons.

ETIO: Seen with alcoholism, rapid correction of hyponatremia (mechanism unknown).

40. What is demyelination with viral encephalitis?

Ans. Seen in progressive multifocal leukoencephalopathy (PML), which is caused by JC virus, a papovavirus. It is commonly seen in AIDS patients. **Virus infects** oligodendroglia causing demyelination. *MORPHO: GROSS:* Demyelination is seen as irregular, gelatinous foci, commonly at the grey-white matter junction. *MICRO:* Demyelination, enlarged astrocytes, enlarged oligodendroglial nuclei having blurred purplish inclusions. Besides JC virus, herpes zoster encephalitis and CMV encephalitis may also cause areas of demyelination.

Nutritional, Metabolic, Toxic Diseases

41. What are the common nutritional and toxic diseases of the nervous system?

Ans. a. *Nutritional:*

1. Vitamin B_1 (thiamine) deficiency.
   a. Wernicke's encephalopathy.
   b. Korsakoff's psychosis.
2. Vitamin B_{12} deficiency (subacute combined degeneration of the spinal cord) and megaloblastic madness.

b. *Associated with systemic diseases:*

1. With hepatic failure.
2. With Wilson's disease.

c. *Associated with industrial toxins:*

1. Metals (arsenic, mercury, lead).
2. Organophosphates.
3. Methyl alcohol.
4. Carbon monoxide.

d. *Associated with therapeutic agents:*

1. Vinca alkaloids.
2. Metronidazole.
3. Methotrexate.

42. What is Wernicke's encephalopathy?

Ans. *DES:* Vitamin B_1 deficiency disease with involvement of brain and peripheral nerves. *ETIO:* Vitamin B_1 (thiamine) deficiency: Commonly seen in chronic alcoholics. *C/Fs:* Rapid onset of confusion, paralysis of extraocular muscles (mainly the lateral rectus), and ataxia which may progress to coma and **death** if untreated, but has good outcome by early treatment with thiamine. *MORPHO:* There is capillary endothelial proliferation with abnormal vascular permeability causing hemorrhages, commonly seen in mamillary bodies and thalamus.

43. What is Korsakoff's psychosis?

Ans. *DEF:* Progressive stage of untreated Wernicke's encephalopathy. *ETIO:* Vitamin B_1 deficiency. *C/Fs:* Inability to remember past events resulting in making up stories to fill the gap in the lost memory **(confabulation)**. Also, person is unable to remember new things. *MORPHO:* Changes are present in the same areas as Wernicke's encephalopathy. These are gliosis and hemosiderin deposition in areas of hemorrhages.

44. What is subacute combined degeneration of the cord?

Ans. *ETIO:* Vitamin B_{12} (cobalamin) deficiency. *MORPHO:* Myelin vacuolation in dorsal and lateral white matter columns of spinal cord. *C/Fs:* Motor and sensory abnormalities with spasticity, weakness, loss of propriosensation. **Megaloblastic madness:** Confusional state with vitamin B_{12} deficiency.

Infectious Diseases

45. What is meningitis/leptomeningitis?

Ans. *DEF:* Inflammation of the leptomeninges *ETIO*: Mostly infectious of 3 types:

1. Acute purulent meningitis—caused by bacteria.
2. Acute lymphocytic meningitis—usually caused by viruses.
3. Chronic meningitis—caused by many different organisms.

46. What is acute purulent meningitis?

Ans. *ETIO:* In neonates: Group B streptococci, *Eschericia coli*, *Listeria monocytogenes*. In children: Neisseria meningitidis (meningococcus), *S. pneumoniae* (pneumococcus). In adults: Pneumococci, meningococci, staphylococci, streptococci, listeria. *GROSS*: Meninges are very congested and opaque due to subarachnoid exudate. *MICRO:* Leptomeninges are hyperemic and infiltrated with PMNs.
C/Fs: Fever, headache, stiff neck, altered mental status photophobia, vomiting.

> Positive signs in meningitis are: **Brudzinskis sign** (flexion of the neck causes flexion of the legs) and **Kernig's sign** (when the thigh is flexed at a right angle, complete extension of the leg is not possible).

CSF: Not clear, containing PMNs, increased protein and decreased glucose. Causative microorganism can be determined by gram stain and culture. *PROG:* Good with immediate **empiric antibiotic treatment, without waiting for culture results, which is mandatory as minutes count to prevent death** which occurs in approximately 1/10 cases even with best care.

47. What is acute lymphocytic (viral) meningitis?

Ans. Viral meningitis is self-limiting and has better prognosis than bacterial meningitis. *ETIO*: Mumps virus, echovirus, coxsackie virus, and Epstein-Barr virus. *MORPHO*: There is lymphocytic infiltrate of the meninges. If encephalitis develops lymphocytic infiltrate is also seen in the Virchow-Robin spaces. *C/Fs:* Similar to bacterial meningitis, except less severe. *CSF:* Cells are mainly lymphocytes. Protein is elevated less than in bacterial meningitis. Glucose level is normal.

48. What is chronic meningitis?

Ans. *ETIO:* Usually by bacteria and fungi, mainly *Mycobacterium tuberculosis*. *Cryptococcus neoformans* (commonly in AIDS). *MORPHO: GROSS:* Leptomeninges are thick. Thick exudate in subarachnoid space is present. This is usually at the base in tuberculosis. *MICRO:* Lymphocytes, plasma cells, and epithelioid histiocytes. Caseous granulomas may be seen in tuberculosis. *C/Fs:* Headache, stiff neck. *CSF:* Increased number of mononuclear cells, increased protein and decreased glucose. In TB: Grossly *CSF* may have a fine fibrin web **(cobweb)**. Cells are mainly lymphocytes. Protein is elevated, but less in comparison to acute bacterial meningitis. Glucose is reduced but less relative to acute bacterial meningitis.

49. What is syphilis of the CNS?

Ans. *Cause: Treponema pallidum. PATHOG:* Congenital or acquired. In acquired: During early stages organism enters CNS. During secondary stage it may cause lymphocytic leptomeningitis. During tertiary stage it may involve meninges, vessels, or CNS parenchyma. Grossly meninges are thick. Microscopically, there is mononuclear infiltrate. Plasma cells are usually seen in syphilis.

50. What is tabes dorsalis?

Ans. Degeneration of dorsal sensory nerve roots and posterior columns of the spinal cord causing loss of vibration, position and pain sense resulting in ataxia and joint injury **(Charcot's joints)**.

51. What is general paresis of the insane (GPI)?

Ans. Brain parenchymal infection by syphilis. There is cortical atrophy, neuronal loss, leading to weakness and dementia.

52. What is encephalitis?

Ans. Infection of the brain parenchyma.

Types:
1. Localized-bacterial abscesses
2. Tuberculoma
3. Toxoplasmosis
4. Generalized viral encephalitis.

53. What is tuberculoma of the brain (brain TB)?

Ans. *PATHOG:* Usually secondary to pulmonary TB via hematogenous spread. May involve meninges or brain parenchyma. Typical tubercular granulomas are present.

54. What do you know about brain toxoplasmosis?

Ans. Causative organism is *Toxoplasma gondii*. Commonly affects AIDS patients. Also, in neonates, is transmitted transplacentally from infected mother. (Part of TORCH test for expecting mothers). It also spreads by ingestion of foods contaminated by animal urine or feces; household pets, especially cats. In neonates, it results in hydrocephalus and mental retardation. X-ray reveals periventricular calcifications. Cerebral cortex, basal ganglia, retina, heart, lungs, liver are involved. Many focal lesions mainly in gray matter are seen in the brain. Microscopically, necrosis and mononuclear cell infiltrate are seen.

55. What is neurocysticercosis?

Ans. It is the infection of the brain by the cysticerci (larva) of *Taenia solium*. *C/Fs:* Based on the number and location of cysts in the brain.

56. What do you know about viral encephalitis?

Ans. Common histologic features are: Perivascular inflammatory cell infiltrate (perivascular cuffing) of lymphocytes, plasma cells and macrophages in the Virchow-Robin spaces; microglial nodules due to proliferation of glial cells. In some cases, intranuclear or intracytoplasmic inclusion bodies, e.g. intracytoplasmic **Negri bodies** in rabies and intranuclear inclusions of CMV.

57. What is herpes simplex encephalitis?

Ans. Most common cause of viral encephalitis. Commonly seen in young adults.

58. What is poliomyelitis?

Ans. Viral infection of the nervous system where the virus causes injury to the cranial nerve motor neurons and lower motor neurons (anterior horn cells of the spinal cord), causing inflammation, degeneration and necrosis leading to wasting and paralysis of the related muscles. Paralysis of respiratory muscles may cause death. Virus is excreted in feces and spreads by fecal-oral route.

59. What is rabies (hydrophobia)?

Ans. Rabies virus is an RNA virus with affinity for salivary glands and nervous tissue. It is present in the saliva of dogs, foxes, squirrels, bats, etc. whose bite transmits it to man. From the wound site virus enters nerves and goes to spinal cord and brain causing severe encephalitis with convulsions and severe muscle contractions upon minimal stimuli. **Once these symptoms develop, it is fatal. If active immunization is given before symptoms develop, it can be cured**. Cause of death is respiratory paralysis and cardiac arrhythmias. Microscopic findings are: neuronal degeneration, perivascular collection of mononuclear cells in the brainstem, spinal cord and intracytoplasmic eosinophilic inclusions **(Negri bodies)** in the hippocampus and Purkinje cells of the cerebellum.

60. What is cytomegalovirus infection of CNS?

Ans. People with immunodeficiency are commonly affected. It causes encephalomyelitis. Also, affects salivary glands, lungs, liver, kidneys. Giant cells are seen with eosinophilic inclusions in cytoplasm and nucleus. Infants with severe congenital infection may have mental retardation, microcephaly, chorioretinitis, hepatosplenomegaly. Periventricular calcification in the brain is seen.

61. What is HIV encephalitis?

Ans. AIDS dementia complex with progressive dementia consisting of disturbances of concentration, memory, thinking, lethargy, depression, personality changes, difficulty with balance, coordination and motor function. HIV virus is carried to the CNS inside monocytes-macrophages, which serve as viral reservoir. Also, HIV can cause aseptic meningitis, vacuolar myelopathy involving posterior and lateral columns of the spinal cord, and peripheral neuropathy.

62. What is St. Louis encephalitis?

Ans. Severity can vary from asymptomatic to very severe. Horses and birds are reservoir. Mosquito is the vector.

63. What is eastern equine encephalitis?

Ans. Has high mortality rate. Horses and birds are reservoir.

64. What is western equine encephalitis?

Ans. It is less severe than eastern equine encephalitis.

65. What is prion disease (spongiform encephalitis)?

Ans. Caused by **prions**, which are protein molecules without any nucleic acids such as DNA or RNA. This idea of a protein able to multiply and cause disease is different from the traditional idea that only an organism with RNA or DNA can multiply and cause disease. Prions propagate in the host by changing normal prion protein (PrPc) into abnormal prion protein (PrPsc) by changing its shape and configuration by acting as a mold. Examples are: CJD (Creutzfeldt-Jacob disease); kuru, scrapie, "mad cow" disease, etc. Spongiform appearance with many small cysts are present in the gray matter. No inflammatory response is seen. For prion disease doctor Prusiner received Nobel prize in 1997. He coined the term "prion" for "proteinaceous infectious particle". The most common form is scrapie, found in sheep and goats, which lose coordination causing inability to stand. They also become irritable and, in some cases, develop an intense itch that leads them to **scrape off their wool or hair (hence the name "scrapie")**. The other most worrisome prion disease affects the cows, the bovine spongiform encephalopathy **(mad cow disease)**. The human prion disease **kuru** has been seen only among the Fore Highlanders of Papua New Guinea, who developed ataxia and dementia due to ritualistic eating brain of their dead, which they do not do anymore with disappearance of this diseases. Another prion disease is **Creutzfeldt-Jakob disease**. It occurs sporadically worldwide and causes dementia. 1 in 10 cases is inherited. Also, a few cases are transmitted iatrogenically by corneal transplantation, use of contaminated surgical instruments, and injection of growth hormone derived from human pituitaries (before recombinant growth hormone became available). **Gerstmann-Straussler-Scheinker disease is inherited and appears in midlife** as ataxia and other signs of damage to the cerebellum. **Fatal familial insomnia** is inherited and appears in midlife with dementia followed by difficulty in sleeping. Mad cow disease is also called new-variant CJD. It is acquired by eating infected tissues of the affected cow.

Neoplasms

66. What is the classification of neoplasms of CNS?

Ans. A. Primary neuroglial intraparenchymal tumors:
  1. Astrocytomas:
     a. Fibrillary (diffuse):
        i. Well-differentiated.
        ii. Anaplastic.
        iii. Glioblastoma multiforme.
     b. Pilocytic.
  2. Oligodendrogliomas.
  3. Ependymomas.

B. Primitive neuroectodermal tumors:
  1. Medulloblastoma.
  2. Neuroblastoma.
  3. Pinealoblastoma.
  4. Ependymoblastoma.

C. Other primary intraparenchymal neoplasms:
  1. Primary lymphomas.
  2. Germ cell neoplasms.
  3. Neuronal neoplasm.
  4. Hemangioblastoma.

D. Meningiomas.

E. Metastatic neoplasms.

67. What are the types of astrocytomas?

Ans. These are mainly of 2 types:

a. Fibrillary b. Pilocytic.

68.a. What are fibrillary (diffuse) astrocytomas?

Ans. Three types:

1. Well-differentiated astrocytoma. 2. Anaplastic astrocytoma.
3. Glioblastoma multiforme.

1. *Well-differentiated astrocytoma: MORPH: GROSS:* These are poorly defined. *MICRO:* Increased number of astrocytes.
2. *Anaplastic astrocytoma: MORPH: GROSS:* Poorly defined like well-differentiated. *MICRO:* Show increased cellularity, nuclear pleomorphism, presence of mitoses, and vascular endothelial proliferation.

3. *Glioblastoma muiltiforme: MORPH: GROSS:* Infiltrative lesions with irregular areas of hemorrhage, necrosis and cystic changes. *MICRO:* Areas of necrosis surrounded by many tumor cells with prominent nuclei (pseudopallisading) are seen. Also, glomeruloid figures. *C/Fs: S/S* of increased intracranial pressure or focal abnormalities.

68.b. What are pilocytic astrocytomas?

Ans. These are more discrete and **less** aggressive. *MORPH: GROSS:* Fairly well-defined. *MICRO:* Astrocytes with long hair-like processes. Eosinophilic structures called **Rosenthal's fibres** are present.

69. What are oligodendrogliomas?

Ans. More common in childhood, usually in cerebral hemispheres. *MORPH: GROSS:* Soft, circumscribed. Calcification is often present and helps in diagnosis by X-ray. *MICRO:* Cells with round uniform nuclei with clear halo around them. *C/Fs:* Prognosis is worse than infiltrating astrocytoma and depends upon the grade.

70. What are ependymomas?

Ans. These are the tumors of the ependymal lining cells of the ventricular cavities of the brain and spinal cord. *MORPH: GROSS:* Well-demarcated, solid, papillary structures. *MICRO:* Elongated cells around blood vessels **(pseudorosettes)** or around a clear lumen **(true ependymal rosettes)**. *C/Fs:* Intracranial ependymomas commonly occur in the IV ventricle and may obstruct *CSF* outflow and cause hydrocephalus and increased intracranial pressure. They can spread via *CSF* within the sub arachnoid space.

71. What are primitive neuroectodermal tumors (PNET)?

Ans. These are tumors that arise from the embryonal cells. Those that arise in the CNS are: medulloblastomas, neuroblastomas, ependymoblastomas, pinealoblastomas. Non-neuronal PNET is **Ewing's** tumor which arises in the bone.

72. What are medulloblastomas?

Ans. Occur mostly in children in cerebellum, commonly located in the vermis of the cerebellum. *MICRO:* Made of small primitive cells with little cytoplasm **(small round blue cells)**.

The neoplastic cells can be present around a central fibrillar core **(Homer Wright pseudorosettes)**. *C/Fs:* These can extend into ventricles and spread along *CSF* causing *CSF* flow obstruction with raised intracranial pressure. So, these present with *S/S* of raised intracranial pressure and also gait abnormalities due to the involvement of the cerebellum.

73. What are other primary intraparenchymal CNS neoplasms?

Ans. i. Non-Hodgkin's lymphomas.

ii. Germ cell neoplasm (germinoma) similar to seminoma and ovarian dysgerminoma.
iii. Nerve cell tumors (neuronal tumor) ganglioglioma, gangliocytoma, neurocytoma.

74. What are meningiomas?

Ans. These are tumors of the meninges. May arise inside the skull or in spinal canal. *MORPH: GROSS:* Firm, discrete mass attached to duramater. *MICRO:* Neoplasm made of compact cells in whorls. **Psammoma bodies** (microscopic bodies with circular calcium in layers). *C/Fs:* Patients may have *S/S* of increased intracranial pressure.

75. What are common metastatic neoplasms of the brain?

Ans. Common metastatic neoplasms are carcinoma and melanomas.

Diseases of the Peripheral Nervous System Neuropathies

76. What is the classification of the diseases of the PNS (peripheral neuropathies)?

Ans. I. Types according to pathophysiology:
1. Wallerian degeneration.
2. Primary axonal degeneration.
3. Segmental demyelination.

II. Types according to causes:
1. *Metabolic and nutritional:* DM, vitamin B_1 deficiency, renal failure.
2. *Toxic:* Lead, arsenic, chemotherapeutic drugs (cisplatin, vincristine).
3. *Inflammatory:* **Guillain-Barre syndrome**, leprosy, sarcoidosis, vasculitis.
4. *Neoplastic:* Paraneoplastic neuropathy.
5. *Miscellaneous:* Amyloidosis.

77. What is Wallerian degeneration?

Ans. Is degeneration of axons distal to the point of injury to the nerve. Seen in trauma and vasculitis with ischemia.

78. What is primary axonal degeneration?

Ans. Is degeneration of axon due to derangement of the nerve cell and occurs from distal to proximally. Seen in nutritional deficiencies and toxins.

79. What is segmental demyelination?

Ans. Here the injury is to the myelin sheath and the axons are normal. Seen in Guillain-Barre syndrome and other inflammatory neuropathies.

80. What is Guillain-Barre syndrome?

Ans. *DES:* It is an acute monophasic (i.e. it does not recur) demyelinating polyneuropathy. It is a **life-threatening disease** of the peripheral nervous system with rapidly progressive ascending motor weakness and failure of respiratory muscles. *ETIO:* Unknown. Possibly immunologic resulting from viral illness, mycoplasma infection, allergic reaction, trauma, surgical procedure. Pathogenesis is possibly autoallergic resulting from **molecular mimicry** due to sharing of liposaccharides of microorganisms and nerve gangliosides. *MORPHO:* Peripheral nerves have inflammation with segmental demyelination. *LAB: CSF* has increased level of protein; but, little cellular reaction.

Neoplasms

81. What are the neoplasms of the PNS?

Ans. a. Schwannomas of VIII cranial nerve: Acoustic neuroma (vestibular schwannoma).

b. Neurofibroma.

82. What are schwannomas?

Ans. *DEF/DES:* Neoplasm of the Schwann sheath of the peripheral nerves. *C/Fs:* Can be hereditary as seen in neurofibromatosis. In these cases schwannomas arise in childhood and are multiple. Seen in cranial nerves (commonly VIII-called acoustic neuroma) or peripheral nerves. *MORPHO: GROSS:* Well-circumscribed mass. *MICRO:* Densely packed spindle cells are present (Antoni A tissue) with some areas of peripheral lining up (palisading of nuclei called **Verocay bodies**). The dense areas (**Antoni A** tissue) are mixed with loose, areas (**Antoni B** tissue). Normal cells are seen pushed to the periphery.

83. What are neurofibromas?

Ans. *DEF/DES:* Neoplasm of peripheral nerves. *ETIO:* Unknown, sometimes seen with hereditary conditions [neurofibromatosis types 1 **(von Recklinghausen's disease)** and 2]. *C/Fs:* In neurofibromatosis these have potential for malignant transformation. *MORPHO: GROSS:* Produce a fusiform enlargement of the nerve. *MICRO:* Interlacing bundles of long cells with thin wavy nuclei. Normal cells are mixed with these neoplastic cells unlike schwannoma. With malignant transformation there is increased cellularity and mitoses.

14 Diseases of the Endocrine System (ES)

OVERVIEW

a. *Pituitary anterior:*
   1. Hyperpituitarism.
   2. Hypopituitarism.

b. *Pituitary posterior:*
   1. ADH increased—SIADH.
   2. ADH decreased—diabetes insipidus.

c. *Thyroid:*
   1. Congenital anomalies—Thyroglossal duct cyst.
   2. Hyperthyroidism.
   3. Hypothyroidism.
   4. Thyroiditis.
   5. Goiter.
   6. Neoplasms.

d. *Parathyroid:*
   1. Hyperparathyroidism.
   2. Hypoparathyroidism/pseudohypoparathyroidism.
   3. Neoplasms.

e. *Adrenal cortex:*
   1. Hyperfunction of cortisol, aldosterone, androgens.
   2. Hypofunction.
   3. Neoplasms.

f. *Adrenal medulla:*
   1. Pheochromocytoma.
   2. Extramedullary pheochromocytoma (paraganglioma).

g. *Endocrine pancreas:*
   1. Diabetes mellitus (DM).
   2. Neoplasms.

h. *Multiple endocrine neoplasia (MEN):* I, IIA, IIB.

Major diseases of the endocrine system are:

1. Increased function.
2. Decreased function.
3. Neoplasms.

Pituitary gland (*Hypophysis:* Anterior = Adenohypophysis, Posterior = Neurohypophysis).

Anterior pituitary increased function (hyperpituitarism) in children causes gigantism and in adults acromegaly. Common cause is pituitary adenomas.

Anterior pituitary decreased function (hypopituitarism) either panhypopituitarism **(Simmond's disease)** or isolated hypopituitarism with manifestations accordingly. Common causes are:

1. Non-secretory tumors.
2. Ischemia (postpartum ischemia with hypopituitarism is known as **Sheehan's syndrome**).

Posterior pituitary: No pathology from decreased or increased oxytocin. Decreased ADH results in diabetes insipidus. Increased ADH (**SIADH**—syndrome of inappropriate ADH secretion) results in hyponatremia, cerebral edema with neurologic dysfunction).

Thyroid Gland

Hyperthyroidism: The commonest cause is Graves' disease.

Hypothyroidism in children causes cretinism and in adult myxedema.

Hashimoto's thyroiditis is autoimmune inflammation of the thyroid causing painless thyroid enlargement with hypothyroidism (sometimes with initial temporary thyrotoxicosis due to inflammatory disruption of thyroid follicles with increased release of thyroid hormone) **(hashitoxicosis)**.

Some other types of thyroiditis are: Subacute granulomatous thyroiditis **(de Quervain)**, Riedel thyroiditis, etc.

Goiter is compensatory enlargement of thyroid due to impaired thyroid hormone synthesis due to iodine deficiency causing increased compensatory secretion of TSH by the anterior pituitary.

Types:

1. Endemic in mountainous regions.
2. Sporadic.

Neoplasms of thyroid gland are:

A. *Benign:* Follicular adenoma.

B. *Malignant:*
   1. Follicular adenocarcinoma.
   2. Papillary adenocarcinoma.
   3. Medullary carcinoma.
   4. Anaplastic adenocarcinoma.

Parathyroid Glands

Types of hyperparathyroidism are:

A. *Primary:*
   1. Adenoma.
   2. Primary hyperplasia.
   3. Adenocarcinoma.

B. *Secondary:*

1. Renal.
2. Gastrointestinal.

C. *Tertiary:*

Types of hypoparathyroidism are:

1. Primary atrophy.
2. Surgical removal.
3. Pseudohypoparathyroidism.

Neoplasms of parathyroid:

1. Benign—adenoma.
2. Malignant—adenocarcinoma.

Adrenal Glands

Types of hyperadrenalism:

1. Hypercortisolism (Cushing's syndrome).
2. Hyperaldosteronism.
3. Adrenogenital syndrome (hyperandrogenism).

Types of hypoadrenalism:

I. *Primary*

1. *Acute:*
   A. Waterhouse-Friderichsen syndrome.
   B. Suddenly stopping long-term steroid treatment.
   C. Acute stress in patients with underlying chronic adrenal insufficiency.
2. *Chronic:*
   A. Autoimmune adrenalitis.
   B. Metastatic diseases.
   C. TB.
   D. Fungal infections.
   E. Sarcoidosis.
   F. Systemic amyloidosis.
   G. Hemochromatosis.

II. *Secondary:* Disroders of hypothalamus or pituitary.

Adrenal neoplasms:

1. *Cortical:*
   A. Benign—adenomas.
   B. Malignant—carcinomas.
2. *Medullary:*
   A. Pheochromocytoma.
   B. Neuroblastoma.
   C. Ganglioneuroma.

Endocrine Pancreas

Diabetes mellitus: A chronic disorder of carbohydrate, fat and protein metabolism with decreased utilization of glucose and hyperglycemia.

Types:

A. *Primary:*
   1. Type I (insulin-dependent).
   2. Type II

B. *Secondary:*
   1. Pancreatectomy.
   2. Mucoviscidosis of pancreas.
   3. Chronic pancreatitis.
   4. Hemochromatosis **(bronze diabetes)**.

Complications:

A. *Acute:*
   1. Hyperglycemia.
   2. Hypoglycemia.
   3. Ketoacidosis.
   4. Hyperosmolar coma.

B. *Chronic:*
   1. Atherosclerosis with ischemic diseases—MI, stroke, gangrene.
   2. Retinopathy.
   3. Nephropathy.
   4. Neuropathy.
   5. Cataract.
   6. Glaucoma.

Insulinoma: Hypoglycemia with hyperinsulinemia.

Gastrinoma: **Zollinger-Ellison syndrome**.

Multiple Endocrine Neoplasia (MEN)

MEN-I:

1. Parathyroid hyperplasia.
2. Pituitary (prolactin or somatotropin secreting adenoma).
3. Pancreas (gastrinoma with **Zollinger-Ellison syndrome**, insulinoma with hypoglycemia).

MEN-IIA:

1. Parathyroid hyperplasia.
2. Thyroid (medullary carcinoma).
3. Adrenal (pheochromocytoma).

MEN-IIB:

1. Thyroid (medullary carcinoma).
2. Adrenal (pheochromocytoma).
3. Ganglioneuroma of GIT.

Pituitary Gland

1. What is the normal structure of pituitary gland?

Ans. It lies at the base of the skull in the pituitary fossa of the sphenoid bone. It has 3 parts:

1. Anterior pituitary (adenohypophysis).
2. Intermediate part (pars intermedia).
3. Posterior pituitary (neurohypophysis).

Anterior pituitary: Chromophil (acidophil and basophil) and chromophobe cells.

Pars intermedia: Part of anterior pituitary derived from cells lining Rathke's pouch lying between anterior and posterior pituitary. Small cysts (remnants of Rathke's pouch) might be present.

Posterior pituitary: Made of nonmyelinated axons of neurosecretory cells of hypothalamus.

2. What are the hormones of the anterior pituitary?

Ans.
1. Somatotrophic hormone (growth hormone).
2. TSH.
3. ACTH.
4. Gonadotrophic hormones:
   a. FSH: This stimulates the development of graafian follicle in the ovary and formation of spermatozoa in the testis.
   b. LH: It regulates the secretion of estrogens and progesterone in the ovary and testosterone in the testis.
   c. Prolactin (luteotrophin): It regulates the secretion of milk and maintains the corpus luteum during pregnancy.

3. What are the hormones of the posterior pituitary (produced by the nerve cells of hypothalamus)?

Ans.
1. *ADH (vasopressin):* This regulates the amount of water passed by the kidneys.
2. *Oxytocin:* It stimulates the contraction of the uterus during birth of the baby and release of milk during feeding the baby.

4. What are the causes of hyperpituitarism?

Ans. *Causes of hyperpituitarism:*

1. Adenomas.
2. Carcinomas.
3. Hyperplasia.
4. Secretion of hormones by non-pituitary tumors, and
5. Some hypothalamic disorders.

5. What are the types of pituitary neoplasms?

Ans. *Types:*

1. Prolactinoma.
2. Growth hormone (somatotroph cell) adenoma.
3. Corticotroph cell adenoma.
4. Gonadotroph-luteinizing hormone (LH) and follicle stimulating hormone (FSH)-producing adenoma.
5. Thyrotroph-thyroid stimulating hormone (TSH)-producing adenoma.
6. Primary adenocarcinomas.

6. What are pituitary adenomas?

Ans. *DEF/DES:* Benign neoplasms of the pituitary gland. *C/Fs:* Pituitary adenomas may be nonfunctional; or functional. Functional cause hyperpituitarism of one particular type since usually they are made of a single cell type therefore, usually produce a single hormone. Nonfunctional may cause hypopituitarism as they compress and destroy adjacent normal anterior pituitary tissue. Also, pituitary adenomas may grow superiorly and compress the optic chiasm causing vision problems with defects in the lateral visual fields (temporal-bitemporal hemianopsia). Also, they can produce signs and symptoms of raised intracranial pressure such as headache, nausea, vomiting. *MORPH: GROSS:* Most of them are encapsulated tumors with smooth surfaces. *MICRO:* These are made of uniform cells arranged in sheets, without reticulin network of normal pituitary. Cytoplasm may be acidophilic (pink) basophilic (blue) or chromophobe (clear) depending upon the hormone present.

7. What is a prolactinoma of the pituitary gland?

Ans. *DEF/DES:* Prolactin secreting benign tumor of the anterior pituitary gland. *C/Fs:* Symptoms are those of hyperprolactinemia such as amenorrhea, galactorrhea, loss of libido, and infertility. *MORPH: GROSS:* Mostly <1 cm. *MICRO:* Most have chromophobe or weakly acidophilic cells.

8. What is growth hormone (somatotroph cell) adenoma of pituitary gland?

Ans. *DEF:* Growth hormone secreting benign tumor of the anterior pituitary gland. *C/Fs:* When these occur in childhood before the closure of the bone epiphyses then it can cause **gigantism** with generalized increase in the size of the body. But, the arms and legs are disproportionately large. When these tumors occur in adults after the closure of the bone epiphyses then it causes a condition called **acromegaly** with increased growth in soft tissues, skin, viscera and in the bones of face, hands, and feet. Jaw enlargement causes it to protrude outwards **(prognathism)**. Increased growth hormone also causes DM, generalized muscle weakness, hypertension, arthritis, osteoporosis, CHF. *MORPHO:* Cells are usually acidophilic.

9. What is corticotroph cell adenoma of pituitary gland?

Ans. *DEF/DES:* Corticosteroids secreting benign tumor of the anterior pituitary gland. *C/Fs:* Excess secretion of the glucocorticoids may result in hypercortisolism **(Cushing's disease)**. *MORPHO: GROSS:* Usually small. *MICRO:* Cells are usually basophilic.

10. What is Nelson syndrome?

Ans. Severe enlargement of corticotroph microadenoma of the pituitary gland after bilateral surgical adrenalectomy for Cushing's syndrome due to lack of inhibitory feedback. This causes mass effect and hyperpigmentation due to melanocyte stimulating hormone.

11. What is panhypopituitarism (Simmond's disease)?

Ans. *DEF/DES:* Decreased pituitary function. *ETIO:* Mainly 2 causes:

1. Pressure atrophy by non-secretary pituitary adenomas.
2. Ischemic necrosis of the pituitary.

1. *Pressure atrophy by non-secreting pituitary adenomas:* Gradual or acute if there is acute hemorrhage in tumor **(pituitary apoplexy can cause sudden death).**
2. *Ischemic necrosis of the pituitary:* Causes:
   a. Postpartum hemorrhage **(Sheehan's syndrome).**
   b. DIC, shock.
   c. Sickle cell anemia.

C/Fs: **Dwarfism** in children, infertility in women, hypothyroidism, hypoadrenalism due to the deficiencies of growth hormone, gonadotropin, TSH and ACTH respectively.

12. What is normal structure and function of posterior pituitary gland (neurohypophysis)?

Ans. It is made of axonal processes of the nerve cell, the bodies of which are present in the hypothalamus. These nerve cell bodies produce 2 hormones:

1. Oxytocin.
2. Antidiuretic hormone (ADH).

1. *Oxytocin:* Stimulates the contraction of pregnant uterus during labor and release of milk during feeding of the baby.
2. *ADH:* Acts on collecting tubules of the kidneys, promoting resorption of water, thereby decreasing its passage in the urine, i.e. decreasing diuresis (antidiuresis). So, when ADH is decreased, decreased amount of water is resorbed and increased amount of water is passed in the urine **(diabetes insipidus)** resulting in increased serum sodium and osmolality requiring drinking of extra water. People who cannot drink enough water to compensate can develop serious dehydration. When ADH is increased, **SIADH (syndrome of inappropriate ADH) secretion,** increased amount of water is resorbed with less passing in urine leading to

increased water in the body resulting in hyponatremia and cerebral edema. This occurs commonly from ectopic ADH secretion by malignant neoplasms, e.g. small cell carcinoma of lung.

13. What are posterior pituitary syndromes?

Ans. No clinical condition occurs with decreased or increased oxytocin secretion. Clinical conditions from decreased ADH secretion is: **Diabetes insipidus** as described above. And, increased ADH secretion (SIADH) is described above.

14. What is craniopharyngioma?

Ans. It is a suprasellar tumor arising from Rathke's pouch, which by pressure effect on adjacent structures may cause retardation of growth or disturbances of vision.

Thyroid Gland

15. Briefly describe normal histology of thyroid gland.

Ans. Thyroid gland has 2 lobes, one on each side of trachea connected by a strip of thyroid tissue, which lies in front of trachea. *Histology:* Vesicles lined by cuboidal epithelium and filled with thyroxine. Also, calcitonin secreting parafollicular cells are present.

16. What is thyrotoxicosis?

Ans. *DEF/DES:* Increase in thyroxine (T_4) and tri-iodothyronine (T_3) with increase in basal metabolic rate (BMR).

ETIO:

A. Due to hyperfunction of thyroid gland:

1. Graves' disease (diffuse hyperfunctional goiter).
2. Hyperfunctional solitary nodular goiter **(Plummer disease/syndrome)** or multinodular goiter.
3. Hyperfunctional thyroid adenoma.
4. TSH secreting pituitary adenoma.

B. Not due to hyperfunction of thyroid gland:

1. Ectopic thyroid in ovarian teratomas **(struma ovarii)** with excess secretion of thyroxine.
2. Temporary, e.g. **hashitoxicosis** in Hashimoto's thyroiditis.
3. Iatrogenic: Excess thyroxine replacement in patients for hypothyroidism.

C/Fs: Increased BMR, intestinal hypermotility with diarrhea, tremors, tachycardia, palpitations, hyperreflexia, irritability, CHF wide staring gaze and lid lag, skin warm, excessive sweating, heat intolerance, weight loss, increased appetite.

DIAG: Decreased thyroid stimulating hormone (TSH) and free T_4 increased.

17. What is thyroid storm?

Ans. A condition of **medical emergency** consisting of acute onset of severe thyrotoxicosis usually in patients with Graves' disease, most likely from increased catecholamine levels. Cardiac arrhythmia causes **death** if not treated immediately. Tests/diagnosis: TSH levels are low (in primary hyperthyroidism). Free T_4 levels are high. T_3 high in patients with T_3 thyrotoxicosis. Radioactive iodine uptake is high in the hyperfunctioning thyroid gland.

18. What is Graves' disease?

Ans. *DEF/DES:* An autoimmune disorder of the thyroid gland with:

1. Hyperfunctional diffuse enlargement of thyroid (most common type of hyperthyroidism).
2. Exophthalmos in approximately 1/2 the patients.
3. Pretibial myxedema in a few patients.

ETIO/PATHOG: Autoimmune (Type II hypersensitivity). Antibodies to TSH receptor, microsomes, thyroglobulin, and thyroid hormones (T_3 and T_4) are present. *C/Fs:* Female more commonly affected. *S/S* are those of thyrotoxicosis, as above. *MORPHO: GROSS:* There is diffuse enlargement of the thyroid gland which is smooth and soft. *MICRO:* Thyroid gland is diffusely enlarged with an intact capsule. There is both diffuse hypertrophy and hyperplasia of the thyroid follicular epithelial cells with crowding of cells causing papillary formation, which do not have a fibrovascular core (in papillary carcinoma papillae have fibrovascular core-helps in *D/D*). Follicles have scalloped margins. Also, there is hypertrophy of the heart, mucopolysaccharides collection in orbit, thickening of dermis.

19. What is hypothyroidism?

Ans. *DEF/DES:* Decreased thyroid hormone production.

ETIO:

A. Primary: Iodine deficiency, post-surgery/radio iodine treatment, Hashimoto's thyroiditis.

B. Secondary (pituitary failure).

C/Fs: Two types:

1. Cretinism (in children) 2. Myxedema (in adults).

20. What is autoimmune hypothyroidism?

Ans. Most common cause of hypothyroidism. Antithyroid antibodies are present causing inflammation, lymphocytic infiltration, atrophy and fibrosis. Can be seen with other autoimmune diseases, e.g. pernicious anemia, etc.

21. What is cretinism?

Ans. Hypothyroidism during infancy and childhood. *ETIO:* Iodine deficiency. Impaired development of skeletal system and CNS. *C/Fs:* Severe mental retardation, coarse facial features, protruding tongue, umbilical hernia.

22. What is myxedema?

Ans. Hypothyroidism in older children and adults. *ETIO/PATHOG:* Iodine deficiency. Mucopolysaccharide collects in skin, subcutaneous tissue and viscera. *C/Fs:* Coarse facial features, enlarged tongue, deepening of voice, constipation, heart failure, mental slowness and cold intolerance. Lab tests: TSH level is high in primary myxedema, T_4 is decreased.

23. What is nontoxic goiter?

Ans. *DEF/DES:* Compensatory enlargement of thyroid due to impaired thyroid hormone synthesis. *ETIO/PATHOG:* Decreased thyroid hormone synthesis, which results in increased TSH secretion leading to hypertrophy and hyperplasia of thyroid gland. *Types:*

1. Endemic
2. Sporadic

1. *Endemic:* In areas with iodine deficiency, e.g. Mountainous regions of the world, e.g. Himalayas, Andes. The reason for this is that natural source of iodine is sea water which is distributed on earth by the rain through the clouds; and, by the time the clouds with rain reach the mountainous regions their iodine content is quite depleted. However, now incidence has decreased due to iodine supplementation in diet.
2. *Sporadic:* This is in some cases due to ingestion of foods which interfere in thyroid hormone synthesis, e.g. cabbage, cauliflower, turnips, etc.

   There are recurrent episodes of stimulation and involution leading to:

   1. Diffuse nontoxic goiter.
   2. Colloid goiter.
   3. Nodular/multinodular goiter.

   C/Fs: *S/S* of mass effects of enlarged thyroid gland, e.g. airway obstruction, dysphagia, compression of large cervical and upper thoracic vessels. Also, a nodule might become hyperfunctioning causing hyperthyroidism **(Pulmmer syndrome)**. Sometimes there might by hypothyroidism.

   MORPHO:

   1. *Diffuse nontoxic goiter:* Follicles are lined by many columnar cells with papillary formation.
   2. *Colloid goiter:* When the demand for thyroid hormone decreases or dietary iodine increases the follicular epithelium involutes to form an enlarged, colloid-filled gland. *GROSS:* Cut surface is brown, glassy and translucent due to the increased presence of colloid. *MICRO:* In early stages the epithelium is hyperplastic and later flattened.
   3. *Nodular/multinodular goiter: GROSS:* Thyroid is asymmetrically enlarged with cut surface showing irregular nodules with brown colloid, focal fibrosis, hemorrhage and calcification. *MICRO:* Some follicles are lined by flat epithelium and contain abundant colliod and some follicles have hypertrophic and hyperplastic epithelium.

24. What is Hashimoto's thyroiditis?

Ans. *DEF/DES:* Autoimmune inflammatory disease of thyroid. *ETIO/PATHOG:* CD4+T lymphocytes are activated, which activate CD8+T cytotoxic lymphocytes and B lymphocytes to produce thyroid antibodies. Cytotoxic T cell injure thyroid tissue causing hypothyroidism. Anti-TSH receptor antibodies block the action of TSH, contributing to hypothyroidism. In early stage due to inflammatory injury follicles release thyroid hormone resulting in temporary thyrotoxicosis **(hashitoxicosis)**. *C/Fs:* More common in females. Gradual onset with slow painless enlargement of thyroid with temporary hyperthyroidism followed by gradual hypothyroidism. *MORPH: GROSS:* Diffuse enlargement of thyroid. Cut surface is pale. *MICRO:* Lymphocytic infiltrate with germinal centers is present. Follicles focally are lined by eosinophilic cytoplasm called **oxyphil** or **Hürthle cells**. Antithyroid antibodies are present in ~90% of the patients and are helpful in the diagnosis of this condition.

25. What is subacute (granulomatous) thyroiditis (de Quervain's disease)?

Ans. *DEF/DES:* Subacute inflammation of the thyroid of unknown etiology. *PATHOG:* Due to injury from inflammation there is extravasation of colloid with foreign body type granuloma formation. *C/Fs:* More common in females with acute onset with pain, fever, and mild enlargement of the thyroid. There is temporary hyperthyroidism from excess release of thyroxine due to inflammatory injury. *PROG:* Spontaneous complete recovery in approximately 2 months.

26. What is Riedel's thyroiditis?

Ans. Inflammation of thyroid of unknown cause with extensive fibrosis making thyroid feel hard.

27. What is the classification of thyromegaly?

Ans. A. *Simple:* Puberty, pregnancy.

B. *Iodine deficiency:* Endemic/sporadic.
   1. Single nodule (solitary nodular).
   2. Many nodules (multinodular).
   3. Colloid.
   4. Diffuse nontoxic.

C. *Inflammatory:*
   1. Infectious:
      a. Suppurative.
      b. Tuberculous.
   2. Autoimmune.
      a. Graves (diffuse hyperthyroid).
      b. Hashimoto (diffuse hypothyroid).
   3. Unknown.

a. de Querain's disease.
b. Reidel (fibrotic hard).
c. Sarcoidosis (non-caseating granulomatous).

D. *Drugs:* Sulphonyl ureas.

E. *Neoplasms:*

1. Adenoma.
2. Adenocarcinoma:
   a. Papillary b. Follicular
   c. Medullary d. Anaplastic.
3. Lymphoma. Also *see* page 299 (thyrotoxicosis).

28. What is the classification of thyroid neoplasms?

Ans. 1. *Benign:* Adenoma.

2. *Malignant:* Carcinomas.
   a. Papillary carcinoma.
   b. Follicular carcinoma.
   c. Medullary carcinoma.
   d. Anaplastic.

29. What is the adenoma of the thyroid gland?

Ans. It is benign neoplasm of thyroid gland. *MORPHO: GROSS:* Single, round, encapsulated tumor. Cut surface is whitish brownish with focal hemorrhage. *MICRO:* Capsule is intact. It is made of follicles which have normal appearance. There are **no papillary changes. If papillary changes seen, encapsulated papillary carcinoma should be suspected**. *C/Fs:* Usually, presentation is with painless mass, sometimes with dysphagia.

30. What is papillary carcinoma of thyroid gland?

Ans. It is a malignant neoplasm of thyroid gland. *C/Fs:* Slow-growing cancer with more than 10 years survival. *MORPHO: GROSS:* Well-circumscribed, sometimes infiltrative. *MICROS:* Papillary structure. Nuclei of cells have very fine dispersed chromatin making them appear clear/ground glass/**Orphan annie** (diagnostic criteria). Concentrically calcified structures **(Psammoma bodies)** are present which help in *D/D* from papillary hyperplasia, where they are not present.

31. What is follicular carcinoma of thyroid gland?

Ans. It is a malignant neoplasm of thyroid gland. Present as single "cold" thyroid nodule. (Rarely "hot"). *GROSS:* Well-circumscribed or infiltrative. *MICRO:* Follicles with colloid in them, which appear like normal thyroid making diagnosis difficult. Capsular and vascular invasion helps in making the diagnosis.

32. What is anaplastic carcinoma of thyroid gland?

Ans. It is a malignant neoplasm of thyroid gland. One of the most aggressive human neoplasms. *GROSS:* Bulky mass, growing beyond thyroid capsule into adjacent neck structures. *MICRO:* Very anaplastic cells, some large giant cells are also present. *C/Fs:* Mostly seen in elderly people. Metastasize early to distant organs causing death in less than one year.

33. What is medullary carcinoma of thyroid?

Ans. It is a malignant neoplasm of thyroid gland. Arises from calcitonin-secreting cells. Sporadic in 3/4 cases and with MEN (multiple endocrine neoplasia) II or III in 1/4 of cases. *GROSS:* Single nodule in sporadic cases and multiple nodules in cases with MEN. *MICRO:* Polygonal and spindle-shaped cells in nests. Stroma has amyloid made from calcitonin. *C/Fs:* Patients usually present with painless thyroid mass, sometimes causing dysphagia. *PROG:* Cases with MEN are aggressive. Sporadic cases are not aggressive.

Parathyroid Glands

34. What are parathyroid glands?

Ans. There are 4 parathyroid glands, 2 behind each thyroid lobe. These secrete parathormone, which regulates calcium metabolism and the amount of calcium in blood and bone.

35. What is classification of hyperparathyroidism?

Ans. 1. Primary 2. Secondary.

36. What is primary hyperparathyroidism?

Ans. *DEF/DES:* Increased parathyroid activity due to cause in the parathyroid gland/s. *ETIO/PATHOG:*

1. Adenoma of the parathyroid gland (commonest).
2. Primary hyperplasia of the parathyroid gland.
3. Adenocarcinoma of the parathyroid gland.

It can occur either sporadically or with MEN type 1 and 2. Parathyroid hormone activates osteoclasts in the bone mobilizing calcium out of the bone into bloodstream causing hypercalcemia, increased reabsorption of calcium from the kidney and absorption in the GIT, and increases conversion of vitamin D to active dihydroxy form in the kidneys and increases urinary phosphate excretion. *C/Fs:* Main feature is increased serum calcium. Increased serum calcium leads to increased excretion of calcium in kidneys causing **kidney stones and deposition in interstitial tissue called nephrocalcinosis**. Increased mobilization of calcium

out of bones make them brittle and prone to fractures. Also there are *S/S* of constipation, nausea, peptic ulcers, pancreatitis, gallstones depression, lethargy, seizures, weakness, hypotonia, polyuria, polydypsia **(renal stones, painful bones, abdominal groans, mental moans)**. Also *see* chapter 16.

37. What is secondary hyperparathyroidism?

Ans. *DEF/DES:* Hyperparathyroidism due to primary disease in some other organ than parathyroid glands. *ETIO/PATHOG:* Function of parathyroid gland is dependent on level of free calcium in the serum and not trophic hormones from hypothalamus or pituitary unlike other endocrine glands. Hypocalcemia stimulates parathyroid gland to increase function and vice versa. Main cause of hypocalcemia is renal failure with retention of phosphates and reduction of serum calcium. *C/Fs:* Similar to primary hyperparathyroidism. *MORPHO:* Parathyroid glands are hyperplastic, but not symmetrically as seen in primary. *MICRO:* Hyperplastic glands have increased number of chief cells, or cells with clear cytoplasm (water clear cells). Bone changes as seen in primary are present. Metastatic calcium deposit may be seen in lungs, heart, BVs. Also *see* chapter 16.

38. What is tertiary hyperparathyroidism?

Ans. It is the development of autonomous parathyroid hyperplasia after long-standing secondary hyperparathyroidism commonly due to renal failure.

39. What is hypoparathyroidism?

Ans. *DEF/DES:* Decreased function of parathyroid glands with decreased serum calcium levels. *ETIO:* Surgical removal or congenital absence of parathyroid glands. *C/Fs:* *S/S* are those of hypocalcemia: Tingling, neuromuscular irritability with positive **Chvostek's** and **Trousseau's signs**, carpopedal spasm and sometimes seizures.

Chvostek's sign is that tapping over the facial nerve causes facial spasm in case of hypocalcemia-tetany.

Trousseau's sign is that carpal spasm is produced by inflating a blood pressure cuff around the arm above the systolic pressure indicating hypocalcemia.

40. What is pseudohypoparathyroidism?

Ans. Parathyroid is normal; however, there is loss of responsiveness to PTH.

41. What is parathyroid adenoma?

Ans. *C/Fs:* Usually in single gland. Other 3 parathyroid glands are usually normal in size or somewhat shrunken owing to feedback inhibition by elevations in serum calcium. (Unlike primary hyperplasia where the other glands are larger in size). *MORPHO: GROSS:* Well-circumscribed nodule. *MICRO:* Uniform, polygonal chief cells with small, normochromic nuclei.

42. What is parathyroid carcinoma?

Ans. *GROSS:* Circumscribed making differentiation with adenoma difficult. MICRO: Composed of uniform benign-appearing tumor cells. Hence, for definite diagnosis of malignancy, local invasion or distant metastasis of tumor is necessary.

Adrenal Glands

43. What are adrenal glands?

Ans. Adrenal gland lies at the upper pole of the kidney, one on each side. Consists of outer cortex and inner medulla. Cortex has 3 layers:

1. Zona glomerulosa (secretes mineralocorticoids).
2. Zona fasiculata (secretes glucocorticoids).
3. Zona reticularis (secretes sex hormones).

Medulla secretes noradrenaline and adrenaline.

44. What is the classification of hyperadrenalism?

Ans. 1. Hypercortisolism (Cushing's syndrome). 2. Hyperaldosteronism. 3. Adrenogenital syndromes (hyperandrogenism).

45. What is classification of hypoadrenalism?

Ans. I. Primary:

a. *Acute:*
   1. Waterhouse-Friderichsen syndrome.
   2. Sudden discontinuation of long-term steroid therapy.
   3. Acute stress in patients with underlying chronic adrenal insufficiency.

b. *Chronic (Addison's disease):*
   1. Autoimmune adrenalitis.
   2. Metastatic diseases.
   3. TB.
   4. Fungal infections.
   5. Sarcoidosis.
   6. Systemic amyloidosis.
   7. Hemochromatosis.

II. Secondary: Disorders of hypothalamus or pituitary.

46. What is Cushing's syndrome (hypercortisolism)?

Ans. *DEF/DES:* Condition due to increased level of glucocorticoids.

ETIO/PATHOG:

1. Primary pituitary disease with increased secretion of ACTH **(Cushing's disease)**.

2. Ectopic ACTH secretion by nonendocrine neoplasms (paraneoplastic syndrome, e.g. small cell carcinoma of the lung).
3. Adrenocortical hyperplasia or neoplasm.
4. Iatrogenic with administration of glucocorticoids.

C/Fs: Onset is gradual. *S/S* are weight gain, hypertension, truncal obesity, moon facies, accumulation of fat in posterior neck and back (buffalo hump), decreased muscle mass, hyperglycemia (due to gluconeogenesis and decreased uptake of glucose by cells), *hypernatremia*, hypokalemia, skin is thin, with easy bruisability, osteoporosis due to bone resorption with increased susceptibility to fractures. Glucocorticoids suppress immune response thereby increasing susceptilbility to infections. Hirsutism, and menstrual abnormalities, mental disturbances. *Tests:* 24-hour urine free cortisol is increased; loss of normal diurnal pattern of cortisol secretion. Localization of cause is done by level of serum ACTH and urinary steroid excretion measurement done by dexamethasone test. *MORPHO:* In Cushing's syndrome due to exogenous glucocorticoids, zona fasciculata and reticularis are atrophied. In endogenous, adrenals are hyperplastic. In pituitary ACTH-producing cells have homogenous light basophilic substance from collection of intermediate cytokeratin filaments. This appearence of the cells is called **Crooke's hyaline change**.

47. What is dexamethasone test?

Ans. This test is done for *D/D* of Cushing's syndrome due to pituitary tumor, ectopic tumor or due to adrenal disease. The test consists of giving high dose of dexamethasone to the patient and then measuring the excretion of steroid in the urine. If the Cushing's syndrome is due to pituitary tumor, urinary corticosteroid excretion will decrease. It would stay the same in Cushing's syndrome due to ectopic tumor and adrenal disease. (However, in ectopic tumor blood ACTH is increased due to ectopic ACTH production. Whereas, in adrenal Cushing's syndrome ACTH is decreased due to feedback inhibition of pituitary ACTH secretion.)

48. What is hyperaldosteronism?

Ans. *DEF/DES:* Increased level of aldosterone causing sodium retention and potassium excretion with hypertension and hypokalemia. *ETIO/PATHOG:* Primary or secondary. *Primary:* Is due to either aldosterone producing adenoma or by primary adrenocortical hyperplasia. Increased aldosterone suppresses renin-angiotensin system and there is decreased plasma renin activity. Mostly are due to aldosterone secreting adenoma called **Conn's syndrome**. *Secondary:* Increased release of aldesterone is due to activation of renin-angiotensin system with increased plasma renin. Seen in decreased renal perfusion, e.g. arteriolar nephrosclerosis, renal artery stenosis, CHF. *C/Fs:* Age of onset of Conn's syndrome is middle age, more common in females. *S/S* are those of hypertension and hypokalemia. *MORPHO:* In Conn's syndrome there is usually one adenoma present. Since increased production of aldosterone does not suppress ACTH secretion remainder of the adrenal cortex of the same side and opposite side are normal. Remainder of the cases are due to primary adrenocortical hyperplasia where there is proliferation of cells in zona glomerulosa.

49. What is adrenogenital syndrome (hyperandrogenism)?

Ans. *DEF/DES:* Virilization due to increased androgenic hormones.

ETIO/PATHOG:

1. *Acquired:* Adrenocortical neoplasm, usually carcinomas.
2. *Congenital:* Due to autosomal recessive hereditary disorder of deficiency in enzymes (mostly 21-hydroxylase deficiency) which are involved in synthesis of cortisol. Decreased cortisol production increases ACTH secretion with resultant adrenal hyperplasia and increased production of cortisol precursor steroids, many having virilizing activity.

C/Fs: In prepubertal females virilization of external genitalia. In post pubertal females oligomenorrhea, hirsutism. In prepubertal males, premature puberty with enlargement of external genitalia. In postpubertal males oligospermia. *MORPHO:* Adrenals are hyperplastic bilaterally, with thickening of adrenal cortex.

50. What is primary acute adrenocortical insufficiency?

Ans. *DEF/DES:* A **life-threatening** condition due to acute deficiency of adrenocortical hormones.

ETIO:

1. Acute on chronic.
2. Massive adrenal hemorrhage, e.g. DIC.
3. **Waterhouse-Friderichsen syndrome**—overwhelming sepsis, e.g. in meningococcal infection.

51. What is Addisons's disease (primary chronic adrenocortical insufficiency)?

Ans. *DEF/DES:* Gradual prolonged decreased adrenocortical function.

ETIO:

1. Autoimmune.
2. TB.
3. Metastatic neoplasms.
4. Amyloidosis.
5. Sarcoidosis.

C/Fs: Weakness, anorexia, nausea, vomiting, weight loss, diarrhea. Hyperpigmentation of skin, hyperkalemia, hyponatremia, volume depletion and hypotension, hypoglycemia. **Stresses, e.g. infection, trauma may precipitate acute adrenal crisis** with vomiting, hypotension, coma and **death may result if not treated immediately**.

52. What is secondary adrenocortical insufficiency?

Ans. Due to disorders of hypothalamus or pituitary. *D/D* with primary adrenocortical insufficiency:

1. Serum ACTH is decreased.

2. Serum aldosterone is normal (because it is primarily regulated by renin-angiotensin system), severe hyperkalemia and hyponatremia are absent.
3. Hyperpigmentation is absent.

53. What is classification of adrenal neoplasms?

Ans. 1. *Cortical:*

A. Benign—adenomas B. Malignant—carcinomas

2. *Medullary:*

A. Pheochromocytoma B. Neuroblastoma C. Ganglioneuroma.

54. What is adenoma of the adrenal cortex?

Ans. It is benign neoplasm of adrenal cortex. *C/Fs:* Most nonfunctional. Usually found incidentally at autopsy. *MORPHO: GROSS:* Well-circumscribed nodule with yellowish cut surface. *MICRO:* Cells are normal appearing.

55. What is carcinoma of the adrenal cortex?

Ans. It is malignant neoplasm of adrenal cortex. More likely to be functional than adenoma, often cause virilism or other features of hyperadrenalism. Invade locally and metastasize by BV and lymphatics. *MORPHO: GROSS:* Large mass with cut surface showing areas of necrosis, and hemorrhage. Invasion of adrenal vessels and inferior vena cava is commonly seen. *MICRO:* Cells well to poorly differentiated.

56. What is pheochromocytoma?

Ans. It is neoplasm of chromaffin cells of adrenal medulla. *C/Fs:* Produce catecholamines with paroxysmal episodes of hypertension. *GROSS:* Small, circumscribed, confined to adrenal to large with cut surface yellow, hemorrhagic. *MICRO:* Polygonal cells with pleomorphic nuclei. Capsular and blood vessel invasion can be seen in benign. Hence, diagnosis of malignancy can be made by certainty by local invasion or dilatant metastasis. Urine shows increased free catecholamines and their metabolites, e.g. vanillyl mandelic acid (VMA). Approximately 10% of pheochromocytoma are: bilateral, arise from extra-adrenal organs, arise as component of multiple endocrine neoplasia (MEN), are malignant, are nonfunctional.

57. What is neuroblastoma?

Ans. It is neoplasm of neuronal cells of adrenal medulla. Seen in infants and children. Commonly arise from adrenal medulla or retroperitoneal sympathetic ganglia from primitive nerve cell, precursor cells. *GROSS:* Tiny nodule to very large mass with cut surface showing smooth white surface to areas of hemorrhage and necrosis. *MICRO:* Small round blue cells in sheet with hyperchromatic nuclei and little cytoplasm. **Homer-Wright pseudorosettes** are also present.

58. What is ganglioneuroma?

Ans. It is neoplasm of adrenal medulla with features of differentiation into: mature ganglion cells, which are large with plenty of pink cytoplasm, large clear nucleus with a large nucleolus.

Endocrine Pancreas

59. What is basic histology and physiology of endocrine pancreas?

Ans. Endocrine pancreas consists of microscopic groups of cells called islets of Langerhans. These cells are mainly of 4 types:

1. Alpha cells which secrete glucagons.
2. Beta cells which secrete insulin.
3. Delta cells which secrete somatostatin.
4. PP (Pancreatic polypeptide) cells which secrete polypeptides which cause stimulation of gastric and intestinal enzymes and decrease intestinal motility.

Functions: Main metabolic function of insulin is to increase the rate of transport of glucose into certain cells of the body, e.g. Skeletal muscle, cardiac muscle, fat cells, fibroblasts. Insulin is secreted in response to glucose level of blood.

60. What is diabetes mellitus?

Ans. *DEF/DES:* It is a chronic disorder of carbohydrate, fat and protein metabolism with decreased utilization of glucose and hyperglycemia.

ETIO/PATHOG:

a. *Secondary:* Postpancreatectomy, chronic pancreatitis, hemochromatosis, pheochromocytoma, etc.

b. *Primary:* There are 2 types of primary diabetes mellitus (DM):
   1. Type I (insulin-dependent).
   2. Type II (non-insulin-dependent).

61. What is type I DM?

Ans. Here there is severe absolute lack of insulin due to decrease in beta cells of the islets of Langerhans. This is caused by:

a. Genetic susceptibility.
b. Autoimmunity.
c. Environmental factors such as viral infection.

62. What is type II DM?

Ans. *Here the pathogenesis is:*

a. Initially abnormal beta cell response to blood glucose level and later mild to moderate permanent reduction in beta cells with decreased insulin blood level.
b. Insulin resistance, i.e. peripheral tissues do not respond to insulin.

63. What are complications of DM?

Ans. Complications of DM are:

a. *Acute:*
   1. Hypoglycemia.
   2. Hyperglycemia.
   3. Hyperosmolar coma.
   4. Diabetic ketoacidosis.

b. *Chronic:*
   1. Microangiopathy.
   2. Retinopathy.
   3. Nephropathy.
   4. Neuropathy.
   5. Atherosclerosis—MI, CVA.
   6. Hypertension.
   7. Foot ulcers/gangrene.
   8. Infections.

Pathogenesis of this is in 2 ways:

1. Nonenzymatic glycosylation with production of AGEs (irreversible advanced glycosylation end products) which collect in the vessel wall with resultant thickening and leakiness of the vessel walls. Also, these help in trapping of LDL promoting atherogenesis [Glycated hemoglobin (HbA1c) is used to test diabetes control during 120-day-period (life of RBC)].
2. Some tissues, e.g. lens, nerves, kidney do not need insulin for glucose transport. So, there is increased intracellular glucose, which metabolizes to sorbitol and fructose which lead to increased intracellular osmolarity with influx of water and injury. In lens this causes opacity, in nerves and retina peripheral neuropathy and retinopathy and retinal microaneurysms.

C/Fs: Type-I: More severe condition where patients have *S/S:* Polyuria, polydypsia, polyphagia, ketoacidosis. Can die of complications such as MI, CVA, renal failure, infections, gangrene, ketoacidosis and hypoglycemia. Type II: Polyuria, polydypsia, polyphagia, weakness, weight loss in spite of increased appetite.

MORPHO:

Pancreas: Type I: Reduced number of islets. Leukocyte infiltrate, mainly lymphocytes.

Type II: Minimal reduction of islets. Amyloid deposit around capillaries and between cells.

BVs: Vessels of all sizes are affected from the aorta to the smallest arterioles to capillaries. Aorta, large- and medium-sized arteries have atherosclerosis with MI, CVA, gangrene. Microangiopathy/hyaline arteriolosclerosis: Diffuse thickening of basement membranes, mainly in capillaries of skin, skeletal muscle, retina, renal glomeruli and renal medullae.

64. What is diabetic nephropathy?

Ans. a. Glomerular lesions:

1. Capillary basement membrane thickening.
2. Mesangial global glomerulosclerosis.
3. Mesangial nodular glomerulosclerosis—KW kidney (Kimmelstiel-Wilson kidney).

b. Hyaline arteriolosclerosis.

c. Pyelonephritis, necrotizing papillitis.

d. Collection of glycogen and fat in convoluted tubular epithelial cells.

65. What are the eye complications of DM?

Ans. Retinopathy, cataract, glaucoma.

66. What are islet cell tumors?

Ans. 1. *Insulinoma:* High serum insulin with Whipple's triad = Hypoglycemia, symptoms of hypoglycemia, relieved by administration of glucose.

2. *Gastrinoma (Zollinger-Ellison syndrome):* Severe peptic ulcers. May be present singly or as part of MEN type I. *HISTO:* In both cases tumors appear as enlarged islets with cytologically typical cells even in malignant tumors.

67. What are MEN (multiple endocrine neoplasia)?

Ans. Inherited as autosomal dominant.

Two types:

MEN-I (Wermer's syndrome): Its components are:

1. Pituitary tumors such as prolactin-secreting adenoma or somatotropin-secreting adenoma with acromegaly.
2. Parathyroid hyperplasia with its manifestations.
3. Tumors of pancreas such as gastrinoma with Zollinger-Ellison syndrome, insulinoma with hypoglycemia.

MEN-IIA (Sipple's syndrome): Its components are:

1. Medullary carcinoma of thyroid.
2. Pheochromocytoma of adrenal gland.
3. Parathyroid gland hyperplasia.

MEN-IIB (Williams syndrome): Its components are:

1. Medullary carcinoma of thyroid.
2. Pheochromocytoma of adrenal gland.
3. Ganglioneuromas of GIT.

15 Diseases of the Reproductive System (REP. S)

OVERVIEW

Male reproductive system

A. *Penis:*
1. Congenital anomalies.
2. Inflammation/infection.
3. Neoplasms.

B. *Scrotum:*
1. Hydrocele.
2. Chylocele.
3. Hematocele.
4. Spermatocele.
5. Varicocele.

C. *Testis:*
1. Congenital anomalies.
2. Inflammation.
3. Neoplasms.

D. *Prostate:*
1. Prostatitis.
2. Nodular hyperplasia.
3. Neoplasms.

Female reproductive system

A. *Breasts:*
1. Inflammation.
2. Fibrocystic diseases.
3. Neoplasms.
4. *Male breasts:* Gynecomastia, neoplasms.

B. *Vulva:*
1. Bartholin cyst.

2. Vulvitis.
3. Leukoplakia.
4. Lichen sclerosus.
5. Condylomas.
6. VIN and invasive carcinoma.
7. **Paget's disease of vulva**.

C. *Vagina:*
1. PID.
2. Neoplasms.

D. *Uterus—cervix:*
1. Cervicitis.
2. Polyps.
3. CIS/carcinoma.

E. *Uterus—body:*
1. Dysfunctional uterine bleeding (DUB).
2. Endometritis.
3. Adenomyosis.
4. Endometriosis.
5. Polyp.
6. Endometrial hyperplasia.
7. Endometrial neoplasms.
8. Myometrial neoplasms.

F. *Fallopian tubes:*
1. Inflammation.
2. Neoplasms.

G. *Ovaries:*
1. Oophoritis.
2. Endometriosis.
3. Non-neoplastic cysts.
4. Neoplasms.

H. *Gestational diseases:*
1. Placental infections.
2. Ectopic pregnancy.
3. Trophoblastic diseases.

MALE REPRODUCTIVE SYSTEM

Penis

Major diseases of penis are: Congenital anomalies (hypospadias and epispadias), inflammation/infections (balanitis, balanoposthitis, phimosis, paraphimosis, Peyronie's disease) and neoplasms (benign condyloma acuminatum) and malignant (CIS—**Bowen's disease, erythroplasia of Queyrat, bowenoid papulosis** and squamous cell carcinoma).

Scrotum

Major diseases of scrotum are: Hydrocele, chylocele, hematocele, (serous fluid, lymph and blood in tunica vaginalis respectively), spermatocele (collection of semen in spermatic cord), varicocele (varicose veins of the pampiniform venous plexus).

Testis

Congenital anomaly of the testis is undescended testis (cryptorchidism) which leads to atrophy and sterility and carries the risk of development of malignancy in the undescended testis and also of the opposite descended testis.

Some of the inflammatory diseases of the testis and epididymis are mumps, tuberculosis and associated with urinary tract infection. *Neoplasms of the testis are:*

A. Germ cell and

B. Sex cord-stromal (Leydig and Sertoli cell tumors).

Germ cell tumors are:

1. Seminoma and
2. Non-seminomatous (Embryonal carcinoma, yolk sac tumor, choriocarcinoma, teratomas).

Prostate

Prostatitis can be acute caused by organisms of urinary tract infection, e.g. *E. coli* and chronic caused by those of the acute prostatitis and Chlamydia, Ureaplasma, *Mycobacterium tuberculosis*, fungi.

Nodular hyperplasia consists of hyperplasia of the epithelial and stromal components with nodule formation.

Neoplasm of the prostate is mainly adenocarcinoma.

FEMALE REPRODUCTIVE SYSTEM

Breasts

Fibrocystic disease consists of epithelial hyperplasia with cysts, atypical hyperplasia, stromal hyperplasia with fibrosis. It has two patterns:

1. *Non-proliferative* consisting of cysts, fibrosis without epithelial cell hyperplasia.
2. *Proliferative:*
   A. *Epithelial:*
      a. Typical without risk of development of carcinoma and
      b. **Atypical with risk of carcinoma development**.
   B. *Sclerosing adenosis* consisting of epithelial cell proliferation and fibrosis with risk of progression to carcinoma much less than atypical hyperplasia.

Acute mastitis usually occurs during nursing usually by staphylocci or streptococci.

Neoplasms of the breast consist of:

A. *Benign:*
   1. Fibroadenoma.
   2. Phyllodes tumor.
   3. Intraductal papilloma.

B. *Malignant:*

1. Ductal carcinoma *in situ*.
2. Lobular carcinoma *in situ*.
3. Invasive ductal carcinoma.
4. Invasive lobular carcinoma.
5. Tubular carcinoma.
6. Colloid carcinoma.
7. Medullary carcinoma.
8. Inflammatory carcinoma.
9. Paget's disease of the breasts.

Vulva

Bartholin cyst is due to Bartholin gland's duct obstruction. Vulvitis is due to infection by HPV, HSV, gonococci, *Treponema palladium*, Candida. Leukoplakia is white plaque seen in several benign and malignant conditions requiring biopsy for correct diagnosis. Lichen sclerosus is stiffening of vulva due to white plaques. **~ 5% can develop to carcinoma**. Condylomas are of 2 types:

1. Lata due to syphilis.
2. Accuminatum due to HPV.

VIN is intraepithelial carcinoma which could progress to invasive squamous cell carcinoma.

Paget's disease is intraepithelial carcinoma with overlying epidermis appearing red-inflammatory. Unlike Paget's disease of the breast there is no underlying ductal carcinoma.

Vagina

Vaginitis is infection of the vagina commonly from Candida and Trichomonas. *Vaginal adenosis* is benign condition consisting of small benign glands in vaginal mucosa. It is due to in utero exposure to diethylstilbestrol (DES). *Clear cell carcinoma* is seen in ~1 in 1000 females exposed in utero to DES. **Sarcoma botryoides** is embryonal rhabdomyosarcoma of the vagina, which grossly appears like a bunch of grapes.

Cervix of the Uterus

Cervicitis is infection of the cervix commonly due to gonococci, herpes virus, *Chlamydia trachomatis*, staphylococci and streptococci. *CIS (Carcinoma in situ)* is intraepithelial carcinoma, which if not treated progresses to invasive squamous cell carcinoma.

Body of the uterus

Endometritis is inflammation of the endometrium which is of two types:

1. Acute due to retained products of conception.
2. Chronic due to retained products of conception, IUDs, gonococcus, tuberculosis.

Adenomyosis is growth of basal layer of endometrium (nonfunctioning) down into myometrium which could lead to menorrhagia, dysmenorrhea.

Endometriosis is presence of endometrial tissue (functional) at sites other than endometrium either in pelvis (ovaries, uterine ligaments, urinary bladder, etc.) or outside pelvis (lungs, heart, bones, etc.).

Abnormal uterine bleeding is of two types:

1. Due to structural lesions, e.g. abortion, ectopic pregnancy, trophoblastic diseases, adenomyosis, hyperplasia, polyps, leiomyoma, leiomyosarcoma, endometrial carcinoma.
2. Dysfunctional without structural lesions.

Endometrial hyperplasia is due to excess of estrogen relative to progesterone caused by failure of ovulation, estrogen-producing ovarian lesion, e.g. granulosa-theca cell tumors, polycystic ovaries.

Endometrial carcinoma is seen with risk factors such as obesity, diabetes mellitus, hypertension, infertility, increased estrogen, persons having breast cancer. Prognosis is good with early diagnosis and poor with late diagnosis.

Leiomyoma is a benign neoplasm of the uterine myometrium. It does not progress to leiomyosarcoma.

Leiomyosarcoma is a malignant neoplasm of the uterine myometrium. It arises directly from myometrial cells and not from leiomyoma.

Fallopian Tubes

Salpingitis is inflammation of salpinx (fallopian tube) commonly due to infection by gonococci, Chlamydia, mycoplasma, *Mycobacterium tuberculosis*, Streptococcus, Staphylococcus. Scarring may lead to sterility.

Ovaries

Oophoritis is inflammation of the ovary usually in association with salpingitis. *Endometriosis* is presence of endometrium in the ovary leading to brown-colored cyst called chocolate cyst. *Follicle and luteal cysts* are due to unruptured graafian follicles or follicles that have ruptured and sealed immediately respectively. *Polycystic ovaries* ***(Stein-Leventhal syndrome)*** are due to excessive production of androgens by ovaries for unknown reason, high levels of luteinizing hormone (LH) and low levels of follicle-stimulating hormone (FSH). Tunica albuginea is thick beneath which are numerous cysts. It causes sterility. *Neoplasms of the ovaries* are from surface epithelium, germ cells, sex cord or metastatic. **These are asymptomatic until late resulting in late diagnosis and hence ~ 50% are fatal**.

Diseases of pregnancy

Placental infections are from ascending infections, e.g. Mycoplasma, Candida, various vaginal flora or hematogenous, e.g. syphilis, tuberculosis, toxoplasmosis, various viruses (rubella, cytomegalo, herpes).

Ectopic pregnancy is implantation of fertilized ovum in any site other than the normal uterine site. Mostly it is in the fallopian tubes due to chronic inflammation and scarring of the tube.

Gestational trophoblastic diseases are:

1. Hydatidiform mole.
2. Invasive mole.
3. Choriocarcinoma.

In all, hCG is produced higher than normal pregnancy; with titer higher in invasive mole than hydatidiform mole and higher in choriocarcinoma than in invasive mole. **Complete** hydatidiform mole is when a **completely** empty ovum is fertilized by two spermatozoa or a diploid sperm. ~ **2% of these develop choriocarcinoma**. Partial hydatidiform mole is when a normal ovum is fertilized by two spermetazoa or a diploid sperm. Very rarely these develop choriocarcinoma. Invasive mole is more aggressive than a benign mole, but less aggressive than choriocarcinoma.

Gestational choriocarcinoma arises from gestational chorionic epithelium—~50% from complete hydatidiform mole, ~25% follow abortion and ~25% follow normal pregnancy. These respond favorably to chemotherapy with 100% cure (unlike choriocarcinomas of the ovaries and testis which respond poorly to chemotherapy and have poor prognosis).

Male
Penis

1. What are the common congenital anomalies of the penis?

Ans. a. Hypospadias: Urethral opening on ventral aspect of the shaft of penis.

b. Epispadias: Urethral opening on dorsal aspect of the shaft of penis.

2. What are the common inflammatory lesions of the penis?

Ans. a. *Balanitis:* Inflammation of glans penis.

b. *Balanoposthitis:* Inflammation of glans penis and overlying prepuce.

c. *Phimosis:* Prepuce cannot be retracted over the glans, common complication of balanoposthitis.

d. *Paraphimosis:* Stenotic prepuce is retracted over the glans penis, circulation to the glans penis may be restricted.

e. *Peyronie's disease:* Fibrous thickening and contracture of the investing fascia of the corpora.

3. What are the common neoplasms of the penis?

Ans. a. *Benign:* Condyloma acuminatum. Cause: HPV. Site commonly at coronal sulcus. *MORPHO*: *GROSS*: Small papillary excrescences. *MICRO*: Branching villi with connective tissue stroma covered by squamous epithelium having hyperkeratosis and acanthosis.

b. *Malignant: ETIO*: Predisposing factors: HPV, smegma.

CIS: Dysplastic cells within epidermis only.

Types:

1. *Bowen's disease:* Commonest. On penile shaft. 1/10 cases develop invasive carcinoma. Visceral malignancies might also be present.
2. *Erythroplasia of Queyrat:* Reddish, located over glans and prepuce, may develop invasive carcinoma like Bowen's disease, but not associated with visceral malignancy.
3. *Bowenoid papulosis:* Rarely invasive carcinoma development. No visceral malignancy.

Invasive carcinoma: Squamous cell carcinoma. Circumcision protects. Sites: Glans, coronal sulcus, inner surface of prepuce.

GROSS: Two types:

1. Flat-papular, may ulcerate.
2. Papillary.

Verrucous carcinoma: Low malignant potential. *PROG*: 5-year survival: Without inguinal metastasis 3/4 cases, with inguinal metastasis 1/4 cases.

Scrotum

4. What are the common pathological conditions of the scrotum?

Ans. *Hydrocele:* Serous fluid in tunica vaginalis. *ETIO:* Idiopathic.
Hematocele: Blood in tunica vaginalis.
Chylocele: Lymph in tunica vaginalis. *ETIO:* Commonly filariasis.
Squamous cell carcinoma: **First cancer recognized due to environmental factors in chimney sweepers by Sir Pott in England in 18th century.**

Epididymis and Testis

5. What are the common developmental anomalies of the testis?

Ans. *Cryptorchidism:* Failure of descent of testis. Leads to atrophy and sterility. *COMPLI:* Risk of malignancy in the undescended testis and also to some degree in the opposite descended testis.

6. What are common inflammatory lesions of the epididymis and testis?

Ans.
1. Associated with urinary tract infection.
2. Mumps: Seen in adults. When severe, there is atrophy of the seminiferous tubules with sterility.
3. Tuberculosis: Granulomatous inflammation with caseating necrosis.

7. What are the neoplasms of testes?

Ans. Classification:

1. Germ cell
2. Sex cord-stromal (Leydig cell and Sertoli cell tumor)

Germ cell tumors:

1. Seminoma—primitive cells differentiating along gonadal lines.
2. *Non-seminomatous:*
   a. Embryonal carcinoma—primitive totipotential cells stay undifferentiated.
   b. Yolk sac tumor—primitive cells differentiate into extra-embryonic tissue.
   c. Choriocarcinoma—same as yolk sac tumor with predominance of trophoblastic tissue.
   d. Teratomas (mature/immature)—primitive cells differentiate into somatic tissues.

C/Fs: Age: ~25 yrs-yolk sac tumor common in children. Predisposing factors: Cryptorchidism. Also, opposite descended testis has some risk. Klinefelter syndrome. More common in siblings. Presents as painless enlargement of testis: **Most important cause of painless enlargement of testis**. Approximately 95% testicular neoplasms are of the germ cell origin. These are all malignant. Remainder arise from Sertoli/Leydig cells, which are generally benign and may give rise to endocrine abnormalities, e.g. Leydig cell tumors.

8. What is differentiation of germ cell tumors?

Ans. Primitive germ cells can differentiate in various ways as follows:

1. Primitive germ cell to mature germ cell to seminoma (dysgerminoma in females).
2. Embryonal differentiation to
   a. Embryonic structure (embryonal cell carcinoma, somatic-teratoma).
   b. Extra-embryonic structure (yolk sac tumor, choriocarcinoma).

9. What is seminoma?

Ans. Malignant neoplasm of the testis of the germ cell origin, where the primitive cells differentiate along gonadal lines. *MORPHO*: *GROSS*: Homogenous cut surface. *MICRO*: Uniform polygonal cells with clear cytoplasm, round nuclei and prominent nucleoli; lymphocytes in the stroma. Tumor markers: **10%** have elevated **hCG**. Large tumor metastasizes to iliac and para-aortic lymph nodes. **S**ensitive to radiation and chemotherapy.

Two types: 1. Classic seminoma—95%.

2. Spermatocytic seminoma—5%. In older age group. *MICRO*: Large and small cells (similar in appearance to secondary spermatocyte and hence the name). Usually no metastasis prognosis is good.

10. What is embryonal carcinoma of testis?

Ans. Age: ~25 yrs. *MORPHO: GROSS:* Cut surface has focal necrosis and hemorrhage. *MICRO:* Large cells in sheets or papillae. Tumor markers: **90%** have elevated **hCG** or **AFP** or **both**.

11. What is yolk sac tumor of testis?

Ans. Age: In children usually below 3 years of age. *MORPHO:* Poorly differentiated cells in sheets, glands, and in configuration resembling primitive glomeruli **(Schiller-Duval bodies)**. Tumor markers: **AFP** elevated in **100%**.

12. What is choriocarcinoma of testis?

Ans. Age: ~25 yrs. *MORPHO: GROSS:* Small mass. *MICRO:* Cytotrophoblast and syncytiotrophoblast without villus formation. Tumor markers: **hCG**-elevated in **100%**.

13. What is teratoma of testis?

Ans. *Age:* All ages. *MORPHO: GROSS:* Cut surface has cysts and cartilage. *MICRO:* Tissues from all 3 germ layers with somatic differentiation. It is of following types:

1. *Mature:* Well differentiated tissue from 1 or more germ cell layers, e.g. neural, bone, cartilage, epithelium.
2. *Immature:* Immature tissues similar to fetus.
3. *With malignant transformation:* Have malignant transformation of teratomatous tissue, e.g. squamous cell carcinoma or adenocarcinoma. **All teratomas in adults are malignant**.

Development of teratomas: Teratomas arise from totipotent germ cells, which appear in mild-line posteriorly in the embryo from where normally they migrate to gonadal ridges where they can give rise to teratomas of testis/ovaries; but, sometimes they do not migrate to gonadal ridges and remain along the mid-line and give rise to teratomas of pineal gland, at the base of the skull, in the posterior mediastinum, retroperitoneal areas and sacrococcygeal region.
Histologically, tissues of embryonic, fetal and adult of all 3 germ layers can be seen. The malignant tumors contain mixture of immature tissue, however, one particular tissue may become frankly malignant and exert more harmful effect than the remainder of the tissues.

14. What is the staging of malignant neoplasms of testis?

Ans. *Stage 1:* Tumor confined to testis, *Stage 2:* Metastases confined to retroperitoneal nodes below the level of diaphragm, *Stage 3:* Metastases beyond retroperitoneal nodes.

Prostate

15. What are common diseases of the prostate?

Ans. 1. Prostatitis.
2. Nodular hyperplasia.
3. Adenocarcinoma.

16. What is prostatitis?

Ans. Inflammation of prostate. *Acute:* Caused by organisms that cause UTI, mainly *E. coli*. *Chronic:* Caused by:
1. Organisms same as in acute cases.
2. *Chlamydia trachomatis*.
3. *Ureaplasma urealyticum*.

Granulomatous: Caused by:
1. Tuberculosis.
2. Sarcoidosis.
3. Fungal infections.

MORPHO: Acute: PMN infiltrate. *Chronic:* Lymphocytic infiltrate, fibroblastic proliferation. *Granulomatous:* Have granulomas. *C/Fs:* Dysuria, frequency, fever. On digital examination, prostate enlarged and tender.

17. What is nodular hyperplasia of prostate?

Ans. *DEF:* Benign hyperplasia of epithelial and stromal components with nodule formation. In the past used to be called BPH (benign prostatic hypertrophy). This term has been abandoned because there is hyperplasia, not hypertrophy and "benign" word is redundant. *MORPHO: GROSS:* Hyperplasia mainly in the peri-urethral glands. Hence, more likely to produce urinary obstruction earlier than carcinoma. (In contrast carcinomas arise in the periphery and hence are palpable easily by rectal digital examination). Prostate enlarged, weighing 100–200 gm (normal 40 gm). Cut surface has mainly circumscribed nodules. Urethra is compressed. *MICRO:* Glands are lined by tall columnar cells with papillary projections and have a peripheral layer of flattened basal cells. Proliferating stroma always surrounds the glands. (In contrast to **carcinoma** where glands lie **back-to-back**). *C/Fs:* Hesitancy (difficulty in starting urination), interruption of urinary stream, frequency, urgency and nocturia.

18. What is carcinoma of prostate?

Ans. *DEF:* It is an adenocarcinoma arising from glands of the prostate. *MORPHO:* Irregular hard mass at the periphery **(therefore, found by digital rectal examination)**. *MICRO:* Well differentiated small glands lying back-to-back without intervening stroma and lined by a single layer of cuboidal cells. *C/Fs:* Age: 60–80 years. Usually asymptomatic. Metastases: Commonly to bone and commonly **osteoblastic**. Osteoclastic less common.

DIAG:

1. PSA (Prostatic specific antigen)—Not a screening tool as it is produced both by normal prostate and nodular hyperplastic prostate (more useful in follow-up).
2. Rectal digital examination.
3. Transrectal sonography.
4. FNA (Fine needle aspiration). Grading: Modified Gleason system uses the spectrum of differentiation present to grade the tumor. Staging: T1: Nonpalpable lesion, T2: Palpable or visible cancer confined to prostate, T3: Local extraprostatic extension, T4: Invasion of contiguous organs/structures (bladder, rectum, pelvic floor, levator ani muscle). N0: No regional lymph nodes, N1: Single regional lymph node <2 cm, N2: Single regional node 2–5 cm (or many nodes <5 cm). N3: Regional nodes >5 cm. M0: No distant metastases, M1: Distant metastases. *PROG:* Almost all patients with early detection survive for at least 10 years.

Female Breasts

19. What are common disorders of the breasts?

Ans. 1. Fibrocystic changes
2. Mastitis
3. Neoplasms.

20. What are fibrocystic changes of the female breast?

Ans. These consist of stromal fibrosis, stromal and epithelial hyperplasia with cysts, atypical hyperplasia.

Two patterns: 1. Non proliferative.

2. Proliferative.
   a. Epithelial hyperplasia—typical and atypical.
   b. Sclerosing adenosis.

Nonproliferative:

Include cysts and/or fibrosis without epithelial cell hyperplasia (simple fibrocystic change). *GROSS*: Cysts 1–5 cm. Unopened they are bluish **(blue dome cyst)**, containing serous fluid. *MICRO*: Cuboidal-columnar multi-layered smaller cysts and flat epithelium in larger cysts. Sometimes lined by large cells with eosinophilic cytoplasm **(apocrine metaplasia—always benign)**.

Proliferative-epithelial hyperplasia: Two types:

1. Mild typical with no risk of carcinoma with ducts having normal appearing cuboidal cells occasionally with gland patterns (fenestrations) and occasionally with papillae (ductal papillomatosis).
2. **Atypical hyperplasia with risk of cancer development** with ducts having dysplastic cells with some pleomorphism and hyperchromatic nuclei. *C/Fs:* There are no discrete lumps. Sometimes, there is nipple discharge.

21. What is sclerosing adenosis of female breast?

Ans. Condition with proliferation of epithelial and myoepithelial cells in small ducts (adenosis) with stromal fibrosis (sclerosing). **This has very little risk to progression to carcinoma (less than atypical hyperplasia).**

22. What is acute mastitis?

Ans. Caused by bacteria entering through fissures in nipples during nursing. Staphylococcal infections cause abscess formation. Streptococcal infections cause generalized inflammation of breast with pain, swelling and tenderness.

23. What is the classification of neoplasms of female breast?

Ans. A. *Benign:*

1. Fibroadenoma.
2. Phyllodes tumor.
3. Intraductal papilloma.

B. *Malignant:*

1. Intraductal carcinoma *in situ*.
2. Lobular carcinoma *in situ*.
3. Invasive ductal carcinoma NOS (not otherwise specified).

4. Invasive lobular carcinoma.
5. Tubular carcinoma.
6. Colloid (mucinous) carcinoma.
7. Medullary carcinoma.
8. Inflammatory carcinoma.
9. Paget's disease of the breast.

24. What is fibroadenoma of the breast?

Ans. Benign tumor of breast. *GROSS*: 1–5 cm firm, encapsulated. Cut surface uniform. *MICRO*: Ducts lined by more than one layer of benign cells surrounded by stroma. In some areas, ducts are round to oval (pericanalicular fibroadenoma). In other areas, ducts are compressed and appear as slits or irregular in shape (intracanalicular fibroadenoma). *C/Fs:* Present as mobile, nonpainful firm mass in a 20 to 40-year female.

25. What is phyllodes tumor of the breast?

Ans. Benign breast tumor with leaf-like cut surface (hence the name Gr. Phyllodes = leaf-like). Very rarely malignant changes. *GROSS*: 4 to >10 cm, smooth round firm. *MICRO*: Similar to fibroadenoma. With malignant transformation there is increased cellularity with anaplasia and infiltration into adjacent breast tissue.

26. What is intraductal papilloma of breast?

Ans. *C/Fs:* Benign neoplastic papillary growth within a duct presents with nipple retraction or nipple discharge. *GROSS:* Single, small cystic. *MICRO:* Papillae made of cuboidal epithelium of more than one layer and myoepithelial cell layer with central stroma.

27. What are the general features of the carcinoma of the breast?

Ans. *Risk factors: Well-established:* Increases with first degree relative with breast cancer, (~3 times increased risk if mother or sister has Ca breast). Age at menarche <12 yrs. Age at menopause >55 yrs, nulliparous, proliferative disease with atypical hyperplasia, lobular CIS. *Less well-established:* Exogenous estrogens, oral contraceptives, obesity, high fat diet, alcohol consumption, cigarette smoking. *Distribution:* Approximately UOQ—50%, Central area—10%, Other 3 Quadrants—10% each, 10% multifocal. 90% arise in ductal epithelium, 10% in lobular epithelium.
Types: A. *Noninvasive:*

1. Intraductal carcinoma.
2. Intraductal carcinoma with Paget's disease.
3. Lobular CIS.

B. *Invasive (infiltrating):*

1a. Invasive ductal carcinoma (NOS).
1b. Invasive ductal carcinoma with Paget's disease.
2. Invasive lobular carcinoma.

3. Medullary carcinoma.
4. Colloid carcinoma (mucinous carcinoma).
5. Tubular carcinoma.

28. What is intraductal carcinoma of breast?

Ans. *MICRO:* Ducts filled with anaplastic tumor cells. In some cases there are glandular spaces **(cribriform pattern)**, central necrosis with calcification is also seen. Sometimes, tumor cells extend into epidermis of nipple and areolar region to produce **Paget's disease**. These cells do not penetrate the basement membrane of duct and so are CIS.

29. What is lobular carcinoma *in situ* of breast?

Ans. Carcinoma arises in terminal ducts and ductules. **Often multifocal and bilateral.** Approximately half develop into invasive carcinoma.

30. What is invasive ductal carcinoma of breast?

Ans. Most common breast cancer. *C/Fs:* Presents as hard, painless mass. *GROSS:* Cut section shows infiltrative tumor retracted below by dense, gritty fibrous tissue (scirrhous). Occasionally, focal white areas of calcification are seen. Dimpling of skin, retraction of nipple may be present, or fixation to chest wall. *MICRO:* Thick fibrosis in which are groups and cords of tumor cells. Round to oval, with uniform small dark nuclei. At the margin tumor shows infiltration of the surrounding tissue.

31. What is Paget's disease of breast?

Ans. Intraductal carcinoma which extends to infiltrate the epidermis of overlying nipple and areola by **Paget's cells**, which are present singly or in groups, and are large cells with hyperchromatic pleomorphic nuclei surrounded by a clear halo. *C/Fs:* Presents with fissuring of areolar and periareolar skin, oozing and sometimes ulceration. Also *C/Fs* of underlying invasive carcinoma which is seen in approximately 50% of the cases.

32. What is medullary carcinoma of breast?

Ans. Consists of large, soft, tumor made of polygonal cells and small amount of stroma with lymphocytic infiltrate.

33. What is colloid (mucinous) carcinoma of breast?

Ans. Consists of very soft, large tumor made of mucus-containing neoplastic cells singly or in glands with mucin in and around them.

34. What is infiltrative lobular carcinoma of breast?

Ans. Often multifocal, bilateral cancer without a well-defined mass. *GROSS*: Poorly circumscribed rubbery to hard in consistency. *MICRO*: Single linear arrangement of small, uniform tumor cells in fibrous stroma **(Indian file)**. Sometimes, tumor cells surround acini or ducts, with a characteristic **bull's eye** pattern.

35. What are the features common to all invasive carcinomas of breast?

Ans. 1. Fixation to underlying chest wall.
2. Adherence to overlying skin with retraction of overlying skin or nipple.
3. Involvement of lymphatics with lymphedema, giving skin the appearance of orange peel **(peau d'orange)**.
4. Sometimes, tumor spreads so fast that it produces an inflammatory reaction with redness and tenderness termed **inflammatory carcinoma**.
5. Spread by lymphatics and hematogenous. UOQ and central tumors spread to axillary and supraclavicular lymph nodes. Inner quadrant tumors spread to internal mammary and supraclavicular lymph nodes. Distant metastases occur to lungs, bone, liver, adrenals and brain.

36. What is the grading of breast cancers?

Ans. On the basis of level of anaplasia: Grades I–III.
Three categories:
1. *Nonmetastasizing:* Intraductal carcinoma without stromal invasion; lobular CIS.
2. *Uncommonly metastasizing:* Colloid carcinoma, medullary carcinoma.
3. *Metastasizing:* All others.

37. What is the staging of breast cancers?

Ans. Prognosis of the breast cancer depends on staging which is based on size of the cancer, lymph node involvement and distant metastases. In general prognosis is best with small size without lymph node involvement and without distant metastases; and worse with large size, lymph node involvement and distant metastases. Also skin invasion with ulceration or skin lymphatics blocking them causing clinically inflammatory appearance or invasion of underlying chest wall with fixation makes prognosis worse.

Diseases of the Vulva

38. What are Bartholin cysts?

Ans. Painful swelling of the Bartholin's glands due to duct obstruction.

39. What are the common causes of vulvitis?

Ans. 1. HPV (Human papilloma virus)—causing condyloma acuminate and VIN (Vulvar intra-epithelial neoplasia).
2. HSV (Herpes simplex virus-2)—causing herpes genitalis. Sometimes HSV-1, which usually causes herpes labialis.
3. Gonococci.
4. Syphilis—causing primary chancre at the site of inoculation.
5. Candida (yeast).

40. What is leukoplakia of vulva?

Ans. White plaque. Seen in:

1. Lichen sclerosus.
2. Lichen simplex chronicus.
3. Vitiligo.
4. Lichen planus.
5. Psoriasis.
6. Paget's disease.
7. CIS.
8. Invasive carcinoma.

Hence, biopsy is a must for correct diagnosis.

41. What is lichen sclerosus of vulva?

Ans. (Gr: Lichen = Papule; Sclerosis = Hardening) Smooth white interconnecting plaques making vulvar surface stiff. *MICRO*: Thinning of the epidermis and disappearance of the rete pegs, superficial hyperkeratosis, dermal fibrosis. **Approximately upto 5% patients develop carcinoma**.

42. What are condylomas?

Ans. Anogenital warts.
Two common types:

1. Condyloma lata.
2. Condyloma acuminata.

Condyloma lata: Caused by secondary syphilis consisting of slightly raised flat wet lesions.

Condyloma acuminata: Small papillary lesions caused by HPV (human papilloma virus). *MICRO*: Papillae lined by stratified epithelium with fibrovascular central stroma. Focally epithelial cells have **koilocytosis** (perinuclear vacuolization), which is characteristic of HPV infection.

43. What are VIN (vulvar intraepithelial neoplasia) and invasive carcinoma of vulva?

Ans. Squamous cell carcinoma, when confined within epithelium, are called VIN and when infiltrating are called invasive carcinoma, which could be exophytic or endophytic with ulceration.

44. What is Paget's disease of vulva?

Ans. Intraepithelial carcinoma within epidermis, clinically appearing red inflammatory (hence, can be mistaken for dermatitis). *MOCRO:* Cancer cells have a clear halo due to collection of PAS positive mucopolysaccharide secreted by them **(Paget's cells)**. There is rarely an underlying gland cancer (unlike Paget's disease of nipple where there is always an underlying ductal cancer).

Diseases of the Vagina

45. What is vaginitis?

Ans. Infection of vagina commonly from Candida, Trichomonas, present as itching and discharge.

46. What is vaginal adenosis/clear cell carcinoma of vagina?

Ans. Vaginal adenosis is a benign condition of vagina consisting of small glands in vaginal mucosa lined by mucus-secreting ciliated columnar cells. *ETIO:* In utero diethyl stilbestrol exposure (pregnant mothers or patients taking it for the management of threatened abortion). Approximately 1 in 30 with in utero DES exposure develop vaginal adenosis and 1 in 1000 develop clear cell carcinoma.

47. What is sarcoma botryoides of vagina?

Ans. (Gr. Botrys = Bunch of grapes) *Nature:* Embryonal rhabdomyosarcoma. Primary vaginal cancer. *C/Fs:* Age: In infants and children under age of 5 yrs. *GROSS*: Soft bunch of grape-like masses. *MICRO:* Small, primitive **round blue cells**. Some have **strap like processes**, as evidence of myoblastic differentiation. Dx: EM: Demonstration of sarcomeres. Immunocytochemistry: Demonstration of muscle-associated antigen, e.g. desmin.

Diseases of the Cervix of the Uterus

48. What is cervicitis?

Ans. Infection of the cervix due to:

1. Gonococci
2. Herpes virus
3. *Chlamydia trachomatis*
4. Staphylococcus/Streptococcus in postpartum women.

Chronic cervicitis has mononuclear inflammatory infiltrate and epithelial cells may be depleted of their normal glycogen content and give a false positive **Schiller test** (Failure to take up applied iodine solution which is **characteristic of glycogen-depleted cancer cells)**. In herpes cells have intranuclear inclusions.

49. What is CIS (carcinoma *in situ*)/invasive carcinoma of the cervix of the uterus?

Ans. CIS is carcinoma of cervix which is confined to full thickness of the cervix. Invasive carcinoma is that which infiltrates through the basement membrane into underlying stroma and beyond.

Risk factors:

1. Early age at first sexual intercourse.
2. Multiple sexual partners.
3. Male partner with previous multiple sexual partners.
4. HPV infection.

Screening: Papanicolaou test, colposcopic exam. **Acetic acid test:** When dilute acetic acid is applied to the ectocervix, areas of abnormal hyperplasia or neoplasia appear paler than the normal mucosa. **Schiller's test:** Cancer cells are glycogen devoid and do not take the applied iodine solution as the normal cells do.

Grades:

1. Mild dysplasia.
2. Moderate dysplasia.
3. Severe dysplasia.
4. CIS.
5. Invasive carcinoma.

MORPHO:

1. *Mild dysplasia:* Cellular atypicality is minimal and confined to basal 1/4 region of the epithelial thickness.
2. *Moderate dysplasia:* Cellular atypicality is moderate and confined to basal 1/2 of the region of the epithelium.
3. *Severe dysplasia:* Cellular atypicality is severe with greater pleomorphism, hyperchromatism of the nuclei, increased nuclear-cytoplasmic ratio and presence of mitotic figures, involving more than 3/4 of basal region of the epithelial thickness but not full thickness.
4. *CIS:* Cellular atypia involves full thickness of the epithelium.
5. *Invasive carcinoma:* Infiltration of the basement membrane is present. 95% of these are squamous cell carcinoma. Remainder are adenocarcinoma [which do not evolve as above, i.e. (1–4)]. These arise from the endocervical columnar cells.

GROSS: Three distinct forms:

1. Fungating.
2. Ulcerative.
3. Infiltrative.

Clinical course: Dysplasia and CIS usually asymptomatic. Invasive carcinoma presents with vaginal bleeding, leukorrhea, painful coitus, dysuria. Progression from CIS to invasive carcinoma takes ~10 yrs. Mortality is from local effects; obstruction of ureters, penetration into bladder or rectum.

Diseases of the Body of the Uterus

50. What is histology of the body of the uterus?

Ans. 1. Mucosal lining—endometrium.

2. Underlying myometrium composed of smooth muscles.
3. Outer serosa.

Endometrium: Is lined by a simple ciliated columnar epithelium supported by a cellular stroma containing numerous simple tubular glands. Composed of 2 parts:

1. Stratum basalis—adjacent to myometrium—undergoes little change during menstrual cycle and is not shed during menstruation.
2. Stratum functionalis—undergoes changes during menstrual cycle and shed during menstruation.

51. What is the menstrual cycle?

Ans. It is of 28 days of 3 phases:

1. *Menstrual phase:* From day 1 to day 5: Bleeding due to withdrawal of progesterone in absence of pregnancy.
2. *Proliferative phase:* From day 6 to day 14: Glands proliferate to form numerous glands. Stroma also proliferates becoming thick and highly vascularized. Proliferative phase is initiated and sustained until ovulation by the increasing production of estrogens from developing ovarian follicles.
3. *Secretory phase:* From day 15 to day 28: Ovulation occurs on day 15 and corpus luteum is formed which secretes progesterone which induces thick glycogen-rich secretion by endometrial glands.

Menstrual phase: In the absence of implantation of fertilized ovum progesterone level diminishes, LH from pituitary is suppressed, involution of corpus luteum occurs, corpus albicans is formed. Withdrawal of progesterone causes spiral arteries of the endometrial stroma to constrict precipitating ischemia leading to shedding of the stratum functionalis thus menstrual bleeding. Thereafter, activation of FSH initiates a new cycle of follicle development with estrogen secretion leading to proliferative phase as above.

52. What is the meaning of the terms—menarche, menopause, postmenopausal bleeding, amenorrhea, oligomenorrhea, cryptomenorrhea, dysmenorrhea, menorrhagia/hypermenorrhea, metrorrhagia, menometrorrhagia, polymenorrhea?

Ans. **Menarche:** Initiation of menstrual periods. **Menopause:** Cessation of menstrual periods. **Postmenopausal bleeding:** Bleeding after 1 yr. of menopause. **Amenorrhea:** Absence of menstruation. **Oligomenorrhea:** Reduction in frequency of menstruation so that the interval between cycles is as long as 40–90 days. **Cryptomenorrhea:** Menstrual bleeding not apparent, e.g. with imperforate hymen. **Dysmenorrhea:** Painful menstruation. **Menorrhagia/hypermenorrhea:** Longer duration or amount of menstruation or both. **Metrorrhagia:** Irregular bleeding between menstrual periods. **Menometrorrhagia:** Irregular heavy bleeding between menstrual periods. **Polymenorrhea:** Too frequent menstrual periods.

53. What is endometritis?

Ans. *Acute:* Due to retained products of conception. *Chronic:* Due to:

1. Gonorrheal pelvic inflammatory disease (PID).
2. Tuberculosis either from miliary or from tuberculous salpingitis.

3. Retained products of conception.
4. IUDs.
5. Idiopathic.

MICRO: Irregular proliferation of endometrial glands with chronic inflammatory cells.

54. What is adenomyosis?

Ans. Growth of basal layer of endometrium **(nonfunctioning)** down into myometrium. *GROSS:* Uterine wall thickened due to presence of endometrial tissue and reactive hypertrophy of myometrium. *MICRO:* Nests of endometrial glands or stroma or both found within the myometrium between smooth muscle bundles. *C/Fs:* Severe involvement may produce menorrhagia, dysmenorrhea and pelvic pain before the onset of menstruation.

55. What is endometriosis?

Ans. Presence of endometrial tissue **(functioning)** at sites other than endometrium, e.g. in pelvis (ovaries, pouch of Douglas, uterine ligaments, fallopian tubes, rectovaginal septum, urinary bladder); in extrapelvic peritoneum, about umbilicus; other remote sites, e.g. lymph nodes, lungs, heart, bone.

ETIO:

1. *Regurgitation theory:* Menstrual backflow through fallopian tubes causing peritoneal implantation.
2. *Metaplastic theory:* Endometrial differentiation of celomic epithelium.
3. Vascular or lymphatic dissemination theory.

C/Fs:

1. Lower abdominal pain.
2. Pain on defecation.
3. Dyspareunia.
4. Dysuria.
5. Dysmenorrhea.
6. Sterility.

GROSS: Small red-brown nodules on serosa. In ovaries, large blood-filled cysts, chocolate-colored due to aging **(chocolate cysts)**. *MICRO:* 2 of 3 following features need to be present to make the diagnosis:

1. Endometrial glands. 2. Stroma. 3. Hemosiderin pigment.

56. What is abnormal uterine bleeding?

Ans. Two types:

1. *Dysfunctional:* Where no uterine lesion is present.
2. *Structural:* Where uterine lesion is present:
   Abortion, ectopic pregnancy, trophoblastic diseases.

Adenomyosis, hyperplasia, polyps, leiomyoma, leiomyosarcoma, endometrial carcinoma.

57. What is endometrial hyperplasia?

Ans. *PATHOG:* Excess of estrogen relative to progesterone.

ETIO: 1. Failure of ovulation.

2. Estrogen-producing ovarian lesions, e.g. granulosa-theca cell tumors, polycystic ovaries (Stein-Leventhal syndrome).

Three categories: 1. *Simple:* With dilatation of glands only.

2. *Complex:* Glands increased in number.

3. *Atypical:* Further increase in number of glands, and the lining cells are mildly atypical. **1/4 cases may develop adenocarcinoma**.

58. What is endometrial carcinoma?

Ans. Risk factors:

1. Obesity
2. DM
3. HTN
4. Infertility
5. Women having breast cancer.

S/S: Leukorrhea and bleeding in postmenopausal women. *GROSS*: Infiltrative or exophytic. It fills the endometrial cavity extends into myometrium and to serosa and to periuterine structures. *MICRO*: Most of these are adenocarcinomas with well-defined glands. Less differentiated are in solid sheets of cells with nuclear atypia and mitotic activity. Some have squamous elements mixed. If squamous elements are not malignant, lesion is called **adenoacanthoma**. If squamous area is malignant **adenosquamous carcinoma**. *Grade:* G1–G3 from well differentiated to poorly differentiated.

Stage: [FIGO]:

I. Confined to uterine corpus.

II. Involvement of Cx.

III. Extension outside uterus but within true pelvis.

IV. Extension beyond III.

PROG: Good in early stage becoming worse with progression of stage.

59. What are the tumors of myometrium?

Ans. 1. Leiomyoma, and 2. Leiomyosarcoma.

60. What is leiomyoma?

Ans. Benign neoplasm of myometrium. *C/Fs:* May be asymptomatic. Most frequent symptom—menorrhagia, metrorrhagia. *GROSS*: Circumscribed, firm grey-white masses with whorled cut surface. Single to multiple. A few mm to several cm. *MICRO:* Whorling bundles of smooth muscle cells.

61. What is leiomyosarcoma?

Ans. Malignant neoplasm of myometrium. *C/Fs:* Arise directly from myometrial cells and not from leiomyoma. *GROSS*: Large single mass infiltrating uterine wall or projecting into uterine lumen. *MICRO:* Similar to leiomyoma. Main difference from leiomyoma is that leiomyosarcoma has atypical cells and many mitoses.

Diseases of the Fallopian Tubes

62. What are common diseases of fallopian tubes?

Ans. 1. Salpingitis
2. Tubal pregnancy
3. Endometriosis
4. Adenocarcinoma.

63. What is salpingitis?

Ans. *DEF:* Inflammation of the fallopian tubes. *ETIO:* Gonorrhea, chlamydia, mycoplasma, tuberculosis, streptococcus, staphylococcus. *C/Fs*: Fever, low-abdominal or pelvic pain, pelvic abscess. Scarring may lead to sterility.

Diseases of the Ovaries

64. What is histology of the ovaries?

Ans. 1. Surface of the ovary is covered by a layer of pluripotent cuboidal epithelium.
2. Below this is a fibrous capsule called tunica albuginea.
3. Below it is cortex. It has numerous follicles in various stages of development, and postovulatory follicles of various kinds: corpora lutea (which produce estrogen and progesterone), corpora albicantes, and degenerate atretic follicles.
4. Below it is medulla. It is highly vascular supplied by ovarian artery (direct branch from aorta) and ovarian branches of the uterine artery, which enter the hilum of ovary from the broad ligament.

65. What are the common diseases of the ovaries?

Ans. 1. Oophoritis.
2. Endometriosis.
3. Follicle and luteal cysts.
4. Polycystic ovaries.
5. Neoplasms/tumors.

Oophoritis: In association with salpingitis: Salpingo-oophoritis.

Endometriosis: Chocolate cysts.

66. What are the follicle and luteal cysts of the ovaries?

Ans. Due to unruptured graafian follicles or quickly sealed ruptured follicles. Usually multiple, 1–2 cm in size. Lined by granulosa or luteal cells. Occasionally these present as **acute abdomen** when they rupture leading to intraperitoneal bleeding.

67. What are polycystic ovaries (Stein-Leventhal syndrome)?

Ans. *PATHOG:* Increased production of estrogens and androgens (by ovaries for unknown reason), high levels of luteinizing hormones (LH) and low levels of follicle-stimulating hormone (FSH). *C/Fs:* Oligomenorrhea, hirsutism, infertility, obesity in young women. *GROSS:* Ovaries are large with a smooth outer cortex, having many ~1 cm subcortical cysts. *MICRO:* Tunica is thick, beneath which are many cysts lined by granulosa cells with hypertrophic luteinized theca interna. Corpora lutea are absent.

68. What are the tumors of the ovaries?

Ans. A. *Surface epithelial-stromal cell tumors:*

1. Serous.
2. Mucinous.
3. Endometroid.
4. Clear cell.
5. Brenner.
6. Cyst adenofibroma.

B. *Germ cell tumors:*

1. Teratoma.
2. Dysgerminoma.
3. Endodermal sinus tumor.
4. Choriocarcinoma.

C. *Sex cord-stromal tumors:*

1. Fibroma.
2. Granulosa-theca cell.
3. Sertoli-Leydig cell.

D. *Metastatic tumors:*

1. From GIT (Krukenberg tumor).
2. Breast.
3. Lung.

69. What are the serous tumors: (cyst adenoma/adenocarcinoma) of the ovaries?

Ans. *C/Fs:* 60% benign, 20% low malignant potential, 20% frankly malignant. *GROSS:* Small (5 cm) to large (40 cm) round cystic. In benign serosal covering is smooth. In malignant nodular irregularities are present due to penetration of tumor. Cut surface of small tumor may show one cavity, larger tumors are usually divided by septa. Spaces are filled with serous fluid with papillary projections seen in some. *MICRO:* Benign tumors have a single layer of tall columnar cell. Circular-layered bodies **(Psammoma bodies)** are present at the tips of the papillae. In malignant tumors papillary projections are multilayered lined by anaplastic cells which invade the underlying axial stroma.

70. What are the mucinous tumors of the ovaries?

Ans. *C/Fs:* 80% benign, 10% low malignant potential, 10% frankly malignant. Prognosis is better than the serous types. **S**erous tumors are **s**evere in their behavior. **M**ucinous tumors are **m**ilder in their behavior. *GROSS:* Look like serous types but the contents of cysts are more mucinous. Benign have few papillae **without Psammoma bodies**. Malignant ones have prominent papillae, serosal penetration and solid areas. *MICRO:* Two types:

1. Endocervix-like (mullerian).
2. Intestinal type—depending on the resemblance to endocervical or colonic epithelium respectively. Rupture or peritoneal metastasis may give rise to **pseudomyxoma peritonei** where peritoneal cavity becomes filled with mucinous material.

71. What are the endometroid tumors of the ovaries?

Ans. *C/Fs:* Usually malignant. *GROSS:* Solid or cystic. *MICRO:* Tubular glands similar to that of endometrium are present.

72. What is Brenner tumor of the ovaries?

Ans. *C/Fs:* Uncommon, unilateral solid ovarian tumor. Mostly benign. *Histogenesis:* May arise from surface epithelium or from urogenital epithelium. *GROSS:* Smooth encapsulated. Cut surface gray-white. *MICRO:* Stroma containing nests of transitional epithelium.

73. What are the germ cell tumors of the ovaries?

Ans.
1. Teratomas
2. Dysgerminoma
3. Choriocarcinoma
4. Yolk sac (endodermal sinus) tumor.

74. What are teratomas of the ovaries?

Ans. *C/Fs:* 90% benign. Arise in first 2 decades of life. **Younger the patient, more the chances of malignancy**.

Benign mature cystic: C/Fs: 90% unilateral and on right side. 10% undergo torsion and present as surgical emergency. Cystic mass <10 cm. Cut section shows cyst filled with sebaceous secretion and matted hair, lined by hair-bearing epidermal lining (hence, also called **dermoid cyst**). Also, bone, cartilage, teeth can be present.

Mature malignant teratoma: Seen in young females of ~20 years. *GROSS:* Large, solid with areas of necrosis on cut section. *MICRO:* Areas of differentiation toward cartilage, bone, muscle, and other structures are seen. **Foci of neuroepithelial differentiation denote aggressive behavior and poor prognosis.**

75. What are specialized teratomas of the ovaries?

Ans. *Struma ovary:* Made of mature thyroid tissue which may be hyperfunctional with hyperthyroidism. *Carcinoid:* Carcinoid syndrome in a few cases.

76. What are the dysgerminoma of the ovaries?

Ans. Counterpart of testicular seminoma and **similarly radiosensitive**. These are malignant but only 1/3 metastasize. *GROSS:* Solid tumor mass. *MICRO:* Sheets of clear cells with some fibrous stroma which may have lymphocytes.

77. What are the choriocarcinoma and yolk sac tumors of the ovaries?

Ans. Similar in appearance to placental choriocarcinoma, however, unlike placental choriocarcinoma, these are resistant to chemotherapy. These secrete human chorionic gonadotropin. Yolk sac tumors are comparable to testicular endodermal sinus tumor and secrete alpha-fetoprotein.

78. What are the sex cord tumors of the ovaries?

Ans.
1. Granulosa-theca cell tumors.
2. Thecoma-fibroma.
3. Sertoli-Leydig cell tumors.

79. What are the granulosa-theca cell tumors of the ovaries?

Ans. These tumors may produce estrogen thereby causing endometrial hyperplasia with predisposition to development of endometrial carcinoma. Granulosa element may be malignant in upto 1/4 cases. *GROSS:* Grayish tumor of varying size. *MICRO:* Cuboidal granulosa cells in sheets and spindle-shaped theca cells. **Call-Exner bodies may be present.**

80. What is the thecoma-fibroma of the ovaries?

Ans. Solid, grayish benign tumors, approximately half of which have associated ascites and hydrothorax **(Meigs' syndrome)**. *MICRO:* Mixture of fibrous and oval theca cells.

81. What is the Sertoli-Leydig cell tumor of the ovaries?

Ans. Small solid brownish tumors having Sertoli or Leydig cells like testis and generally are masculinizing or defeminizing.

82. What are the common sites of metastatic tumors to the ovaries?

Ans. Breast, lung, and GIT **(Krukenberg tumor)**.

83. What are the clinical features common to all ovarian tumors?

Ans. *C/Fs:* Asymptomatic until late. Therefore, **50% fatal**. *S/S*: Similar for all ovarian tumors: Pain, GIT symptoms, urinary frequency, ascites, hormonal changes. CA 125 elevation in approximately 3/4 cases, which is also elevated in several benign conditions and nonovarian cancers. Therefore, only useful in follow-up and not for diagnosis. Do not respond to treatment resulting in poor prognosis.

Diseases of Pregnancy

84. What are the general problems from the diseases of the pregnancy and placenta?

Ans. Diseases of pregnancy and placenta are important causes of intrauterine and perinatal death, premature birth, congenital malformations, intrauterine growth retardation, maternal death and other morbidities for mom and baby.

85. What are the placental inflammations and infections?

Ans. Two pathways:

1. Ascending.
2. Hematogenous (transplacental).

1. *Ascending infections: ETIO:* Mycoplasmas, candida, various vaginal flora. *PATHOG:* Due to premature birth or premature rupture of membranes. *MORPHO*: Chorioamnion has PMN infiltrate with edema, and congestion of blood vessels (chorioamnionitis). It may extend to umbilical cord causing vasculitis.
2. *Hematogenous spread:* May affect the fetus and cause TORCHS complex: Toxoplasmosis, rubella, cytomegalovirus, herpes simplex, syphilis. *MORPHO:* Villi have inflammation (villitis).

86. What is ectopic pregnancy?

Ans. *DEF:* Implantation of fertilized ovum in any site other than normal uterine site. Mostly in tubes (tubal pregnancy). Other sites are ovaries, abdominal cavity, intrauterine portion of the tubes (interstitial pregnancy). *PATHOG:* Any hindrance in the passage of ovum.

ETIO:

1. Chronic inflammation of tubes.
2. Intrauterine tumors.
3. Endometriosis.

Course: Until rupture asymptomatic. Rupture presents with acute abdomen.

87. What are gestational trophoblastic diseases?

Ans. 1. Hydatidiform mole.

2. Invasive mole.
3. Choriocarcinoma.

In all, hCG (human chorionic gonadotrophin) is produced higher than in normal pregnancy, with titre being higher in invasive mole than hydatidiform mole and higher in choriocarcinoma than in invasive mole.

88. What is hydatidiform mole: complete and partial?

Ans. *Complete:* Karyotype: Diploid as an **completely empty ovum** is fertilized by 2 spermatozoa or a diploid sperm. (46, XX or 46, XY). Villous edema is of all villi. Trophoblast proliferation is diffuse circumferential. Atypia is often present. Serum hCG: elevated. Tissue hCG is markedly increased. Fetal parts are always absent because embryogenesis not possible. **2% develop choriocarcinoma**.

Partial: Karyotype is triploid as a **normal ovum** is fertilized by 2 sperms or a diploid sperm (69, XXY or 69, XXX). Villous edema is seen in some villi only. Trophoblast proliferation is focal and slight. Atypia is absent. Serum hCG is less elevated. Tissue hCG is mild. Fetal parts are present as compatible with early embryo formation. Choriocarcinoma develops only rarely.

89. What is invasive mole?

Ans. *C/Fs:* In between a benign mole and choriocarcinoma. Invasive locally but does **not** have the aggressive metastatic potential of choriocarcinoma. *GROSS:* Hydropic villi, which penetrate the uterine wall deeply, sometimes causing rupture and life-threatening hemorrhage. *MICRO:* Epithelium of the villi has hyperplastic and atypical changes with proliferation of cuboidal and syncytial components. *TRT:* Chemotherapy is curative.

90. What is gestational choriocarcinoma?

Ans. *C/Fs:* Arises from gestational chorionic epithelium. Approximately 1/2 arise from complete hydatidiform mole, 1/4 arise after an abortion, 1/4 arise after normal pregnancy **(CAN)**. *S/S:* Bloody-brownish discharge. *GROSS:* Hemorrhagic necrotic masses. *MICRO:* Chorionic villi are absent. Anaplastic cytotrophoblast and syncytiotrophoblast are seen. **Excellent response to chemotherapy with 100% cure. (Unlike choriocarcinomas of ovaries and testis which respond poorly to chemotherapy)**.

16 Diseases of the Musculoskeletal System (MSS)

OVERVIEW

Bones

1. Congenital diseases.
2. Fracture.
3. Osteoporosis.
4. Osteomalacia/rickets.
5. Bone disease due to hyperparathyroidism and chronic renal failure.
6. Paget's disease of the bone.
7. Osteonecrosis.
8. Infection.
9. Neoplasms.

Joints (arthritides)

1. Osteoarthritis.
2. Infectious arthritis.
3. Rheumatoid arthritis.
4. Seronegative arthritis.
5. Metabolic arthritis.
6. Miscellaneous.

Skeletal muscles

1. *Diseases of the neuromuscular junction:*
   A. Myasthenia gravis.
   B. Eaton-Lambert syndrome.
2. *Genetic dystrophies:*
   A. Duchenne.
   B. Becker.
3. *Autoimmune myositis:*
   A. Polymyositis.
   B. Dermatomyositis.
4. *Neoplasms:* Rhabdomyosarcoma.

Smooth muscles
Neoplasms: Benign (leiomyoma) and malignant (leiomyosarcoma).

Soft tissues

1. Reactive diseases.
2. Neoplasm.

Diseases of the bones
Some of the congenital diseases of the bone are:

1. *Achondroplasia* where the cartilage maturation is impaired in the developing growth plate causing dwarfism.
2. *Osteogenesis imperfecta* **(brittle bone disease)** where there is abnormal development of the type I collagen causing weak (brittle) bones and multiple fractures and **blue sclera.**
3. Osteopetrosis **(marble bone disease)** where the osteoclast function is defective causing decreased bone resorption and increased bone deposition which is weak and breaks easily like chalk; and, it also encroaches upon the bone marrow causing anemia, leucopenia and thrombocytopenia resulting in weakness, susceptibility to infections and easy bleeding.

Fracture is the break in the continuity of a bone. These are of different types. Fractures heal in step-wise fashion; and, there are various factors which hinder in the healing.

Osteoporosis consists of decreased quantity of the normally mineralized total bone mass causing increased susceptibility to fracture. It is caused by various conditions.

Rickets and *osteomalacia* which occur in children and adults respectively are diseases of the bone consisting of poor quality of the bone due to decreased mineralization of the bone as opposed to osteoporosis which consists of decreased quantity of normally mineralized bone.

Bone disease due to hyperparathyroidism consists of increased resorption of calcium from the bone by the action of increased parathyroid hormone making the bone thin with compensatory fibrosis and susceptibility to fracture, hemorrhage and cystic changes, called **osteitis fibrosa cystica (von Recklinghausen's disease of bone)**.

Renal osteodystrophy is bone changes such as osteitis fibrosa cystica, osteomalacia due to chronic renal failure.

Paget's disease of the bone ***(osteitis deformans)*** is of unknown origin consisting of increased osteoclastic action causing increased bone resorption followed by increased osteoblastic activity causing new bone formation of abnormal architecture **(mosaic pattern)** which is weak and easily breakable **("chalk stick fracture")** and increased blood flow to the bone which could lead to **high output cardiac failure. Another complication is development of osteogenic sarcoma.**

Osteomyelitis is infection of the bone which could be acute or chronic; pyogenic due to infection by group B streptococci, staphylococci, *E. coli*, Salmonella, etc. or tuberculous due to infection by *Mycobacterium tuberculosis*.

Neoplasms of the bone are:

a. Benign or
b. Malignant.

Some of the benign neoplasms are **osteoma, giant cell tumor (osteoclastoma).** Amongst the malignant neoplasms **secondary neoplasms are more common than the primary neoplasm.** Common primary sites for the secondary neoplasm are thyroid, lungs, breasts, prostate

(osteoblastic) and kidney **(osteoclastic)**. Amongst the primary malignant bone neoplasms some of the common ones are osteogenic sarcoma, chondrosarcoma, Ewing's tumor, **most common is multiple myeloma**.

Diseases of the joints

Osteoarthritis (OA) is a chronic noninflammatory degenerative joint disease due to wear and tear usually seen in elderly people.

Acute suppurative arthritis is commonly due to infection by gonococci, staphylococci, streptococci, *Hemophilus influenzae*, gram-negative rods, Salmonella, etc. Lyme disease is infectious arthritis due to infection by *Borrelia burgdorferi* transmitted by deer ticks from rodent to people.

Rheumatoid arthritis (RA) is noninfectious inflammatory arthritis most likely due to autoimmune type III hypersensitivity where majority of the patients have IgM antibody against body's own IgG **(rheumatoid factor—RF)** in their blood and synovial fluid. **Felty's syndrome** is a variant of RA where the patients have splenomegaly and neutropenia. *Juvenile rheumatoid arthritis* is a variant of RA seen in younger patients where the RF is absent. **Still's disease** is a variant of RA where the onset is acute with fever, increased WBCs, hepatosplenomegaly and lymphadenopathy. *Seronegative arthritis are:*

1. Reiter' syndrome.
2. Psoriatic arthritis.
3. Enteropathic arthritis.
4. Ankylosing spondylitis.

RF is absent and HLA-B27 antigen is usually present.

Gout is a metabolic arthritis due to urate deposition in the joints.

Pseudogout is arthritis due to calcium pyrophosphate deposition in the joints.

Miscellaneous conditions cause joint disorders/arthritis/arthropathies, e.g. hereditary hemochromatosis with arthritis, bronchogenic carcinoma with hypertrophic osteoarthropathy, **Charcot's joints** (neuropathic joints caused by joint trauma due to sensory loss seen in tabes dorsalis, diabetes mellitus, leprosy, syringomyelia), hemophilia, sickle cell crises, etc.

Diseases of the skeletal muscles

Myasthenia gravis is an acquired disease of the skeletal muscle with weakness due to autoimmune destruction of acetyl choline receptors (AChR) at the motor end plate.

Eaton-Lambert syndrome is acquired myasthenia gravis-like syndrome due to autoantibodies to calcium channel causing interference to release of acetyl choline at the motor nerve terminal. It is one of the paraneoplastic syndromes seen with small cell carcinoma of the lung.

Duchenne muscular dystrophy is an X-linked recessive hereditary muscular dystrophy in male children where genetic absence of dystrophin impairs contractility of cardiac and skeletal muscles causing death by ~20 years of age due to respiratory failure/pneumonia.

Becker's muscular dystrophy is X-linked recessive hereditary muscular dystrophy in male children in whom partial absence of dystrophin causes muscle abnormalities which are less severe than Duchenne muscular atrophy. *Rhabdomyosarcoma* is a malignant mesenchymal neoplasm with skeletal muscle differentiation.

Diseases of the smooth muscles

Leiomyoma is benign neoplasm of the smooth muscle commonly seen in the body of the uterus.

Leiomyosarcoma is malignant neoplasm of the smooth muscle, common site being uterus where it arises new and not as malignant transformation of the benign leiomyoma.

Diseases of the soft tissues

Nodular fascitis is reactive fibroblastic proliferation, occasionally post-traumatic.

Fibromatosis is reactive fibroblastic proliferation which tends to recur. Its superficial types are palmer **(Dupuytren's contracture)**, plantar, penile **(Pyronie's disease)**. Its deep type is **desmoid tumor**. *Fibroma* is a benign tumor of fibroblast, commonly seen in ovaries. Fibrosarcoma is a malignant neoplasm of fibroblasts growing in a **herringbone pattern**. Malignant fibrous histiocytoma is malignant neoplasm of fibroblast and histiocytes with spindle cells in a **storiform pattern**. *Lipoma* is a benign neoplasm of the fatty tissue. *Liposarcoma* is a malignant neoplasm of the fatty tissue.

Diseases of the Bones

1. What is achondroplasia?

Ans. *DEF/DES:* It is a congenital bone disorder with autosomal dominant inheritance in 1/4 and spontaneous mutation in 3/4 cases where in the developing growth plate the cartilage maturation is impaired. *C/Fs:* **Dwarfism**. Proximal limbs are short, legs are bowed. *MORPHO:* Chondrocytes in the cartilaginous growth plates are disorganized.

2. What is osteogenesis imperfecta (brittle bone disease)?

Ans. *DEF/DES:* Inherited, commonly as autosomal dominant bone disorder causing abnormal development of type I collagen resulting in weakness of bone. *C/Fs:* **Multiple bone fractures. Blue sclera** (since type I collagen is also present in sclera).

3. What is osteopetrosis (marble bone disease)?

Ans. It is a hereditary bone disease inherited as autosomal dominant and autosomal recessive. Osteoclast function is defective with decreased bone resorption and increased bone deposition, which is not strong and **breaks as easily as chalk stick**. Also, the increased amount of bone tissue takes up the marrow space leading to decreased RBC, WBC and platelet production resulting in anemia, leucopenia with susceptibility to infections, and thrombocytopenia with bleeding tendency. Recessive form can lead to early death due to these complications.

4. What is a fracture?

Ans. *DEF:* Break in the continuity of a bone. *Pathologic fracture:* When break occurs in a bone, which is already altered by a disease process it is called pathologic fracture, e.g. osteoporosis, osteomalacia, neoplasia, infection, etc. *Non-pathological fracture:* When break occurs in a healthy bone.

Types of fracture:

1. *Closed (simple):* When the overlying tissue is intact.
2. *Compound (open):* When there is break in continuity of the overlying skin. When the fracture site communicates with the skin surface.
3. *Comminuted:* When the bone breaks into more than two parts.
4. *Stress (fatigue):* Slowly developing fracture following a period of increased physical activity in which the bone is subjected to new repetitive stress, e.g. sports training, marching in military camps, etc.

Fracture healing: Steps:

1. Following a fracture hematoma develops at the site.
2. Primitive mesenchymal cells differentiate into primitive osteoblasts and proliferate.
3. The early primitive bone produced is called **fracture callus**.
4. If motion persists fibrous scar develops **fibrous nonunion**.

5. If there is no motion fracture callus gets mineralized and normal fracture healing occurs.

   Complications:

   1. Soft tissue contracture.
   2. Delayed union.
   3. Non-union, e.g. **fibrous nonunion**.
   4. Avascular necrosis.
   5. Pseudoarthrosis (fracture surfaces become lined by synovial-like cells creating a false joint.

Factors interfering with healing of fracture:

1. Infection.
2. Inadequate levels of calcium or phosphorus.
3. Vitamin deficiency.
4. Diabetes mellitus.
5. Vascular insufficiency.

5. What is osteoporosis?

Ans. *DEF:* Acquired disorder of the bone involving the quantity of the bone which is decreased with decrease in total bone mass and thinning of microscopic bone tissue leading to increased risk of fractures. *ETIO: Localized:* It could be localized due to immobilization (disuse atrophy) of a particular bone/limb. *Generalized:* It could be generalized, *risk factors of which are following:*

6. What are risk factors for osteoporosis?

Ans. A. *Primary:*

1. Senile.
2. Postmenopausal.

B. *Secondary:*

1. *Nutritional:*
   a. Malnutrition.
   b. Malabsorption.
2. *Endocrine disorders:*
   a. Hyperparathyroidism.
   b. Hyper/hypothyroidism.
   c. Hypogonadism.
   d. Acromegaly.
   e. Cushing's syndrome.
   f. Addison's disease.
   g. Diabetes (type I).
3. *Neoplasms:*
   a. Multiple myeloma.
   b. Carcinomatosis.

4. *Drugs:*
   a. Corticosteroids.
   b. Chemotherapeutic agents.
5. *Miscellaneous:*
   a. Immobilization.
   b. Anemia.
   c. COPD.
   d. Osteogenesis imperfecta.
   e. Smoking and alcohol.

PATHOG: Bone mass is dependent on many factors, e.g. genetic, gender, age, physical activity, nutrition, hormones. *Diet:* Vitamin D and calcium in diet. *Age:* Bone is being lost and new bone made on a continual basis. After age 30 osteoblastic activity decreases and same amount of new born is not formed as is lost and this results in decreased amount of bone with increasing age (like graying of hair). *Hormone:* Estrogens decrease bone loss (by decreased osteoclast function) and increase bone formation (by increased osteoblast function). Estrogen level decreases after menopause. Therefore, after menopause females develop osteoporosis. *Mechanical factors/physical activity:* Increased physical activity and weight bearing increases bone mass, and decreased physical activity decreases it. *C/Fs:* Initially no symptoms. In later stages, susceptibility to fractures mainly of vertebrae, pelvis, femur. *MORPHO:* Bony trabeculae are thin and wider apart. Entire skeleton is affected, but certain bones are more affected, e.g. vertebrae. *TRT:* Estrogens to menopausal females, vitamin D, calcium fluoride, calcitonin, exercise (weight bearing) are helpful in management of osteoporosis. Harmful effects of estrogen therapy consist of increased risk of breast and endometrial cancers and of thromboembolism due to induction of increased production of coagulation factors by the liver.

7. What are the diseases associated with abnormal mineral homeostasis?

Ans. 1. Rickets.
2. Osteomalacia.
3. Hyperparathyroidism.
4. Renal osteodystrophy.

8. What are rickets and osteomalacia?

Ans. *DEF/DES:* Bone disorder where the **quality of bone is affected** with decreased mineralization of bone (as opposed to osteoporosis where the quantity of bone is reduced; but, the quality of the remaining bone is normal with normal mineralization). In rickets this decreased mineralization is of the developing bones in children. In osteomalacia decreased mineralization is of the bones which have completed development—during their remodeling process. *ETIO:* Vitamin D deficiency.

Metabolism of vitamin D:

1. Absorption in the small intestine or synthesis in sun with help of sunlight.
2. Binding to alpha-1 globulin and transport to liver.
3. In liver—conversion to 25-hydroxy vitamin D [25 (OH) D] by 25 hydroxylase.
4. In kidney—conversion to 1,25 dihydroxy vitamin D [1,25 (OH) 2D] (most active form of vitamin D) by alpha-1 hydroxylase.

Role of vitamin D in maintenance of normal plasma levels of calcium and phosphorus: 1,25 (OH) 2D maintains normal levels of serum calcium and phosphorus involving actions of intestines, bones and kidneys as follows:

1. Stimulates absorption of calcium and phosphorus in the small intestine.
2. Helps parathyroid hormone in resorption of calcium in distal renal tubules.
3. Helps parathyroid hormone in moving calcium out of the bone.

Etiology of Rickets/Osteomalacia

1. *Vitamin D deficiency:* Dietary.
2. *Vitamin D deficiency:* Decreased absorption:
   a. Cholestatic liver disease.
   b. Biliary tract obstruction
   c. Pancreatic insufficiency.
   d. Celiac sprue.
   e. Small intestinal disease.
3. *Vitamin D deficiency of synthesis:* Inadequate sunlight exposure.
4. *Vitamin D deficiency due to renal disease:* Decreased synthesis of 1,25 (OH) 2D.
5. *Phosphate deficiency* due to decreased GIT absorption due to binding with aluminium hydroxide in people with chronic use of antacids.

Morphology in Rickets and Osteomalacia

Basic problem is increased unmineralized bone matrix (osteoid tissue).

In rickets:

a. Craniotabes (small unossified areas in membranous bones of the skull which get depressed when pressure is applied and assume normal position when pressure is released).
b. Frontal bossing.
c. Rickety rosary (swelling of the ribs costochondral junctions).
d. Pigeon breast deformity [protrusion of the breast bone (sternum) anteriorly due to pull by the respiratory muscles on the soft ribs].
e. Harrison's groove (due to inward pull at the margin of the diaphragm).
f. Bowing of the legs.

In osteomalacia

Osteoid is normal. Mineralization is deficient, therefore, bone is weak and is susceptible to fractures.

9. What are bone diseases associated with hyperparathyroidism?

Ans. Parathyroid hormone (PTH) plays the main role in calcium homeostasis in our body as follows:

1. *In the bone:* It activates the osteoclasts with increased resorption of calcium from the bone into the blood.
2. *In the kidneys:* It increases the resorption of calcium by the renal tubules.
3. *In GIT:* Increases calcium absorption.

MORPHO: Increased resorption of calcium from the bone makes trabecular bone thin with compensatory increase in fibrous tissue and make them easily break with hemorrhage and cystic changes. This is traditionally known as **osteitis fibrosa cystica (von Recklinghausen disease of bone)** although **there is no inflammation** (osteitis). Due to focal collection of osteoclasts, reactive giant cells, fibroblasts, and hemorrhage a brownish mass is formed, which is traditionally known as **brown tumor** of hyperparathyroidism (although **there is no tumor**, i.e. neoplasm).

10. What is renal osteodystrophy?

Ans. Chronic renal failure resulting in bone changes such as osteomalacia, osteitis fibrosa cystica.

11. What is Paget's disease of the bone (osteitis deformans)?

Ans. *DEF/DES:* Bone disease where the bone becomes weak and easily breakable. *ETIO:* Unknown. *PATHOG:* First, there is increased osteoclastic action with bone resorption. Then there is compensatory increased osteoblastic action with new weak bone formation with abnormal architecture **(mosaic pattern)**, which is easily breakable **(chalk-stick fracture)**, and there is increased blood flow to the bone. *C/Fs:* Increase in head circumference, bone pain. Either one bone is involved (monostotic) or many (polyostotic).

COMPLI: **PHONED**

1. **P**athological fractures.
2. **High output cardiac failure** due to increased blood flow.
3. **Osteogenic sarcoma, development of**.
4. **N**erve compression due to increased new bone.
5. **E**ye-vision problems.
6. **D**eafness.

12. How does the serum calcium, phosphate and alkaline phosphatase level differ in osteoporosis, osteomalacia, Paget's disease of bone, primary hyperparathyroidism, secondary hyperparathyroidism and hypoparathyroidism which help in their *D/D*?

Ans. 1. *In osteoporosis:* These are normal.
2. *In osteomalacia:* Alkaline phosphatase is increased, calcium is decreased, phosphate is normal.
3. *In Paget's disease of bone:* Alkaline phosphatase is increased, calcium and phosphate are normal.
4. *In primary hyperparathyroidism:* Alkaline phosphatase is normal, calcium is increased, phosphate is decreased.
5. *In secondary hyperparathyroidism:* Alkaline phosphatase is increased, calcium is decreased, phosphate is normal.
6. *In hypoparathyroidism:* Alkaline phosphatase is decreased, calcium is decreased, phosphate is increased.

13. What is osteomyelitis?

Ans. *DEF/DES:* Infection of the bone and marrow.
ETIO/PATHOG: Etiologic classification:
1. Pyogenic.
   a. Acute
   b. Chronic.
2. Tuberculous.

14. What is pyogenic osteomyelitis?

Ans. This is caused by bacteria: Group B strep, staphylococci, *E. coli*, Salmonella (more common in patients with sickle cell anemia due to unknown reason). Route of infection is:
1. Direct extension from infection in adjacent soft or joint tissue.
2. Hematogenous spread.
3. Traumatic implantation. *C/Fs: S/S:* Local pain, swelling, redness, fever, malaise. *COMPLI:* Pathologic fracture, endocarditis, sepsis, systemic amyloidosis, cancer in sinus tracts. *MORPHO:* Metaphyseal plate is more common site in kids, in adults it can occur anywhere in the bone. In acute PMN infiltrate, necrosis infection spreads to periosteal area with formation of subperiosteal abscess. It may spread into soft tissue by sinus formation. If not healed, develops **chronic osteomyelitis** with chronic inflammatory cell infiltrate, and new bone formation. Residual necrotic bone is called **sequestrum**, which may be surrounded by a rim of sclerotic bone called **involucrum**. Rim of sclerotic bone may also surround an abscess called **Brodie's abscess**.

15. What is tuberculous osteomyelitis?

Ans. Caused by *Mycobacterium tuberculosis* commonly by hematogenous spread from tuberculosis of lungs or GIT. Common sites are vertebrae and long bones. Tuberculosis of the vertebrae is called **Pott's disease**. It causes collapse of vertebrae, with secondary neurologic deficit. Infection spreads from here to the adjacent soft tissue and forms an abscess in the psoas muscle of the back called **cold abscess** in psoas.

16. What is the classification of neoplasms of the bones?

Ans. **Metastatic tumors to bones are more common than primary bone tumors.** Common primary sites are thyroid, lungs, breasts, prostate (osteoblastic) and kidneys (osteolytic).

Classification of primary bone tumors:

a. *Hematogenous:* Benign: None. Malignant: Myeloma.

b. *Cartilaginous:* Benign: Chondroma, osteochondroma. Malignant: Chondrosarcoma.

c. *Osteogenic:* Benign: Osteoma, osteoid osteoma. Malignant: Osteogenic sarcoma.

d. *Unknown origin:* Benign: Giant cell tumor. Malignant: Malignant giant cell tumor. Ewing's tumor.

17. What is osteoma?

Ans. *DEF:* Benign neoplasm of the bone. Does not have the potential to become malignant. *MORPHO: GROSS:* Bones of the skull, face and long bones. Exophytic, smooth, round. *MICRO:* Appear like normal mature bone. **Gardner's syndrome:** Intestinal polyps with multiple osteomas mainly of mandible, skull and long bones.

18. What is giant cell tumor (osteoclastoma)?

Ans. *DEF:* Benign tumor of bone. *ETIO:* Unknown. *C/Fs:* Present with local pain. *Age:* 20–40. *Site:* Epiphysis of long bone (lower end of femur, upper end of tibia, upper end of humerus, lower end of radius). *MORPHO: GROSS:* Lytic lesions which erode cortex. *MICRO:* Round oval mononuclear cells, which are the neoplastic cells. Osteoclast-like giant cells formed by fusion of reactive monocytes. **X-ray: Soap bubble appearance**. *TRT:* Curettage—Approximately 50% local recurrence rate. **10% cases become frankly malignant with metastasis by bloodstream**.

19. What is osteogenic sarcoma?

Ans. *Age:* 10–20 years and 50–60 years (secondary to radiation, complication of Paget's diseases of bone). *Sites:* Ends of long bones. Metaphysis of distal femur, proximal tibia and humerus. *MORPH: GROSS:* Grow outward lifting periosteum and inward into marrow. *MICRO:* Malignant cells form osteoid (therefore, called "osteogenic", i.e. generating osteoid—opposed to bronchogenic carcinoma, which means generated or arising from the bronchus). Cartilage could also be formed. Appearance variable pleomorphism. Tumor giant cells. Spindle-shaped connective tissue. New bone formation. *C/Fs:* May present with painful swelling or pathologic fracture. X-ray: Cortex appears to have been "burst open". There is evidence of new bone formation under the corners of raised periosteum **(Codman's triangle)**. Well-marked radiating spicules of new bone are seen within the tumor **(sun-ray appearance)**. Behavior: Metastases early by blood, commonly to lung. Osteogenic sarcoma may also be seen with familial retinoblastoma.

20. What is chondrosarcoma?

Ans. *DEF:* Malignant neoplasm of the cartilage. *C/Fs: Age:* Middle age. *Site:* Bones of shoulder, ribs, pelvis and proximal femur. *MORPHO: GROSS:* Arise within medullary cavity. They erode the cartilage. *MICRO:* Either well-differentiated with mature cartilage-like appearance or anaplastic hypercellular with anaplastic chondrocytes with pleomorphism, tumor giant cells, mitoses.

21. What is Ewing's tumor?

Ans. *DEF:* Malignant neoplasm of the bone. *MORPHO: GROSS:* Arise in medullary cavity as soft-gray tumor. *MICRO:* Sheets of uniform small round blue cells. Cells contain increased glycogen. Origin of cell (histogenesis): Neuroectodermal. Therefore, also called PNET (primitive neuroectodermal tumor). *C/Fs: Age:* 10–20. *Site:* Diaphysis of long bones. Presents as a painful, enlarging mass, often tender, warm and swollen, **(giving the misleading suggestion of infection). X-ray: Onion-skin appearance**.

22. What are common metastatic (secondary) neoplasms of the bone?

Ans. Osteoblastic: Prostate, lung, breast, thyroid. Osteolytic: Kidney.

Diseases of the Joints

23. What is the classification of diseases of the joints?

Ans. One way to classify diseases of the joints is as follows: **DIM²S**

1. **D**egenerative
2. **I**nflammatory
3. **M**etabolic
4. **S**eronegative
5. **M**iscellaneous.

24. What is osteoarthritis (OA)?

Ans. *DEF:* It is a chronic, noninflammatory, **degenerative** (of articular cartilage) joint disease. Most common arthritis. "Itis" means inflammation. This is misleading because osteoarthritis is not primarily an inflammatory disease but primarily a degenerative disease. However, inflammation occurs secondarily, and it may play a role in the progression of the disease.

Types: 1. *Primary:* When osteoarthritis occurs without a predisposing cause.

2. *Secondary:* When joint degeneration occurs in a previously deformed joint or together with another disease, e.g. diabetes mellitus. *PATHOG:* Main feature is degeneration of the articular cartilage, which is due to old age and mechanical effects.

MORPHO:

1. Fissure formation on the cartilage surface.
2. Fissures slowly extend into subchondral bone with complete erosion of the cartilage.
3. This exposes the subchondral bone which becomes thick and polished like ivory (hence called **eburnation**).

4. Also, fragments of cartilage and bone become dislodged and freely float in the joint cavity and are called **joint mice**.
5. Synovial fluid leaks through the resultant defects in the cartilage and underlying bone to form **cysts** in the bone.
6. From the margins of underlying bone small bone spurs grow **(osteophytes)**. These at the distal interphalangeal joints are called **Heberden's nodes** and at the proximal interphalangeal joints called **Bouchard's nodes**.
7. These changes cause injury and inflammation of the synovial membrane. *C/Fs: S/S* gradual onset involving hip, knee, lower lumbar and cervical vertebrae, proximal and distal interphalangeal joints of the fingers. Common symptoms are: Joint stiffness and deep aching pain, **mainly in the morning**. In late stages, joints may be deformed but they do not fuse together (unlike in rheumatoid arthritis).

25. What are inflammatory arthritides?

Ans. a. Infectious; and

b. Autoimmune (rheumatoid arthritis).

26. What are infectious arthritides?

Ans. These are:

1. Acute suppurative arthritis.
2. Lyme disease.

27. What you know about acute suppurative arthritis?

Ans. *DEF:* Arthritis caused by pus-forming bacteria. *ETIO:* Gonococci, staphylococci, streptococci, *Haemophilus influenzae*, gram-negative rods, Salmonella (more common in patients with sickle cell disease for unknown reason). *C/Fs:* Pain, fever, swelling, erythema. *DIAG:* Gram stain and culture of the aspirate, which is purulent.

It is a medical emergency and diagnosis should be made urgently and appropriate treatment given immediately which should be begun empirically before culture and sensitivity results to prevent severe permanent joint destruction which can occur within only a few days.

28. What is Lyme disease?

Ans. *DEF/DES:* Infectious arthritis. First found in town named Lyme in the state of Connecticut in USA. *ETIO:* Spirochete *Borrelia burgdorferi*, which is transmitted from rodents to people by deer ticks. *C/Fs:* Affects several organs of the body. *Has 3 stages:* Stage 1. Organisms multiply at the site of tick bite with skin developing a temporary (lasting a few weeks) red indurated area **(erythema chronicum migrans)**. Stage 2. Organisms spread by blood causing myalgia, lymphadenopathy, cardiac arrhythmia, meningitis, cranial nerve involvement. Stage 3. Arthritis involving large joints, e.g. knee, shoulder, elbow, encephalitis. *MORPHO: MICRO:* Lymphocytes and plasma cells are seen in skin lesions, synovium of involved joints, and CSF during meningitis. Synovitis appears similar to rheumatoid arthritis with formation of villi and lymphocyte plasma cell infiltrate. Onion-skin like arteritis may also be seen.

29. What is rheumatoid arthritis?

Ans. *DEF:* It is a **chronic systemic inflammatory disorder mainly involving** joints causing synovitis and destruction of the articular cartilage, mainly of peripheral joints in a symmetrical polyarthritis pattern, and may also involve skin, heart, lungs, etc. Common in females of 20–40 years. *PATHOG:* Genetic predisposition (HLADR4). Most likely **autoimmune (Type III hypersensitivity reaction). IgM with anti-IgG Fc specificity, called rheumatoid factor, is seen in blood and synovial fluid.**

MORPHO of the joint:

1. First, there is acute inflammatory reaction with infiltrate by neutrophils, lymphocytes and plasma cells.
2. Hyperplasia and hypertrophy of synovial lining cells form fingerlike villi with underlying granulation tissue **(pannus)**.
3. Extension of pannus to subchondral bone causes erosion and cyst formation, with deformities of cartilage and bone.
4. Finally, the pannus fills the joint space causing fibrosis, calcification and ankylosis.
5. Extension of inflammation to ligaments, tendons and bursae lead to scarring, contracture, and deformity (characteristic radial deviation of the wrist, ulnar deviation of the fingers, fixed hyperextension **swan-neck deformity)**, fixed flexion **(buttonhole** or **boutonniere deformity)** of PIP joint of hands.

Subcutaneous rheumatoid nodule: These are seen at the extensor surface of the elbow, lungs, heart, spleen. These are nontender, round masses having a **fibrinoid necrosis**, surrounded by macrophages and granulation tissue.

C/Fs: Fatigue, malaise, anorexia, weight loss, fever, myalgia, swelling of joints and stiffness especially in the morning or after inactivity, polyarticular joint involvement mainly of proximal interphalangeal and metacarpophalangeal joints of hands, ulnar deviation of fingers, radial deviation of the wrist, normochromic normocytic anemia, **Caplan's syndrome** (RA with pneumoconiosis by silica, asbestos, coal), **Raynaud's syndrome, Sjogren's syndrome, nephrotic syndrome** due to amyloidosis, lymphadenopathy, splenomegaly **(Felty's syndrome)**, pericarditis, pleural effusion, fibrosing alveolitis, rarely atlanto-axial subluxation causing spinal cord compression.

30. What are variants of rheumatoid arthritis?

Ans. These are:

1. Felty's syndrome.
2. Juvenile rheumatoid arthritis.

31. What is Felty's syndrome?

Ans. Rheumatoid arthritis with splenomegaly and neutropenia.

32. What is juvenile rheumatoid arthritis?

Ans. Rheumatoid arthritis in younger age group. Rheumatoid factor (RF) is absent. There are a few variants, e.g.

1. *Pauci articular:* Where fewer larger joints (ankle, knee, elbow) are involved.
2. *Still's disease:* Where the onset is acute with fever, increased WBC count, enlarged liver, spleen and lymph nodes, quickly fading skin rash.

33. What is gout?

Ans. *DEF:* Increased serum uric acid (urate) with urate deposition in joint (causing repeated attacks of arthritis), on pinna of ear with fibrosis and foreign body giant cells **(tophi)**, deposition in interstitial kidney tissue **(nephropathy)** and in kidney tubules **(renal calculi)**.

Types: 1. *Primary:* Cause unknown. Commonly seen in middle-aged males with family history of gout.

2. *Secondary:* Increased production of uric acid, e.g. chronic myelogenous leukemia (CML) or decreased excretion, e.g. diuretic therapy or due to X-linked hypoxanthine guanine phosphoribosyl transferase (HGPRT) deficiency **(Lesch-Nyhan syndrome)**. *PATHOG* and *MORPHO:* There is acute inflammation with phagocytosis of urate crystals by neutrophils with release of proteolytic enzymes causing injury with painful arthritis and bursitis. Most common joint involved is metatarsophalangeal joint of the great toe **(podagra)**.

34. What is pseudogout (chondrocalcinosis)?

Ans. Caused by deposition of calcium pyrophosphate dihydrate crystals with inflammatory reaction in the cartilage. Clinically resembles gout.

35. What is the *D/D* of OA/RA/gout?

Ans. *RA:* Frequent site: Hands, knees, feet, metacarpal/proximal interphalangeal joints. *ETIO:* Autoimmune. Incidence: Female 20–50 yrs. Special features: **RA factor** (anti-IgG), subcutaneous nodules. *OA:* Frequent sites: Weight-bearing joints, distal IP joints. *ETIO:* Wear and tear. Incidence: Females >50. Special features: **Heberden's and bouchard nodes, osteophytes, joint mice**. *Gout:* Frequent sites: Metacarpal phalangeal joints of big toe. *ETIO:* Hyperuricemia. Incidence: Male >30. Special features: **Tophi, kidney stones, renal damage**.

36. What are seronegative arthritis?

Ans. These are arthritis in which serum is negative for rheumatoid factor (RF). HLA-B27 antigen is usually present. Examples are: Reiter's syndrome, ankylosing spondyloarthritis **(Marie-Strumpell disease)**, psoriatic arthritis, enteropathic arthritis, etc.

37. What is Reiter's syndrome?

Ans. It consists of polyarthritis, conjunctivitis, uveitis and nongonococcal urethritis (often due to *Chlamydia trachomatis, Ureaplasma urealyticum*).

38. What is ankylosing spondylitis?

Ans. Ankylos = fusion or bent; spondylos = vertebra. It is inflammatory disease of spine with erosion of bone at the intervertebral and sacroiliac regions with new bone formation causing fusion **(bamboo spine)** leading to stiffness and limitation of flexion of spine. Costovertebral joints also fuse causing limitation of chest movements. Uveitis is also present. HLA-B27 is positive in almost all cases.

39. What are some of the miscellaneous systemic diseases which cause joint disorders?

Ans. Hereditary hemochromatosis causes arthritis; bronchogenic carcinoma causes hypertrophic osteoarthropathy; tabes dorsalis, diabetes mellitus, syringomyelia **Charcot's joints** (neuropathic joints due to sensory loss and consequent joint trauma); hemophilia; sickle cell crises, etc.

Diseases of the Skeletal Muscle

40. What is the classification of skeletal muscle diseases?

Ans. 1. Diseases of neuromuscular junction:
   A. Myasthenia gravis   B. Eaton-Lambert syndrome
2. Genetic dystrophies:
   A. Duchenne   B. Becker   C. Myotonic dystrophy
   D. Facioscapulohumeral muscular dystrophy   E. Limb girdle dystrophy
3. Autoimmune myositis:
   A. Polymyositis.   B. Dermatomyositis
4. Neoplasms:
   A. Rhabdomyoma.   B. Rhabdomyosarcoma.

41. What is myasthenia gravis (MG)?

Ans. *DEF:* Muscle weakness due to autoimmune destruction of acetyl choline receptors (AChR) at motor end plate. Approximately 60% and 20% patients have thymic hyperplasia and thymoma respectively. *MORPHO:* Muscle appears normal. Collection of lymphocytes **(lymphorrhea)** may be present in connective tissue. *C/Fs:* Gradual onset of muscle weakness in the evening because it is worse after repeated use. Eyelid and eyeball muscles are commonly affected causing drooping of eyelids **(ptosis)** and double vision. Respiratory muscle involvement will cause **respiratory failure in untreated cases**. *DIAG:* Serum has antibodies to AChR in almost all cases. Repeated motor nerve stimuli show decreased muscle contractions.

42. What is Eaton-Lambert syndrome?

Ans. It is acquired myasthenia-like syndrome due to autoantibodies to calcium channel causing interference in release of acetyl choline at the motor nerve terminal. It is one of the paraneoplastic syndromes of the small cell carcinoma of the lung. *DIAG:* Repeated motor nerve stimuli show increased muscle contractions (unlike MG). Serum has antibodies to calcium channels in almost all cases.

43. What are muscular dystrophies?

Ans. *General:* Group of muscular disorders having following features:

1. Inherited.
2. Progressive degeneration of skeletal muscle fibers with wasting and weakness.
3. Increased serum creatinine phosphokinase (CPK).
4. Degenerative changes on muscle biopsy.

Types:

1. Duchenne muscular dystrophy.
2. Becker's muscular dystrophy.
3. Myotonic dystrophy.
4. Facioscapulohumeral muscular dystrophy.
5. Limb-girdle dystrophy.

44. What is Duchenne muscular dystrophy?

Ans. X-linked recessive muscular dystrophy, therefore, occurring in male children. Molecular basis: Dystrophin gene is affected causing absent dystrophin, which is normally present in all muscles and it helps in normal contractility of the myocyte. Consequently, its absence causes impaired contractility of cardiac and skeletal muscles. *MORPHO:* There is variation in size of the muscle fibres due to atrophy and compensatory hypertrophy. Also, there is compensatory increased fibrous and fatty tissue **(pseudohypertrophy)**. *S/S:* Begin at approximately 1–5 years of age with clumsiness followed by weakness followed by wasting, contracture, immobilization with wheel-chair existence by 10 years of age and death by 20 years of age from respiratory failure/pneumonia. Patient may also suffer from cardiac arrhythmia. *DIAG:* Elevated serum CPK, muscle biopsy.

45. What is Becker's muscular dystrophy?

Ans. *Inheritance:* X-linked recessive. Mutation of dystrophin gene resulting in dystrophin which is present as less functional leading to muscle abnormalities and clinical features which are less severe than Duchenne muscular atrophy.

46. What is myotonic dystrophy?

Ans. *Inheritance:* Autosomal dominant. *C/Fs:* Weakness with myotonia (i.e. inability to relax muscles once contracted). Associated with cataracts, testicular atrophy and baldness in males.

47. What is facioscapulohumeral muscular dystrophy?

Ans. *Inheritance:* Autosomal dominant. *C/Fs:* Involves muscles of face, scapular area and humerus. Slowly progressive, nondisabling. Life expectancy is normal.

48. What is limb girdle dystrophy?

Ans. *Inheritance:* Autosomal recessive. *C/Fs:* Involves the proximal muscles of shoulder girdle or pelvic girdle or both.

49. What do you know about rhabdomyosarcoma?

Ans. *DEF/DES:* Malignant mesenchymal neoplasm with skeletal muscle differentiation. *C/Fs:* Peak incidence first decade. Infancy and childhood. *Common sites:* Head, neck, genitourinary tract, retroperitoneum.

Types: **PEA**

1. **Pleomorphic** 2. **Embryonal** (botryoides) 3. **Alveolar**

MORPHO: GROSS: Varies. Those arising in the mucosal surfaces of the genitourinary tract and head neck area have soft, grape-like masses called **sarcoma botryoides**. *MICRO:* Embryonal (*sarcoma botryoides*). **Small round blue cell tumor,** some might have eosinophilic **straplike** processes as feature of myoblastic differentiation, without which it might be very difficult to *D/D* from other small round blue cell tumors. *Alveolar:* Neoplastic cells have fibrous septa forming pulmonary alveolar-like spaces. *Pleomorphic:* Here the cells are very pleomorphic including irregular neoplastic giant cells.

Diseases of the Smooth Muscle

50. What is leiomyoma?

Ans. *DEF:* Benign neoplasm of smooth muscles. Most common site is uterus, can arise at any other site which has smooth muscles, e.g. GIT. *MORPHO: GROSS:* Same as in uterus. *MICRO*: Same as in uterus.

51. What is leiomyosarcoma?

Ans. *DEF:* Malignant neoplasm of the smooth muscle. *Common sites:* Uterus, GIT. Arise new and not as malignant transformation of the leiomyomas. *MORPHO: GROSS:* Infiltrative lesions. *MICRO:* Cellular lesions of pleomorphic spindle-shaped cells with atypical nuclei. Most important differentiating feature from their benign counterpart leiomyoma is the increased number of mitotic figures.

Diseases of the Soft Tissue

52. What is nodular fascitis?

Ans. *DEF:* Reactive fibroblastic proliferation. In some cases, post-traumatic. Commonly in the upper extremities in subcutaneous tissue, deep fascia or muscle. *MORPHO: GROSS:* Unencapsulated, circumscribed mass. *MICRO*: Benign-appearing fibroblasts arranged in small fascicles.

53. What is fibromatosis?

Ans. *DEF:* Reactive fibroblastic proliferation with a tendency to recur.

Types:

1. *Superficial:* Palmer **(Dupuytren's contracture)**, plantar, penile **(Pyronie's disease)**.
2. *Deep:* **Desmoid tumors**. Superficial fibromatosis cause local contractures. Deep fibromatosis is located in muscles of abdomen, trunk and extremities. These have a tendency to infiltrate locally and to recur. *MICRO*: Uniform bundles of fibroblasts.

54. What is fibroma?

Ans. Benign tumor of fibroblast. Can occur in various sites of the body, commonly in ovaries.

55. What is fibrosarcoma?

Ans. *DEF:* Malignant neoplasm of fibroblasts. Common sites deep tissues of trunk, thigh. Slow growing. May recur after resection. Can also metastasize. *MORPHO: GROSS:* Infiltrative mass. *MICRO:* Fibroblast in interlacing bundles, sometimes, in a **herringbone pattern**.

56. What is fibrous histiocytoma?

Ans. *DEF:* Benign neoplasm of fibroblast and histiocytes. Common sites are dermis or subcutaneous tissue. *MORPHO: GROSS:* Circumscribed nodules. *MICRO:* Spindle cells in interlacing bundles with foamy histiocyte-like cells.

57. What is malignant fibrous histiocytoma?

Ans. *DEF:* Malignant neoplasm of fibroblasts and histiocytes. Common sites are deep in muscles of the limbs, or retroperitoneum. Behavior: Aggressive, with metastasis in approximately 50% cases. *MORPHO: GROSS:* Circumscribed-appearing mass. *MICRO:* Infiltrative spindle cells arranged in a **storiform pattern**.

58. What is lipoma?

Ans. *DEF:* Benign neoplasm of the fatty tissue. Most common soft tissue neoplasm. *MORPHO: GROSS:* Well-circumscribed, soft-yellow mass. *MICRO:* Fat cells similar to mature fatty tissue. Some variants are: *Fibrolipoma*, which contains fibrous tissue, *angiolipoma*, which contains increased number of blood vessels. *Angiomyolipoma*, which contains increased blood vessels and smooth muscle, is seen in kidneys in patients of **tuberous sclerosis**.

59. What is liposarcoma?

Ans. *DEF:* Malignant neoplasm of the fatty tissue. Common sites are mainly intra-abdominal and limbs. *MORPHO: GROSS:* Well-circumscribed soft-yellow mass. *MICRO:* Well-differentiated to pleomorphic types. Well-differentiated are difficult to distinguish from benign lipoma and are less aggressive than the pleomorphic types.

17

Diseases of the Skin (S)

OVERVIEW

A. *Diseases of the epidermis:*
   1. Pemphigus vulgaris.
   2. Psoriasis.

B. *Diseases of the epidermal-dermal interface:*
   1. Bullous pemphigoid.
   2. Erythema multiforme.
   3. Lichen planus.
   4. Dermatitis herpetiformis.

C. *Diseases of the dermis:* Urticaria.

D. Diseases of the epidermis and dermis:
   1. Acute dermatitis.
   2. Eczema.
   3. Erythema marginatum.

E. *Diseases of the subcutaneous tissue:* Erythema nodosum.

F. *Neoplasms:*
   a. *Benign:*
      1. Seborrheic keratosis.
      2. Keratoacanthoma.
      3. Verrucae.
      4. Actinic keratosis.
      5. Nevocellular nevi.
   b. *Malignant:*
      1. Squamous cell carcinoma.
      2. Basal cell carcinoma.
      3. Melanoma.

G. *Infection:* Leprosy.

Pemphigus vulgaris is an autoimmune severe bullous dermatitis due to type II hypersensitivity reaction mediated by IgG antibodies against intercellular cement substance of the skin and mucous membrane and causing blisters in superficial epidermis.

Psoriasis is an idiopathic chronic dermatitis causing plaques covered by silver-white scales, common sites being extensor surfaces of elbows, knees, scalp, glans penis, etc.

Bullous pemphigoid is an autoimmune dermatitis due to type II hypersensitivity reaction mediated by antibodies against lamina lucida of epidermis and hemidesmosomes of basal cells causing blisters beneath the basal epidermis or mucosal epithelium.

Erythema multiforme is an acute self-limiting dermatitis with multi-form lesions, e.g. macules, papules, vesicles, bullae seen in various conditions, e.g. infections, allergic drug reactions, malignancies, collagen vascular diseases.

Stevens-Johnson syndrome is a variant of severe degree involving skin and mucosal surfaces. Toxic epidermal necrolyis (TEN) is another serious variant with generalized mucocutaneous involvement and clinically appear like 3rd degree burn.

Lichen planus is an idiopathic condition having self-limiting multiple itchy papules over the skin and mucus membranes.

Dermatitis herpetiformis is an autoimmune bullous disorder with bullae resembling herpes mediated by IgA and IgG antibodies against epidermal-dermal junctional reticulin.

Urticaria (hives) is an IgE-mediated acute dermatitis causing localized edema and itching.

Acute dermatitis is due to type IV hypersensitivity reaction due to contact with allergic agent such as poison ivy, oak, etc.

Eczema is a skin disease with red, papulovesicular oozing lesions in early stage and scaly plaques in later stage caused by type IV hypersensitivity reaction to poison ivy, oak, etc. and exposure to certain drugs, sun light, etc.

Erythema marginatum: It is one of the **5 major Jones criteria** for the diagnosis of acute rheumatic fever. It consists of erythematous macules with pale center seen usually over the inner surfaces of the arms. Microscopically epidermal spongiosis and parakeratosis is present and in the dermis perivascular lymphocytic infiltrate is seen.

Erythema nodosum: It consists of tender red nodules usually over the shins. It can be idiopathic or can be seen with streptococcal infection, sarcoidosis, drug reaction, e.g. sulphonamides. Microscopically, panniculitis is present consisting of infiltration of the subcutaneous fat by lymphocytes and macrophages.

Seborrheic keratosis is a benign epidermal tumor seen in middle-aged people on trunk, limbs, head and neck.

Keratoacanthoma is a benign epidermal neoplasm seen in sun-exposed areas of the body which heal spontaneously.

Verrucae (warts) are self-limiting benign epidermal neoplasms caused by human papilloma virus (HPV) of 4 types:

1. Verruca vulgaris.
2. Verruca plana.
3. Verruca palmaris and plantaris.
4. Condyloma acuminatum **(venereal wart)**.

Actinic keratosis are lesions seen in chronic sun-exposed areas (face, arms, dorsal surface of the hands) consisting of excess deposition of keratin in the dermis. These are nonneoplastic lesions, however, **these can progress to CIS and infiltrating squamous cell carcinoma.**

Squamous cell carcinoma is the most common skin cancer. It arises in old age in sun-exposed areas and is locally invasive. ~ 5% metastasize by lymphatics.

Basal cell carcinoma is a malignant tumor of the epidermis, arising in sun-exposed areas. It invades locally and burrows deep into tissue like a rodent; and, hence is also called **rodent ulcer**.

Lesions of melanocytes are benign nevus and malignant melanoma. *Dysplastic nevus* is one of the types of nevi. **It has the potential to become melanoma.**

Melanoma arise in sun-exposed areas. It has two growth phases:

1. Laterally (initial).
2. Vertically (later), when it grows deeper into the skin and can metastasize.

Types of melanoma are:

1. Superficial spreading.
2. Lentigo maligna melanoma.
3. Acral lentiginous melanoma.
4. Nodular melanoma, **which has the poorest prognosis**.

Leprosy **(Hansen disease)** is a slowly progressive infection by *Mycobacterium leprae*. It mainly affects skin and peripheral nerves, causing deformities by type IV hypersensitivity. It has three main types:

1. Tuberculoid.
2. Intermediate (borderline).
3. Lepromatous.

Tuberculoid is the **less severe** form due to good immune response of our body. Lepromatous is **more severe** form due to poor immune response of our body.

1. Classify diseases of the skin. Give a few examples of each.

Ans. There are many ways the diseases of the skin can be classified. One way with a few examples is:

1. Diseases of the epidermis:
   a. Acute dermatitis.
   b. Pemphigus vulgaris.
   c. Psoriasis.
   d. Eczema.
2. Diseases of the epidermal-dermal interface:
   a. Bullous pemphigoid.
   b. Erythema multiforme.
   c. Lichen planus.
   d. Dermatitis herpetiformis.
3. Diseases of the dermis: Urticaria.
4. Diseases of epidermis and dermis: Erythema marginatum.
5. Diseases of the subcutaneous fat: Erythema nodosum.
6. Neoplasms:
   a. Benign and premalignant.
   b. Malignant: Squamous cell carcinoma, basal cell carcinoma, melanoma.
7. Infection: Leprosy.

Diseases of the Epidermis

2. What is acute dermatitis?

Ans. *DEF:* Dermatitis due to reaction from contact with some allergic agent. *ETIO:* Poison ivy, poison oak, etc. *PATHOG:* Type IV hypersensitivity reaction. *MORPHO: GROSS:* Swelling, redness, vesiculation of the skin. *MICRO*: Vesicles are intra-epidermal, formed due to necrosis of the cells of the epidermis. Superficial dermis has edema, capillary dilatation and perivascular infiltration with neutrophils, eosinophils and lymphocytes. *C/Fs:* Severe itching and burning.

3. What is pemphigus vulgaris?

Ans. *DEF:* It is an autoimmune severe **bullous dermatitis**. There are 4 types of pemphigus. The most common type is pemphigus vulgaris (vulgar = common). *ETIO:* It is type II hypersensitivity reaction mediated by IgG antibodies against intercellular cement substance of skin and mucous membrane. This is seen by direct immunofluorescence as a characteristic **fishnet-like pattern** of intercellular IgG deposit at the site of acantholysis. *MORPHO: MICRO:* Main feature is acantholysis. *C/Fs:* Age: 50–60 years. *S/S*: Axilla and groin are common sites. Itching and burning. Blisters are very superficial and rupture very easily leaving shallow erosions. Degenerated squamous cells, called **Tzanck cells**, are seen in the bullae.

4. What is psoriasis?

Ans. *DEF:* Chronic dermatitis with well-demarcated pink plaque covered by silver-white scales. *ETIO:* Unknown. *MORPHO: MICRO:* Acanthosis with hyperkeratosis and parakeratosis. Within the parakeratotic corneal layer is focal small collection of neutrophils **(Munro's micro-abscesses)**. Granular layer is thin to absent. Thinning of the part of the epidermal layer which is over the dermal papillae with dilated blood vessels within these papillae, which bleed easily upon lifting of the plaque. *C/Fs:* Common sites are extensor surfaces of the elbows, knees, scalp, lumbosacral area, intergluteal cleft, glans penis. **Sometimes, associated with arthritis**. Also, nail can become yellowish and have pitting.

5. What is eczema?

Ans. *DEF:* Clinical condition initially consisting of red vesicular, oozing lesions and later of raised scaling plaques.

ETIO: 1. Allergic reaction from contact with poison ivy, poison oak etc. This is type IV hypersensitivity mediated by T lymphocytes.
2. Drugs.
3. Sunlight.
4. Atopic.

Diseases of the Epidermal-Dermal Interface

6. What is bullous pemphigoid?

Ans. *DEF:* An autoimmune bullous disorder due to detachment of the basal layer of the epidermis from the underlying dermis. *ETIO:* It is caused by type II hypersensitivity with antibodies against antigen of lamina lucida and hemidesmosomes (the attachment between basal cells and the underlying basement membrane). This leads to linear deposition of antibodies and complement in this area. Complement activation results in tissue injury via attracted neutrophils and eosinophils. *MORPHO:* Vesicle is beneath the basal layer of the epidermis/mucosal epithelium.

7. What is erythema multiforme?

Ans. *DEF:* Acute self-limiting dermatitis with multi form lesions, e.g. macules, papules, vesicles, bullae, **target lesions** consisting of a red macule or papule with a pale center looking like a target.

ETIO: 1. *Infection:* Typhoid, leprosy, herpes simplex, mycoplasma, histoplasmosis, etc.
2. *Allergic reaction to some drugs:* Sulfonamides, penicillin, salicylates, etc.
3. *Malignancies:* Carcinomas, lymphomas.
4. *Collagen vascular diseases:* SLE, PAN, dermatomyositis.

Steven-Johnson syndrome is a variant of severe degree involving skin and mucosal surfaces. **Toxic epidermal necrolysis (TEN)** is another serious variant with generalized mucocutaneous involvement and clinically appear similar to 3rd degree burn.

8. What is lichen planus?

Ans. *DEF:* Multiple, self-limiting pruritic, papules over the skin and mucus membranes. *ETIO:* Unknown. *MORPHO:* Thick lymphocytic infiltrate at the dermo-epidermal junction is present giving the dermo-epidermal junction a zig-zag **(saw tooth)** appearance. Some apoptotic basal cells are present in papillary dermis called **colloid** or **civatte bodies**. *C/Fs:* Common sites: Wrists, elbows, glans penis.

9. What is dermatitis herpetiformis?

Ans. *DEF:* An autoimmune bullous disorder due to IgA and IgG antibodies against reticulin that attaches the epidermal basement membrane to the underlying dermis. The bullae are in groups similar to bullae in infection with herpes virus. Therefore, this condition is called **herpetiformis**. However, **herpes virus is not involved in this condition**. *ETIO:* Unknown, except some cases are seen with celiac disease because IgA and IgG antibodies to gluten of the wheat cross react with the above stated reticulin. These people are cured by gluten-free diet. *MORPHO:* Granular deposits of IgA are seen between epidermal basement membrane and the underlying dermis by direct immunofluorescence.

Diseases of the Dermis

10. What is urticaria (hives)?

Ans. It is an IgE-mediated acute dermatitis, causing degranulation of mast cells releasing chemical mediators, e.g. histamine resulting in increased permeability of the small blood vessels leading to localized edema and itching.

Diseases of the Epidermis and Dermis

11. What is erythema marginatum?

Ans. It consists of erythematous macule with pale center. It is seen in conditions such as acute rheumatic fever **(one of the 5 Jones major criteria)**. *MICRO:* Epidermal spongiosis and parakeratosis. In the dermis, dermal edema and perivascular lymphocytic infiltrate is seen.

Diseases of Subcutaneous Fat

12. What is erythema nodosum?

Ans. It consists of tender red nodules usually over the shins. *ETIO:* Idiopathic, streptococcal infection, sarcoidosis, drugs, e.g. sulphonamides.
MICRO: Panniculitis consisting of infiltration by lymphocytes and macrophages.

Neoplasms: Benign and Premalignant

13. What is seborrheic keratosis?

Ans. *DEF:* Benign epidermal tumor. *MORPHO: GROSS:* Round, flat, plaque a few millimeters to a few centimeters in diameter. *MICRO:* Exophytic lesion composed of sheets of small cells with hyperkeratosis at the surface with small keratin-filled cysts **(horn cysts)** and down growth of keratin into main tumor mass **(pseudohorn cyst)**. *C/Fs:* Seen in middle-aged people on trunk, limbs, head and neck.

14. What is keratoacanthoma?

Ans. *DEF:* Benign neoplasm of epidermis in sun-exposed areas of body which heal spontaneously. *ETIO:* Unknown. *MORHO: GROSS:* Dome-shaped nodule with a cup-like central depression filled with keratin. *MICRO:* Proliferation of keratin in a cup-like shape with central cavity filled with keratin. Epithelial cells are large, with reactive cytological atypia and glassy eosinophilic cytoplasm.

15. What is verrucae (warts)?

Ans. *DEF:* Self-limiting benign epidermal neoplasms caused by HPV (human papilloma virus).

MORPHO: GROSS: Depending on the type (4):

1. *Verruca vulgaris (commonest):* Light brown-colored papules 0.1 to 1 cm with a rough surface.
2. *Verruca plana (flat wart):* Flat papules, with smooth surface.
3. *Verruca palmaris and plantaris:* On the palm and sole of feet, scaly lesions.
4. *Condyloma acuminatum (venereal wart):* On penis, female genitalia, urethra, perianal areas and rectum. Soft, light brown, cauliflower-like growths. *MICRO:* Epidermal hyperplasia in papillary finger-like formation. Cytoplasm of superficial cells have clear halos around nuclei **(koilocytes)**.

16. What is actinic keratosis?

Ans. *DEF:* Lesions in chronic sun-exposed areas (face, arms, dorsal surface of hands) leading to excess deposition of keratin and hence the term: "Actinic (= sun-related) keratoses (keratin deposition)". *MORPHO: GROSS:* Commonly brownish 1 cm in diameter. Some may produce so much keratin that a **cutaneous horn** develops. *MICRO:* In the dermis, there is blue-gray elastic fibers (elastosis). In the epidermis, There is cytologic atypia seen in the lowermost layers of the epidermis. Stratum corneum is thickened with retained nuclei (parakeratosis). Some of the lesions progress to full thickness atypia **(CIS), which may progress to infiltrating squamous cell carcinoma.**

17. What is a nevus (pleural nevi)?

Ans. Nevus means congenital lesion of the skin. Nevocellular nevus are congenital or acquired neoplasm of melanocytes.

Types of nevocellular nevi:

1. Congenital.
2. Blue.
3. Spindle and epithelioid cell (Spitz).
4. Halo.
5. Dysplastic **(Potential to become malignant melanoma)**.

MORPHO: GROSS: Uniform light brown small papules.

MICRO: Three stages:

1. Junctional. 2. Compound. 3. Dermal

1. *Junctional:* Melanocytes are present at the dermo-epidermal junction. Melanocytes are benign appearing, uniform, normochromic arranged in small nests.
2. *Compound:* Later, junctional nevi grow into underlying dermis as nests and cords of cells.
3. *Dermal:* Eventually, the epidermal nests may be lost entirely to leave pure dermal nevi. The **nevus cells undergo maturation, becoming hypopigmented (melanoma cells do not do so)**.

Neoplasms. Malignant

18. What are the common malignant neoplasms of the skin?

Ans. 1. Squamous cell carcinoma.
2. Basal cell carcinoma; and
3. Malignant melanoma.

19. What is the commonest risk factor for these 3 neoplasms?

Ans. Ultraviolet light exposure.

20. What is squamous cell carcinoma?

Ans. It is the most common skin cancer. It arises in sun-exposed skin. Usually, in old age. Most are locally invasive and approximately 5% metastasize, usually to regional lymph nodes. *Predisposing factors:* Ultraviolet light exposure in the sunlight, industrial carcinogens (tars, oils), chronic ulcers, draining osteomyelitis, old burn scars, ingestion of arsenicals, ionizing radiation. *MORPHO: GROSS:* Scaling, indurated, ulcerated nodule. *MICRO:* Sheets and islands of neoplastic polygonal squamous cells with keratinization, usually with **keratin pearls**.

21. What is basal cell carcinoma? What is its other name (why)?

Ans. Slow-growing malignant tumor of the epidermis which invades locally and ulcerates. It burrows deep into underlying tissue like a rodent. Therefore, this neoplasm is also called **rodent ulcer**. These rarely metastasize. *Predisposing factors:* Exposure to ultraviolet light in sunlight. *MORPHO: GROSS:* Common site is face. Early lesion is a papule. Later ulceration with deep invasion of underlying bone. *MORPHO: MICRO:* Tumor cells resemble those in the normal basal cell layer of the epidermis. *Two microscopic (histologic) patterns are present:*

1. Multifocal superficial type
2. Nodular type.

Multifocal superficial types extend along the basal layer of the skin surface. Nodular types grow downward deeply into dermis as cords and groups of basophilic cells with hyperchromatic nuclei in a mucinous matrix. Cells at the periphery of the groups of tumor cells are placed in parallel configuration **(palisading)**.

22. What is a malignant melanoma?

Ans. It is a malignant neoplasm. It arises from melanocytes. Its common site is skin. Ultraviolet sunlight exposure predisposes to it. It can also be seen in uvea, vulva. *Growth phases: It has two growth phases:*

1. Radial (initial).
2. Vertical (later).
   a. *Radial phase:* Growth is mainly laterally within the epidermis and papillary zone of the dermis. Melanomas in the radial growth phase do not metastasize and can be cured by local excision.
   b. *Vertical phase:* Growth extends into reticular dermis or deeper. Prognosis varies with thickness of the lesion. Lymphatic or hematogenous metastasis may occur. Malignant melanomas have a better prognosis when they have a long period of radial growth than when they have an early vertical growth phase.

Clinical variants:

1. *Superficial spreading melanoma:* Most common. Consists of radial growth phase. Most common sites are trunk and limbs. Irregularly bordered having various colors. This does not metastasize. So, prognosis is good.
2. *Nodular melanoma:* Begins with the vertical growth phase. Has the **poorest prognosis**. Prognosis is based on depth of invasion: 1.5 mm or less = good prognosis, 1.5 mm to 3 mm = fair prognosis, 3 mm or more = poor prognosis.
3. *Acral-lentiginous melanoma:* Most often occurs on the hands, feet and mucosal surfaces of dark-skinned persons.
4. *Lentigo maligna melanoma:* It has a long radial growth phase before it becomes invasive. Its precursor lesion is lentigo maligna **(Hutchinson's melanotic freckle)**. (*in situ* lesion). It is most common in elderly people in sun-exposed areas of the body, mainly the face.

MORPHO: GROSS: Most important gross feature is a change in color or size in a pigmented lesion. Unlike benign nevi (non-dysplastic), malignant melanomas have irregular borders and variation in color consisting of black, brown, red, dark blue and gray. *MICRO:* Melanoma cells are quite larger than nevus cells. The nuclei are

irregular hyperchromatic with prominent nucleoli. These are present in epidermis and dermis and show no maturation in deeper layers as of dermis unlike nevi. (This helps in *D/D* with nevus). Deeper the melanoma cells are in dermis, worse is the prognosis. *C/Ts:* Usually asymptomatic. Sometimes there is itching.
Clinically warning signs are:
1. Enlargement of a preexisting mole.
2. Itching or pain in a preexisting mole.
3. Development of a new pigmented lesion during adult life.
4. Irregular borders of a pigmented lesion.
5. Different colors in a pigmented lesion.
6. Appearance of new pigmented lesion.

Infection: Leprosy

23. What is leprosy (Hansen's disease)?

Ans. *ETIO:* Infection by *Mycobacterium leprae. Microbiology: Mycobacterium leprae* is an obligate intracellular bacteria. It is acid-fast. It grows very poorly in culture; but, it can be grown in the armadillo. It grows more slowly than other mycobacteria. It grows best at 32 to 34°C. It secretes no toxin. Its virulence is based on properties of its cell wall. This causes injury by inducing type IV hypersensitivity reaction in our body (cell-mediated immune reaction—delayed type hypersensitivity). This is seen when dermal injection of bacterial extract (lepromin) is done.

Pathology/PATHOG: It is a slowly progressive infection. Its communicability is low. Incubation period is 2 to 6 years. It mainly affects the skin and peripheral nerves. This leads to disabling deformities. It can also affect respiratory tract and other systems of the body. It can be transmitted from one person to other by aerosols from lesions in the upper respiratory tract. Thereafter, the inhaled *M. leprae* are taken up by the alveolar macrophages and spread via the blood. But, *M. leprae* grow only in the cool tissues of skin and limbs.

Types:
1. Tuberculoid
2. Lepromatous (anergic).
3. Borderline (intermediate).

Based on these, the spectrum of disease is of 5 subtypes:

a. *TL (Tuberculoid leprosy):* Here, there is increased cell-mediated immunity making it a **less severe form** of leprosy. Therefore, the lesions are localized. Lesions are hypopigmented, anesthetic, (both due to nerve involvement) well-outlined with central healing and atrophy. Main sites are face, buttocks and limbs. Cutaneous nerves of these areas are thick and tender. Muscles supplied by these are atrophied. Outcome is good. Lesions heal spontaneously.
b. *BT (Borderline tuberculoid leprosy):* Similar to TL; but, lesions are many. Instead of cutaneous nerves, peripheral nerves are involved. There is deformity of hands and feet.

c. *BB (Borderline leprosy):* Skin lesions are many. Size and form of these vary from macule to papule to plaques. Annular lesions with hypopigmented anesthetic center is characteristic. Many nerves are involved with limb deformity.

d. *BL (Borderline lepromatous leprosy):* Many skin lesions of different forms with many AFBs present in them.

e. *LL (Lepromatous leprosy):* This is **more severe form** of leprosy as there is unresponsiveness of host immune response. So, it is called **anergic leprosy**. Lesions are similar as BL with many lesions of different forms with many AFBs present. Ear lobes are large. Eyebrows are thin. Facial skin infiltration gives a **leonine facies**. Mucus membrane involved with stuffiness of the nose, laryngitis, nasal septal perforation with collapse of nasal cartilage giving a saddle shape to the nose. Glove and stocking type of anesthesia. Testes atrophied with gynecomastia. Neurotrophic atrophy leads to gradual disappearance of the fingers. Nerve involvement is less than TT. Nervous system is damaged by invasion of lepra bacilli of the Schwann cells and into endoneural and perineural macrophages. Macrophages containing many lepra bacilli **(lepra cells)** are present in the lesions. Lepra bacilli are present in sputum and blood.

18 Diseases of the Eyes and Ears (E and E)

OVERVIEW

Selected diseases of the eyes

1. Trachoma.
2. Glaucoma.
3. Sympathetic ophthalmitis.
4. Cataract.
5. Retrolental fibroplasia.
6. Retinoblastoma.
7. Ocular melanoma.

Trachoma is **one of the world's leading preventable causes of blindness**. It is not a neoplasm although its name ends with "oma". It is an infectious disease caused by *Chlamydia trachomatis* primarily affecting conjunctiva and cornea finally leading to scarring and opacification of cornea resulting in blindness. This happens in 4 stages. If treated in early stage, the blindness is preventable. WHO has a goal to eradicate it by 2020 by its **SAFE** program consisting of **S**urgery, **A**ntibiotics, **F**acial cleanliness and **E**nvironmental improvement.

Glaucoma is **also one of the world's leading causes of blindness**. It is not a neoplasm although its name ends in "oma". It is a disease with increased intraocular pressure due to obstruction to the drainage of the aqueous humor through the angle of the anterior chamber of the eye and at the pupil. Its types are congenital or acquired. The main acquired types are:

1. Primary which is of 2 types:
   a. Open angle (simple, chronic glaucoma) due to sclerosis of the trabecular meshwork. Additionally, the endothelial lining of the canal of Schlemn may be closed.
   b. Narrow angle (closed angle, angle closure) due to narrow or closed angle of the anterior chamber of the eye. **It is an ophthalmic emergency as patient can become completely blind within a few days if not treated promptly**.
2. Secondary from obstruction of aqueous drainage due to complications of uveitis, trauma, dislocation of lens.

Sympathetic ophthalmitis where the opposite normal eye develops autoimmune granulomatous inflammation in ~ 10% of cases following traumatic autoimmune granulomatous inflammation of the affected eye. **Timely enucleation of the traumatic eye can prevent this**.

Cataract is one of the world's leading causes of preventable blindness due to opacification of the lens.

Retrolental fibroplasia is an iatrogenic degeneration of retinal arterioles and capillaries together with proliferation of adjacent vessels in the premature infants who are treated with high tension oxygen therapy.

Retinoblastoma is a malignant eye tumor of childhood. It can be familial or sporadic. In both cases, there is loss of function mutation of one of the cancer suppressor genes. It causes blindness and if untreated is fatal. However, patient can be cured by early treatment with enucleation, chemo- and radiotherapy.

Ocular melanoma is a malignant neoplasm of the eye arising from the melanocytes of the uvea. It causes blindness. It can metastasize and be fatal. Timely enucleation or radiotherapy might prevent this outcome.

Selected diseases of the ears

1. Infections.
2. Chloesteatoma
3. Otosclerosis.
4. Acoustic neuroma (vestibular schwannoma).

Common infections of the ear are: Otitis externa and otitis media, which are usually seen in infants and children and cause complications of infection of the mastoid bone and rupture of tympanic membrane.

Cholesteatoma is not a neoplasm although its name ends with "oma". It is seen in the middle ear with otitis media as a cystic lesion sometimes having spicules of cholesterol and hence the name "chole".

Otosclerosis is a disease which causes deafness due to sclerosis and ankylosis of the foot plate of stapes bone thereby interfering with transmission of sound to the inner ear.

Acoustic neuroma (vestibular schwannoma): It is a benign, slow-growing tumor which arises from the Schwann cells of the vestibular division of the 8th cranial nerve in the internal auditory canal, which it gradually erodes and appears in the cerebellopontine angle.

Selected Diseases of the Eyes (E)

1. What is trachoma?

Ans. It is an infectious disease of the eye. (It is not a neoplasm, even though its name ends with "oma"). **It is one of the world's leading causes of preventable blindness**. *ETIO:* It is caused by *Chlamydia trachomatis*. *PATHOG:* It primarily affects conjunctiva and corneal epithelium finally leading to cicatrization of the tissue. Its course is in 4 stages:

Stage I: Clinically: There is formation of conjunctival follicles (subepithelial conjunctival inflammatory infiltrates) and diffuse punctate inflammation of the cornea. Subsequently, there is growth of fibrovascular tissue in the substantia propria of the conjunctiva and the cornea **(pannus)**. *MICRO:* Corneal epithelium contains cytoplasmic **inclusion bodies** composed of microcolonies of **elementary bodies** and larger basophilic **initial bodies**. Corneal and conjunctival epithelium is infiltrated by neutrophils. Subepithelial tissue is infiltrated by lymphocytes and plasma cells.

Stage II: Clinically: Inflammation worsens with further formation of follicles and epithelial thickening. Corneal pannus becomes more extensive. *MICRO:* Large macrophages with phagocytized debris **(Leber's cells)** are seen in the conjunctiva. Conjunctival epithelium is hyperplastic and has round cell infiltration and subepithelial edema.

Stage III: Clinically: Follicles disappear. Cicatrization occurs. Cicatrization causes inversion of the upper eyelid (cicatricial **entropion**) with eyelashes bent inwards **(trichiasis)**. *MICRO:* There is subepithelial scar tissue. Some lymphocytes and plasma cells are still present.

Stage IV: Clinically: There is spontaneous arrest of the disease. Residual entropion and trichiasis lead to continuing corneal damage thereby denuding the corneal epithelium and predisposing the cornea to infection and further **opacification** as a result of scarring, leading to **blindness**.

Trachoma is completely preventable. WHO has a goal to eradicate it by 2020 by its **SAFE** program consisting of **S**urgery, **A**ntibiotics, **F**acial cleanliness and **E**nvironmental improvement.

2. What is glaucoma?

Ans. *DEF:* Increase in the intraocular pressure due to obstruction to the drainage of the aqueous humor through the angle of the anterior chamber and at the pupil enough to cause degeneration of the optic disk and nerve. **It is one of the world's major causes of blindness**. It is not a neoplasm even though its name ends with "oma".

CLASSI: A. *Congenital (least common):* Isolated or with **aniridia, neurofibromatosis, Marfan's syndrome**.

B. *Acquired:*

1. Primary (very common):
   a. Wide (open) angle (simple or chronic glaucoma)—90% of primary glaucoma.
   b. Narrow angle (closed angle, angle closure)—10% of primary glaucoma.

2. Secondary (less common):
   a. Uveitis with anterior synechiae.
   b. Trauma.
   c. Dislocation of lens.

Acquired Primary Wide (Open) Angle Glaucoma

People with myopia and diabetes mellitus are more susceptible to developing this. Aqueous humor does not flow out of the eye through the angle causing increased intraocular pressure. Mild degeneration with sclerosis adjacent to the canal of Schlemm may be present. **Onset is slow and not noticed** in people of over 40 years of age. It is slowly progressive with slow increase in intraocular pressure leading to progressive degeneration of the optic disc. This causes increase in the size of blind spot (scotoma) and loss of the peripheral visual field. Fundoscopic examination shows optic cup as deep and large. **Visual loss can be stopped, if treated** with pupillary constrictors (mioptics) such as pilocarpine, laser trabeculoplasty, surgery.

Acquired Primary Narrow (Angle Closure) Angle Glaucoma

This is due to narrow or closed angle of the anterior chamber. People with shallow anterior chamber, e.g. hyperopic, are susceptible to developing this. Onset is acute with rapid increase of intraocular pressure with acute red eye, severe pain, vomiting and rapid visual impairment. **It is an ophthalmic emergency. Complete blindness can occur within a few days if not treated promptly. Acute attack may be precipitated by dilation of pupil,** e.g. for fundoscopic examination. Treatment for acute phase is osmotic agents and pupillary constrictors started immediately. Peripheral iridectomy can help in acute relief of symptoms and also in prevention of future episodes.

3. What is sympathetic ophthalmitis?

Ans. *DEF/DES:* When there is a penetrating wound to an eye with injury to the uvea, a granulomatous autoimmune reaction can develop in that eye. **If this eye is not timely enucleated**, in approximately 10% of the cases the opposite eye can develop similar autoimmune granulomatous inflammation with blindness (in "sympathy" to the sister-traumatized eye). *MORPHO: MICRO:* Infiltration by lymphocytes, eosinophils and clusters of epithelioid cells are present. *C/Fs:* **Mild visual impairment and photophobia, which should alert the physician to immediately remove the injured eye to prevent blindness in the uninjured eye.**

4. What is a cataract?

Ans. *DEF:* Opacity of the lens is called cataract (cataract in English means a large water fall, which obscures the view beyond it). **It is one of the world's major causes of preventable blindness.**

ETIO:

1. Degeneration in old age (most common).
2. Congenital.
3. Trauma.
4. Infrared radiation.

5. Diabetes mellitus, etc.

COMPLI: Glaucoma due to interference with flow of the intraocular fluid. Endophthalmitis due to autoimmune reaction to release of sequestrated lens protein.

5. What is retrolental fibroplasia?

Ans. *DEF:* Degeneration of retinal arterioles and capillaries due to high tension oxygen therapy in premature infants whose peripheral retina is not completely vascularized. *PATHOG:* Therapeutic oxygen at high tension causes closing, obliteration and degeneration of arterioles and capillaries in premature infants leading to proliferation of adjacent vessels, which penetrate the inner membrane of the retina and grow into vitreous with formation of organized mass behind the lens (hence the name) leading to blindness.

6. What is retinoblastoma?

Ans. Retinoblastoma is a malignant tumor of the retina. *It has several unique features:*

1. It is the most common malignant eye tumor of childhood.
2. It can undergo spontaneous regression.
3. It can be multifocal and bilateral.
4. It frequently occurs as congenital tumor.
5. Its incidence decreases with age and is uncommon after 4 years of age
6. Patients have high incidence of second primary tumors, e.g. osteogenic sarcoma.
7. It can occur in both familial and sporadic pattern.
8. Familial cases typically develop multiple tumors that are bilateral.
9. Sporadic, nonfamilial tumors are all unilateral and unifocal.
10. Patients with familial retinoblastoma are at increased risk for developing **osteosarcoma** and **other soft tissue tumors**.
11. There is genetic abnormality consisting of recessive, loss of function mutation of one of the cancer suppressor genes (Rb = Retinoblastoma gene).

MORPHO: GROSS: Nodular mass.

MICRO:

a. Small, round cells with large hyperchromatic nuclei and little cytoplasm.
b. **Flexner-Wintersteiner rosettes:** These consist of clusters of cuboidal or short columnar cells arranged around a central lumen **(true rosettes)**. *C/Fs:* May be present at birth, but most commonly it presents at 2 years of age with poor vision, strabismus, pain and tenderness. Pupil appears whitish and a yellow reflex is seen behind the pupil when light is shone into it **(amaurotic cat's eye reflex)**. Metastases may be seen in brain, skull, lymph nodes. *PROG:* **Untreated tumors are usually fatal. But, patient can be cured by early treatment with enucleation, chemotherapy and radiotherapy**.

7. What is ocular melanoma?

Ans. *DEF:* Melanoma arising from the melanocytes of the uvea (iris, ciliary body, choroids). *MORPHO: GROSS:* Pigmented mass. Choroidal melanoma may spread to the surface of the eyeball and present as episcleral mass and spread to periorbital tissue. *MICRO:* Cells are spindle-shaped, nuclei are large with prominent nucleoli. *C/Fs:* Iris melanoma may spread intraocularly and cause pain and loss of vision. Choroidal melanoma may develop hepatic metastasis through blood. Timely enucleation or radiation might prevent this.

Selected Diseases of the Ears (E)

8. What is otosclerosis?

Ans. It is a condition where the foot plate of the stapes bone between fenestra ovale and cochlea becomes gradually sclerotic with ankylosis, which interferes with the transmission of sound waves to the perilymph of cochlea producing progressive deafness. Etiology is unknown.

9. What is cholesteatoma?

Ans. It is a cystic lesion seen with chronic otitis media. It is about 1 to 4 cm in diameter. It is lined by keratinizing squamous epithelium and filled with debris, sometimes having spicules of cholesterol. Even though this term ends with "oma", it is not a neoplasm (just like granuloma, trachoma, glaucoma, ameboma, tuberculoma, etc. which are not neoplasms). *C/Fs:* It might present with foul-smelling discharge from the ear (otorrhea). Examination might show ruptured tympanic membrane. *COMPLI:* Erosion of facial nerve or extension intracranially therefore, it should be removed by mastoid surgery.

10. What is otitis media?

Ans. *DEF:* It is infection of the middle ear. *ETIO: Hemophilus influenzae,* beta hemolytic streptococci and *Streptococcus pneumoniae. C/Fs:* Happens usually in infants and young children. *COMPLI:* Infection of the mastoid bone. Recurrent infection can cause perforation of the tympanic membrane.

11. What is acoustic neuroma (vestibular schwannoma)?

Ans. It is benign, slow-growing neoplasm, which arises from the Schwann cells of the vestibular division of the VII cranial nerve in the internal auditory canal, which it slowly erodes and appears in the cerebellopontine angle and represents ~1/10 of all the intracranial neoplasms. It can be part of the autosomal dominant inherited **neurofibromatosis type 2**, when it is bilateral. *MORPHO:* On gross examination, it is encapsulated, well-circumscribed tumor. Microscopically, it has cellular area consisting of spindle-shaped cells with long nuclei **(antoni A)**, where nuclei are arranged in palisades (parallel) **(Verocay bodies)** and less cellular loose myxoid areas (antoni B). *C/Fs:* Sensory neural hearing loss with tinnitus. V, VII, IX, X cranial nerves may be involved. Brainstem and cerebellum may be also involved.

Appendix 1

Some Mnemonics

A

Adaptations: **H²AM**

1. **H**ypertrophy
2. **H**yperplasia
3. **A**trophy
4. **M**etaplasia.

Alzheimer's disease, microscopic features:
He is **s**enile, has **n**o **g**rasp, **n**o **a**wareness of **l**ife.

1. **H**irano bodies
2. **S**enile plaques
3. **N**eurofibrillary tangles
4. **G**ranulovacuolar degeneration
5. **N**euronal loss
6. **A**myloid angiopathy
7. **L**ewy bodies.

Aneurysm complications: **ROPE**

1. **R**upture
2. **O**bstruction
3. **P**ressure
4. **E**mbolism.

Atherosclerosis, major modifiable risk factors: **↑S^4**

1. **S**weet blood (diabetes mellitus)
2. **S**alty blood (NaCl) (hypertension)
3. **S**ticky blood (hyperlipidemia)
4. **S**moky blood (smoking).

Atherosclerosis, minor modifiable risk factors: **↑S^4**

1. **S**tarchy diet
2. **S**edantary life
3. **S**exy life (oral contraceptives)
4. **S**tressed life.

Atherosclerosis, nonmodifiable risk factors: **S3**

1. **S**enior age
2. **S**ex male
3. **S**iblings/same family.

B

Blood vessels, congenital anomalies: **C^2AB**

1. **C**avernous and **c**apillary hemangiomas
2. **A**rteriovenous fistulas
3. **B**erry aneurysm of the circle of Willis.

Brain herniations: **CUT**

1. **C**ingulate gyrus (subfalcine)
2. **U**ncinate (transtentorial, mesial, temporal)
3. **T**onsillar.

C

Carcinoid syndrome: **VANISH**

1. **V**asomotor: Flushes and apparent cyanosis
2. **A**sthma
3. **N**iacin deficiency (due to niacin being used up in serotonin synthesis)
4. **I**ntestinal: diarrhea, cramps, nausea, vomiting
5. **S**ystemic fibrosis: Right ventricle endocardial surface, tricuspid and pulmonary valve thickening and stenosis
6. **H**epatomegaly with nodular metastases.

Cardiac death, sudden, causes: **CAME**

1. **C**AD (coronary artery disease)
2. **A**rrhythmia, conduction problems
3. **M**yocardial diseases
4. **E**ndocardial diseases (endocarditis, aortic stenosis, mitral valve prolapse).

Cellular events in acute inflammation: **RATE**

1. **R**olling
2. **A**dhesion
3. **T**ransmigration
4. **E**ating (phagocytosis).

Coronary syndromes, acute: **SAC**

1. **S**udden cardiac death
2. **A**cute myocardial infarction
3. **C**rescendo angina (unstable, pre-infarction angina pectoris).

Choriocarcinomas gestational approximately arise from: **CAN**

1. **C**omplete, mole 1/2
2. **A**bortion 1/4
3. **N**ormal pregnancy 1/4.

D

Disseminated intravascular coagulation: **DIC and M**

1. **D**elivery-related (septic abortion, amniotic fluid embolization, retained products of conception, abruptio placenta, etc.)
2. **I**nfections (septicemia, meningococcemia)
3. **C**ancer (acute promyelocytic leukemia, carcinoma of lung, pancreas, prostate, stomach)
4. **M**iscellaneous (shock, severe trauma).

G

Gastritis, acute, causative factors: **HANS^3**

1. **H**. pylori
2. **A**lcohol
3. **N**SAIDs (NO_2 steroidal anti-inflammatory drugs)
4. **S**hock
5. **S**tress
6. **S**moking.

Gastroenteritis, chronic, causative factors: **HA^{2}DS**

1. **H**. pylori
2. **A**utonomic destruction of parietal cells
3. **A**lcohol
4. **D**uodenogastric reflux
5. **S**moking.

H

Hypertension, secondary, causes: **CRANE**

1. **C**ardiovascular:
   a. **C**oarctation of aorta
   b. **I**ncreased cardiac output
   c. **I**ncreased intravascular volume
   d. **P**AN.
2. **R**enal:
   a. Renal artery stenosis
   b. Acute glomerulonephritis
   c. Chronic renal failure
   d. Polycystic kidney disease.
3. **A**ssorted (miscellaneous):
   a. Toxemia of pregnancy
   b. Drugs, e.g. steroids, sympathomimetics, amphetamines.
4. *Neurologic:* Increased intracranial pressure due to hydrocephalus, edema, neoplasm, abscess, etc.
5. *Endocrine:*
   a. Primary aldosteronism (Conn's syndrome)
   b. Cushing's syndrome
   c. Pheochromocytoma
   d. Acromegaly
   e. Hyperthyroidism.

I

Ischemic heart disease, pathogenetic factors affecting coronary arteries/myocardium:

Four main factors: **APTS**

1. **A**therosclerosis, severe
2. **P**laque changes, acute
3. **T**hrombosis
4. **S**pasm

Three other factors: **DIE**

1. **D**ecreased blood supply (sudden drop in BP)
2. **I**ncreased myocardial demand (hypertrophy)
3. **E**mboli

L

Lymphadenopathy, causes: **LI²MA**

1. **L**ipid storage disease
   a. Gaucher's disease
   b. Niemann-Pick disease
2. **I**nfections:
   a. Viral, e.g. infectious mononucleosis, AIDS, rubella, varicella zoster
   b. Bacterial (see page 116)
3. **I**mmunologic diseases:
   a. SLE
   b. RA
4. **M**alignancies:
   a. Primary, e.g. Hodgkin's and non-Hodgkin's lymphomas
   b. Leukemias
5. **A**ssorted (miscellaneous):
   a. Sarcoidosis
   b. Sinus histiocytosis
   c. Mucocutaneous lymph node syndrome (Kawasaki disease).

M

Malignant hypertension, characteristics: **>120 CREEP**

1. **>120** = Diastolic pressure over 120 mmHg.
2. **C**ardiovascular abnormalities
2. **R**enal failure
3. **E**mergency
4. **E**ncephalopathy
5. **P**apilledema.

Myocardial infarction, complications: **VAMP²IRES**

1. **V**entricular **a**rrhythmia
2. **M**yocardial rupture (cardiac tamponade)
3. **P**ulmonary edema
4. **P**ericarditis
5. **I**mmunologic—Dressler's syndrome
6. **R**upture of papillary muscles
7. **E**mbolization ← thrombosis
8. **S**hock.

N

Necrosis: Necrosis is changes of dead cells/tissue which can only be seen in a living organism/person/fellow. These changes are: **L**iving **f**ellow **c**an **c**reate

1. **L**iquefactive
2. **F**ibrinoid
3. **C**aseous
4. **C**oagulative.

Neoplasm, genes involved in the development of: **ABCD**

1. **A**poptosis regulating genes
2. **B**ring about growth genes (growth-promoting proto-oncogenes—converted to oncogenes
3. **C**ut down growth genes (growth-inhibiting tumor suppressor genes)
4. **D**NA repair genes.

Neoplasm, proto-oncogenes converted to oncogenes in 4 ways: **TAPE**

1. **T**ranslocation
2. **A**mplification
3. **P**oint mutation
4. (**E**xtra) over expression.

Neoplasm, chromosome changes associated with neoplastic mutations of the genes: **TB**

1. **T**ranslocation
2. (**B**y) Deletion.

Neuropathies, peripheral causes: **MINT**

1. **M**etabolic: (**R**enal failure, **A**lcoholism, **D**iabetes mellitus) **RAD**
2. **I**nflammatory: Guillain-Barre syndrome, leprosy, sarcoidosis
3. **N**utritional: Deficiencies of vitamins B_1 (thiamine), B_6 (pyridoxine)
4. **T**oxic: (**S**olvents, **L**ead, **A**rsenic, **C**isplatin). **SLAC**

P

Paraneoplastic syndrome: **CONES**

1. **C**oagulation abnormalities (Trousseau's syndrome with migratory thrombophlebitis in carcinoma of the head of pancreas, and other visceral malignancies)
2. **O**sseous (hypertrophic osteopathy and clubbing of fingers in cancer of lung)
3. **Neurologic** (Lambert-Eaton myasthenic syndrome in small cell carcinoma of the lung)
4. **E**ndocrine—endocrinopathies, e.g.

a. Cushing's syndrome due to production of ACTH-like substance in small cell carcinoma of lung, renal cell carcinoma
b. Hyperthyroidism due to production of TSH-like substance in some lung neoplasms, hydatidiform mole and choriocarcinoma
c. Hypercalcemia due to production of parathormone-like substance in squamous cell carcinoma of the lung
d. Hypoglycemia due to production of insulin-like substance in hepatocellular carcinoma, mesothelioma and some sarcomas
e. Polycythemia due to production of erythropoietin in renal cell carcinoma and some other neoplasms
f. Dilutional hyponatremia with concentrated urine due to production of ADH in small cell carcinoma of the lung and some other neoplasms

5. **S**kin conditions: For example, dermatomyositis or acanthosis nigricans in various visceral malignancies.

Peptic ulcer, microscopic layers: DIGS

1. **D**ebris necrotic
2. **I**nflammation
3. **G**ranulation tissue
4. **S**car.

Peptic ulcer, common complications: HOP

1. **H**emorrhage
2. **O**bstruction
3. **P**erforation.

Not ***CHOP*** (*Cancer*, hemorrhage, obstruction, perforation), because cancer is *a rare complication*.

Pulmonary diseases, obstructive, causes: C^2AB^2

1. **C**OPD chronic obstructive pulmonary diseases (chronic bronchitis and emphysema)
2. **C**ystic fibrosis (mucoviscidosis, fibrocystic disease of pancreas)
3. **A**sthma
4. **B**ronchiectasis
5. **B**ronchiolitis.

Pulmonary diseases, restrictive, causes: MONK-SHIP CAT

A. **M**usculoskeletal (extrapulmonary):
   1. **O**besity
   2. **N**eurogenic, e.g. *Guillain-Barre syndrome*
   3. **K**yphoscoliosis

B. Pulmonary:

1. **S**arcoidosis
2. **H**emorrhage, diffuse alveolar syndrome, e.g. *Goodpasture's syndrome*
3. **I**diopathic pulmonary fibrosis
4. **P**neumoconiosis, e.g. (**S**ilicosis, **A**sbestosis, **C**oal worker's lung) **SAC**
5. **C**ollagen vascular diseases, e.g. SLE, RA
6. **A**ngittis and granulomatosis, e.g. *Wegener granulomatosis*
7. **T**reatment with busulfan, bleomycin, methotraxate.

R

Rhabdomyosarcoma, types: **PEA**

1. **P**leomorphic
2. **E**mbryonal (botryoid)
3. **A**lveolar.

S

Small round blue cell tumors:

Some **m**en are **e**asy **r**unners and **c**an **r**un **w**ell via **n**arrow **l**anes:

1. **S**mall cell carcinoma of the lung
2. **M**edulloblastoma
3. **E**wing's tumor
4. **R**habdomyosarcoma
5. **C**arcinoid
6. **R**etinoblastoma
7. **W**ilms' tumor
8. **N**euroblastoma
9. **L**ymphoma.

Splenomegaly etiologic classification: **MACHINES**

1. **M**iscellaneous
   a. Sarcoidosis
   b. Amyloidosis
   c. Gaucher's disease
   d. Niemann-Pick disease
2. **A**utoimmune
   a. RA (Still's disease)
   b. SLE
   c. ITP
3. **C**ongestion
   a. Cirrhosis

b. Portal hypertension
c. Portal vein thrombosis
4. **H**ematologic
a. Hemolytic anemias (hereditary spherocytosis, autoimmune, thalassemia)
b. Extramedullary erythropoiesis
c. Myeloid metaplasia with myelofibrosis
5. **I**nfections
a. Infectious mononucleosis (EB virus)
b. Typhoid
c. Malaria
d. TB
e. Infective endocarditis
f. Sepsis
6. **N**eoplasia
a. CLL
b. Hairy cell leukemia
c. CML
d. Lymphomas (Hodgkin's and non-Hodgkin's)
e. Polycythemia rubra vera
f. Acute leukemias
g. Histiocytosis X
7. **E**tiologic classification of
8. **S**plenomegaly.

T

Thrombus formation, predisposing conditions (Virchow's triad): **SHE**

1. **S**tasis
2. **H**ypercoagulability
3. **E**ndothelial/endocardial injury

Or

ABC

1. **A**bnormal (injured) surfaces of the blood vessels and heart
2. **B**lood flow abnormal (stasis or turbulence)
3. **C**oagulation abnormal.

Thrombus, fate: **DOPE**

1. **D**issolution
2. **O**rganization and recanalization

3. Propagation
4. Embolization.

Thyroid cancers: Folded **MAP**

1. Follicular carcinoma
2. **M**edullary carcinoma
3. **A**naplastic carcinoma
4. **P**apillary carcinoma.

Thrombolysis (which re-opens the flow of blood) is achieved by: **TAP**

1. **T**issue plasminogen activator
2. **A**ntithrombin III
3. **P**rotein S and C.

V

Valvular heart diseases, complications: **PAVE IT**

1. **P**ressure overload
2. **A**rrhythmia
3. **V**olume overload
4. **E**ndocarditis
5. **I**schemia: Angina, MI, syncope, stroke
6. **T**hrombosis.

Appendix

2

Some Selected Definitions

A

Achalasia of the esophagus: Incomplete relaxation of lower esophageal sphincter in response to swallowing.

Acute coronary syndromes: Three acute serious conditions of coronary artery disease (ischemic heart disease):

1. Unstable or crescendo, preinfarction angina pectoris
2. Acute myocardial infarction (MI)
3. Sudden cardiac death.

Acute tubular necrosis: Clinicopathological condition of destruction of tubular epithelial cells with acute suppression of renal function. Etiologically, it is of 2 types:

1. Ischemic.
2. Nephrotoxic.

Acute inflammation: It is early response to injury lasting a short duration. Its main cell is polymorphonuclear leukocyte (PMN). It is characterized by calor (heat), dolor (pain), rubor (redness), tumor (swelling) and functio laesa (loss of function).

Acute respiratory distress syndrome (ARDS)/acute lung injury: Acute onset of diffuse alveolar damage involving both the alveolar epithelium and capillary endothelium.

Adaptation: Normally, the cells stay the same and do not change. Under certain circumstances (stimuli), physiologic or pathologic, in order to meet the functional demand or stay alive, the cells adjust by some change. This phenomenon is known as adaptation. According to the circumstances (stimuli), these adaptations are of the following 4 types:

1. Atrophy
2. Hypertrophy
3. Hyperplasia
4. Metaplasia.

Aleukemic leukemia: Acute leukemia when there is pancytopenia and no or very few blasts are present in the peripheral blood; but, only in the bone marrow, which is full of blast cells. (This helps to differentiate it from aplastic anemia).

Amyloidosis: Conditions in which amyloid is extracellularly deposited in various tissues/organs of the body. *Nature of amyloid:* Group of proteins form a similar structure with similar amorphous eosinophilic appearance similar to carbohydrate or amylum, which are, therefore, called amyloid.

Anemia: Decrease in oxygen-transporting capacity of blood due to decreased total circulating red cell mass, seen as low hemoglobin concentration and low hematocrit.

Aneurysm: Aneurysm is an abnormal dilatation of an artery or a vein.

Angina pectoris: Episodic chest pain due to inadequate oxygen supply to the heart caused by **reversible** ischemia. Relieved by nitroglycerin.

Angina, stable (typical): Pain occurs upon exertion and is relieved by rest or by vasodilator drugs. Due to severe atherosclerotic narrowing of coronary arteries, which cannot meet the increased demand of exertion. Commonest type of angina.

Angina, unstable (crescendo, preinfarction): History of stable angina developing angina upon rest or less exertion, more severe or lasts longer or recurs more frequently.

Angina, variant (Prinzmetal): Chest pain is at rest from the beginning. Here there is no atherosclerosis, but chest pain is thought to be due to spasm of coronary arteries.

Aplastic anemia: Suppression of multipotent marrow stem cell resulting in pancytopenia (anemia, thrombocytopenia, leukopenia).

Apoptosis: It is programmed death of single or small group of cells.

Anaplasia: Lack of differentiation. The changes present here are those present in CIS or infiltrating carcinoma but in more severe degree as follows:

1. In anaplasia the lack of architectural and cellular differentiation (atypia) is of the most severe degree. There is a total loss of the normal architecture and the neoplastic cells are present in sheets with marked loss of polarity. Atypia is also of the most severe degree and giant cells may be present called tumor giant cells.
2. Mitotic figures are markedly increased in number.
3. Mitotic figures may be abnormal, i.e. instead of normal bipolar, tripolar or quadripolar mitotic figures might be present.

Arteriosclerosis: Arteriosclerosis is thickening of arteries with loss of elasticity consisting of 3 types:

1. Atherosclerosis.
2. Arteriolosclerosis.
3. Monckeberg's medial calcific sclerosis.

Arteriolosclerosis: Thickening of the arterioles.

Atelactasis: Collapse. Loss of lung volume due to inadequate expansion of air spaces. Results in shunting of inadequately oxygenated blood from pulmonary arteries into veins with ventilation-perfusion imbalance and hypoxia.

Atherosclerosis: In Greek language, "athera" means porridge. Atherosclerosis consists of intimal lesion made of fibrofatty plaque with a central porridge-like core which is rich in lipid. This plaque is called atheroma.

Atresia of the small intestine: Complete failure of development of intestinal lumen is atresia. Only narrowing is **stenosis**.

Atrophy is reduced size of cell and the organ.

Atypia means when the cells are not typical to the normal cells. This lack of typicality could be in the following ways:

1. Loss of uniformity—cells may differ from each other in size and shape (called pleomorphism).
2. The nuclei become bigger and the ratio of the nucleus to cytoplasm increases.
3. Nuclei become darker in color (deeply stained—hyperchromatic).
4. The nuclear chromatin becomes clumped focally, i.e. in some places.
5. Nucleoli become larger and dark-colored and more than one may be present.

B

Bronchial asthma: Episodic reversible bronchospasm and airway narrowing due to increased bronchial smooth muscle spasmodic and inflammatory response to various stimuli.

Bronchiectasis: Permanent dilation of bronchi and bronchioles due to destruction of the muscle and elastic supporting tissue, resulting from or associated with chronic necrotizing infections. It is *not* a primary disease; but, secondary to:

1. Infection
2. Obstruction
3. Congenital or hereditary conditions.

Bulla: Grossly seen skin lesion that is filled with fluid measuring >5 mm.

C

Carcinoid: Tumor of cells of neuroendocrine/enterochromaffin origin which sometimes secrete hormones/endocrine polypeptides causing carcinoid syndrome (q.v.).

Carcinogenesis: It is a multistep process at phenotypic and genetic level. Phenotypic characteristics are excessive growth, local invasiveness, ability to form distant metastases. Genetic characteristics are collection of genetic lesions, which, in some cases, are helped by defects in DNA repair.

Carcinogenesis main factor: Nonlethal genetic damage is the main factor of carcinogenesis.

CCF (Congestive cardiac failure): It is a condition when heart cannot eject the blood delivered to it by the venous system due to decreased capacity of the heart or in some cases due to increased demand for the blood by the tissues **(high output failure)**.

Cardiac shunts (congenital):

1. *Left-to-right:* Flow of the blood from the left side of the heart to the right without going through the systemic circulation, e.g. in ASD, VSD, PDA.
2. *Right-to-left (reversed shunt, Eisenmenger's complex or syndrome):* Flow of the blood from the right side of the heart to the left without going through the lungs, e.g. in ASD, VSD, PDA due to development of pulmonary hypertension resulting from the left-to-right shunt.

Choriocarcinoma, gestational, incidence: **MAN**

1. **M**ole, complete hydatidiform—~50%
2. **A**bortion—~25%
3. **N**ormal pregnancy—~25%.

Choristoma: It is not a neoplasm, therefore, it should not be called "oma". It is small area of normal tissue of one organ misplaced within another organ such as normal area of pancreatic tissue in the wall of the stomach.

Chronic bronchitis: Persistent productive cough for at least 3 consecutive months in at least 2 consecutive years (definition based on clinical findings).

Chronic inflammation: Chronic inflammation is characterized by:

1. Lasts weeks to months or years
2. *Infiltration by chronic inflammatory cells:* Mononuclear cells: Lymphocytes, plasma cells, macrophages
3. Tissue destruction
4. Repair by new vessels proliferation (angiogenesis) and fibrosis.

CIS (carcinoma—*in situ*): Carcinoma *in situ* means cancer confined to the full thickness of the epithelium or epidermis, i.e. it has not broken through the basal layer and gone into **(infiltrated)** the deeper tissue beneath the basal layer of the epithelium. The changes present here are those present in dysplasia with following differences:

1. The changes involve the **full thickness of the epithelium**
2. The changes are **of more severe degree** than in dysplasia
3. These changes **are not reversible** unlike in dysplasia.

Cirrhosis: End stage of liver disease. Its three characteristics are as follows:

1. Scarring with replacement of normal liver architecture with fibrosis forming fibrous septae.
2. Parenchymal nodules formed by regeneration of encircled hepatocytes (<3 mm = micronodular cirrhosis; >3 mm = macronodular cirrhosis).
3. Entire liver architecture is disrupted.

Concussion: Due to blunt injury to the skull there is transient loss of consciousness and widespread paralysis and sometimes seizures followed by recovery within a few hours to days. There is loss of memory about the episode. There is no other residual effect of this event. There is no anatomic lesion. Transient injury to the reticular activating system is thought to be the cause of this.

Congenital diseases: Diseases present at the time of birth.

Hyperemia: Is an active process. It results from increased tissue inflow of blood due to arteriolar dilation, e.g. sites of inflammation. The affected tissue is redder due to engorgement with oxygenated blood.

Congestion: Is a passive process. It results from impaired venous outflow from a tissue, e.g. systemic—such as cardiac failure or local—such as isolated venous obstruction. The affected tissue is of bluish-red color (cyanosis) due to deoxygenated blood.

D

Diarrhea and dysentery

Diarrhea: Loose watery stools with increased amount and frequency.

Dysentery: Painful, bloody diarrhea.

DIC (Disseminated intravascular coagulation) (consumption coagulopathy)

DIC is *not a disease*; but, a potential complication of any condition associated with widespread activation of thrombin. This causes widespread formation of fibrin thrombi in the microcirculation, which is only visible microscopically, which can cause diffuse circulatory insufficiency by blockage, e.g. brain, lungs, heart, kidneys, etc. With development of multlple thrombi there is rapid consumption of platelets and coagulation proteins. Hence, it is also called *consumption coagulopathy*. Simultaneously, fibrinolytic mechanisms are activated. So, the initial thrombotic disorder ends as a serious bleeding disorder.

Causes **DIC and M**

1. **D:** Delivery-related: Amniotic fluid embolism, septic abortion, retained dead fetus, toxemia, abruptio placenta
2. **I:** Infections: Septicemia, meningococcemia
3. **C:** Cancer: Acute promyelocytic leukemia, carcinoma of lung, pancreas, prostate, stomach
4. **M**iscellaneous: Severe trauma, shock.

Dysplasia: Dysplasia is disorderly proliferation of cells where there is:

1. Loss in the orientation of cells, i.e. the cells are not arranged in an orderly fashion known as **loss of** polarity.
2. Loss of orderly maturation of cells, i.e. the cells do not mature in the normal order from the tall cells in the bottom basal layer of the epithelium to the flattened squamous cells in the top superficial layer of the epithelium; but, a disorderly scrambling of dark basal-appearing cells is present within the epithelium.
3. Atypia of the cells is present.
4. Mitotic figures are more in number than usual.

5. Mitotic figures appear in abnormal locations, i.e. they are not confined to the normal location of the basal layer; but, are seen in all layers of the cell.
6. In dysplasia these changes do **not** occupy the full thickness of the epithelium; but, **only the partial thickness of the epithelium**.
7. In dysplasia, these changes are reversible, i.e. when the stimuli which evoked these changes are removed these changes revert to normal.
8. Dysplasia can progress to malignancy, as is seen in dysplasia of metaplastic squamous epithelium of cervix progresses to squamous cell carcinoma of the cervix.

E

Edema: A local or generalized condition in which there is excessive amount of fluid in the tissues of our body.

Embolus: Embolus is a detached intravascular solid, liquid, or gaseous mass that is carried by the blood to a site distant from its point of origin. ~99% of the emboli are dislodged thrombi. Hence, the term thromboembolism.

Emphysema: Permanent enlargement of airspaces distal to the terminal bronchioles accompanied by destruction of their walls (definition based on morphologic changes).

Epidural hematoma and lucid interval: Hematoma above the dura mater usually due to the rupture of the meningeal artery or its branch between squamous portion of temporal bone and dura mater with fracture of the bone. Hematoma is formed beneath the bone above the dura. *If not drained immediately, it will compress the underlying brain and cause uncal and cerebellar tonsillar herniation, brainstem compression and **death**.* Immediately after the injury many patients have a brief period of unconsciousness due to concussion. Then, the patient recovers consciousness for a short interval of time. This short recovery of consciousness is known as *lucid interval*. This recovery can give a false sense of security and well-being. After a few minutes or hours, due to continuous bleeding and increase in the size of hematoma there is progressively increased intracranial pressure ***leading to progressive loss of consciousness, coma and death if not promptly treated.***

Erythroplasia of the oral cavity: Red, velvety, granular circumscribed areas, sometimes elevated, with poorly defined irregular boundaries. Microscopically, always almost have marked epithelial dysplasia. **Malignant transformation is >50%.**

F

Fracture: Break in the continuity of a bone.

Free radicals: Free radicals are high-energy atoms, molecules, or group of molecules with single unpaired electron in their outermost orbit. Therefore, they are "free" to give or take an electron.

G

Goiter: Enlargement of the thyroid gland.

Grading: I to IV of neoplasms to determine their aggressive potential. It is determined by microscopic examination of the neoplastic cells based on cytological differentiation and mitoses (number and shape). (**Clinical staging** based on the size and the extent of spread of the tumor (TNM = Tumor size, lymph node involvement and distant metastases) has been known to give better prognostic information than microscopic/morphologic grading).

Granulation tissue: Grossly, it is pink, soft granular-appearing tissue formed during repair of injured tissue. Microscopically, it consists of proliferation fibroblasts, and new thin-walled capillaries in a loose extracellular matrix (ECM).

Granuloma: When the body is not able to eliminate the offending organism/substance, the **activated macrophages** which look like epithelial cells (therefore, are called epithelioid cells) surround the area to isolate it from the rest of the body. *This collection of epithelioid cells is called a granuloma* (granuloma in Latin means a small grain or granule).

H

Hamartoma: It is not a neoplasm, therefore, it should not be called "oma". It is a collection of cells normally found in an organ but not organized in a normal pattern of that organ.

Hemolytic anemia: Shortened lifespan of RBCs (normal 120 days). Marrow cannot keep pace with RBC destruction.

Hemostasis: Hemostasis means maintaining blood in a free-flowing, clot-free fluid state in normal vessels and rapid formation of a hemostatic plug at the site of breach in the continuity of the vessel to prevent bleeding. *This depends on normal:*

a. Vessel wall (structure and function)
b. Platelets (number, structure and function) and
c. Coagulation cascade (components and function).

Hemorrhage: Extravasation of blood due to rupture of a blood vessel.

Hemochromatosis: Deposition of excess iron in the tissue with injury to structure and function.

Hemosiderosis: Deposition of excess iron in the tissues without affecting the structure or function.

Hernia: Protrusion of a part of an organ or tissue through an abnormal opening.

Hiatal hernia: Protrusion of a portion of stomach through separation of the diaphragmatic crura or widening of space between muscular crura and esophageal wall into thorax.

Herniation of brain: Displacement of a part of the brain due to increased intracranial pressure.

Hydrocephalus: Increased CSF in the cranial cavity.

Hyperemia: Is an active process. It results from increased tissue inflow of blood due to arteriolar dilation, e.g. sites of inflammation. The affected tissue is redder due to engorgement with oxygenated blood.

Hyperkeratosis: Microscopically seen skin lesion that has thickened stratum corneum.

Hyperplasia: Increase in the size of the organ due to increase in the number of cells.

Hypertensive heart disease: Left ventricular hypertrophy in a person who has chronic hypertension and does *not* have other conditions which could cause left ventricular hypertrophy such as aortic stenosis, hypertrophic cardiomyopathy.

Hypertension: Arterial pressure greater than 140/90 mmHg on at least 3 consecutive visits to the doctor's office.

Hypertrophy: Increase in size of organ or tissue due to increase in the size of cells.

I

Icterus: Yellow color of sclera due to elevated serum bilirubin at 2 to 2.5 mg/dl (normal is approximately half of this). Increased serum carotene also makes skin color yellow **but not of sclera**.

Immunity: Immunity means freedom or protection from any injury.

Infarction: Area of ischemic necrosis caused by occlusion of either arterial supply or the venous drainage in a particular tissue, e.g. MI, CVA, pulmonary, bowel, limbs. ~ 99% infarcts are from thrombotic/embolic events and almost all are from arterial occlusion.

Inflammation: Complex reaction in vascularized connective tissue caused by various exogenous and endogenous stimuli that can cause direct cell injury.

Ischemia: Reduced blood supply to an organ or part of the body. (In Greek, Isch = restriction, hemia = blood, restricted blood supply).

Inferior vena cava syndrome: It is the obstruction of the inferior vena cava.

Ischemic heart disease: Decreased blood supply to meet the demands of the heart.

J

Jaundice: Yellow color of skin and icterus (yellow color of sclera) due to elevated serum bilirubin at 2 to 2.5 mg/dl (normal is approximately half of this). Incresed serum carotene also makes skin color yellow but not of sclera.

K

Kernicterus: Deep yellow staining of the basal nuclei of the brain with neurologic signs and symptoms due to high serum bilirubin seen in newborns with severe hemolytic anemia usually when baby is Rh positive and mother is Rh negative.

L

Leukoplakia of the oral cavity: A whitish, well-defined mucosal patch caused by epidermal thickening or hyperkeratosis, ~10% progress to squamous cell carcinoma.

Lymphangitis: Inflammation of the lymphatics.

Lymphoid neoplasms: Arise from multipotent stem cells which give rise to T, B, NK cells.

Types:

A. Non-Hodgkin's lymphoma

B. Lymphocytic leukemias

C. Hodgkin's lymphoma.

A. **Non-Hodgkin's lymphoma:** Neoplastic proliferation of lymphoid cells as discrete masses in lymph nodes, spleen or other sites (~ 2/3 arise in lymph nodes and 1/3 in lymphoid tissue at other sites).

B. **Lymphatic leukemias:** Malignant lymphoid neoplasms present with generalized bone marrow involvement usually with large number of tumor cells in peripheral blood. Essentially, the difference between non-Hodgkin's lymphoma and leukemia is like ice and water and in the tissue distribution when initially seen.

C. **Hodgkin's lymphoma:** Hodgkin's lymphoma is now thought to be a lymphoma of B cell origin, the diagnosis of which is made by biopsy of lymph node or extranodal lymphoid tissue showing Reed-Sternberg cell within the appropriate cellular background of lymphocytes, eosinophils, histiocytes, neutrophils, plasma cells, fibroblasts and collagen fibers.

Lymphedema: It is edema due to impaired lymphatic flow.

M

Macule: Grossly, a flat circumscribed area of the skin having a different color than surrounding skin.

Malignant hypertension: It is severe (diastolic blood pressure > 120 mmHg), rapid rise of blood pressure. It can be a complication of either primary or secondary hypertension. It has rapid clinical course with early death from CVA, renal failure, LVH, left ventricular failure. Retinopathy with focal retinal hemorrhage and papilledema.

Metaplasia: Reversible change in which in the place of one normal adult cell type (epithelial or mesenchymal) another adult cell type is produced.

Metastasis: Development of secondary implants (metastases) discontinuous with the primary tumor, possibly in remote tissues. [Metastasis (singular), Metastases (plural)].

Myocardial infarction (MI): Irreversible ischemia with necrosis of myocardium due to blockage in the blood supply.

N

Necrosis: Morphologic changes in living tissue after cell death.

Neoplasm: An abnormal mass of tissue the growth of which exceeds and is uncoordinated with that of normal tissues and persists in the same excessive manner after the cessation of stimuli which evoked the change.

Nephritic syndrome: *Consists of:*

1. *Hematuria:* Due to inflammatory leakage of the glomerular capillaries with bleeding into Bowman's space. RBCs can collect in renal tubules and together with proteinaceous material acquire shape of the renal tubules to form RBC casts.
2. Oliguria.
3. Azotemia (increased BUN and creatinine)
4. Hypertension.

Seen in:

1. Alport's syndrome (hereditary nephritis)
2. Goodpasture's syndrome
3. RPGN
4. IgA nephropathy (Berger's disease)
5. Poststreptococcal GN
6. SLE.

Nephrosclerosis: Arteriolosclerosis of the renal arterioles.

Types:

1. Hyaline
2. Hyperplastic.

Nephrotic syndrome: *Consists of:*

1. Massive proteinuria (>4 gm per day), (due to increased basement membrane permeability).
2. Hypoalbuminemia, (serum albumin reduced to < 3 gm/ 100 mls.) (due to massive proteinuria).
3. Generalized edema, (due to hypoalbuminemia with decreased plasma oncotic pressure) and hypernatremia (due to reduced renal flow and concomitant increased aldosterone) with accompanying increased water and hydrostatic pressure.
4. Hyperlipidemia (due to increased lipid synthesis by the liver).

Nodule: Grossly seen skin lesion that is elevated solid area of >5 mm.

P

Papilloma: Benign tumor of epithelium with finger-like configuration. Epithelium can be squamous skin, larynx, tongue or columnar of GIT tract or any gland or transitional of the urinary bladder, ureter, or renal pelvis.

Papule: Grossly seen skin lesion that is solid, measuring up to 5 mm.

Parakeratosis: Microscopically seen skin lesion that shows nuclei in the stratum corneum.

Plaque: Grossly seen skin lesion that is elevated, flat measuring >5 mm.

Phlebothrombosis/thrombophlebitis: Formation of thrombus in veins is phlebothrombosis. This causes inflammation of vein (thrombophlebitis).

Paradoxical embolism: With ASD or VSD the venous embolus instead of going into lungs might go into systemic circulation.

Paraneoplastic syndromes: Symptom complex other than cachexia that appear in patients with cancer and that cannot be readily explained either by local or distant spread of the tumor or by the elaboration of hormones indigenous to the tissue of origin of the tumor. These can be first *S/S* of tumor, may mimic metastases, or can cause complications which could result in the patient's death.

Pneumonia: Infection of the lungs.

Pneumonia, broncho (bronchopneumonia): Patchy consolidation of lung near inflamed bronchioles.

Pneumonia, lobar: Alveolar inflammation with consolidation involving large continuous areas of lung.

Pneumonia, community-acquired atypical: Called "atypical" because: no physical findings of consolidation, not much sputum production, WBC not much elevated, no bacteria could be found.

Pneumonitis, acute interstitial: Inflammation of the alveolar septae.

Pneumoconiosis: Disorders caused by inhalation of any aerosol, fumes, vapors, inorganic mineral dusts or organic dusts.

Polycythemia (erythrocytosis): Increase in concentration of RBCs and Hb level.

Polyp: Tumor projecting from the surface. *Sessile* = Without a stalk. *Pedunculated* = With a stalk.

Portal hypertension: Increased pressure in portal circulation.

Pyelonephritis: Suppurative inflammation of the pelvis of the kidney and kidney proper.
Types:
1. Acute
2. Chronic.

R

Renal failure: Loss of kidneys' ability to maintain the volume and composition of the body fluids under conditions of normal dietary intake. Is always associated with **azotemia** (increased serum creatinine and/or urea of renal origin). In advanced stages results in **uremia** (biochemical plus clinical syndrome seen in symptomatic renal disease).

Restrictive lung diseases: Reduced compliance (stiff lungs) with increased pressure required to expand the lungs with less amount of air in the lungs. Total lung capacity and FVC are reduced. But, the expiratory flow rate is normal or only reduced equally. So, **the ratio of FEV1/FVC is normal.**

Repair: Healing of injured tissue.

Types:

1. Regeneration.
2. Fibrosis:

1. **Regeneration:** Repair by growth of the same type of cells.
2. **Fibrosis:** Repair by connective tissue.

S

Shock: Systemic hypoperfusion due to reduction either in cardiac output or in the *effective* circulating blood volume resulting in hypotension, impaired tissue perfusion and hypoxia.

Staging of neoplasms: It is a clinical method based on the size of the primary lesion, its extent of spread to the regional lymph nodes and the presence or absence of distant metastases to quantify probable clinical aggressiveness of a given neoplasm, its apparent extent and spread in an individual patient in order to plan treatment and predict probable outcome. **Has greater clinical value than grading.**

Types:

1. TNM (Tumor size, node involvement, presence of metastasis).
2. AJC (American Joint Committee).

Superior vena cava syndrome: Obstruction of the superior vena cava.

T

Thrombosis: Formation of blood clot (thrombus) in the noninterrupted vascular system (blood vessels and cardiac chamber). *It is pathologic blood clotting* with several pathologic problems as opposed to **hemostasis** where there is *physiologic blood clotting* with formation of blood clot *in an interrupted (broken) blood vessel to prevent bleeding.*

Transient ischemic attack (TIA): Transient episodes of neurologic dysfunction lasting from several minutes to several hours (maximum 24 hours) due to self-limited episodes of vascular obstruction by atheromatous emboli and/or platelet-fibrin aggregates. Usually, onset of brain infarction is fairly sudden but often preceded by TIAs. *TIAs are important predictor of subsequent infarcts, as approximately 1/3 of patients with TIAs develop significant infarcts within 5 years.*

U

Ulcer: Breach in the continuity of a surface.

Uremia: Biochemical plus clinical syndrome characteristic of symptomatic renal disease.

V

Vasculitis: Inflammation of the walls of the vessels (arteries, arterioles, capillaries and venules).

Vericose veins: Abnormally dilated tortuous veins.

Vesicle: Grossly seen skin lesion that is filled with fluid, measuring up to 5 mm.

Appendix 3

Some of the Changes in the Cells in Various Disorders

Axonal spheroids: Swelling of axons of neurons seen in diffuse axonal injury.

Anitschkow cell: Macrophage with a caterpillar-like nucleus in Aschoff body in heart seen in rheumatic carditis.

Ballooned cells/degeneration: Large nerve cells in Pick's diseases (Pick's cells); swollen liver cell in injury.

Bunina bodies: Small eosinophilic intracytoplasmic structures in normal spinal motor neurons in ALS.

Civatte bodies: Colloid bodies.

Cloudy swelling: With mild intracellular water collection.

Colloid bodies: Apoptotic cells of epidermis in papillary dermis in lichen planus.

Councilman bodies: Apoptotic liver cells seen as anuclear eosinophilic round bodies in yellow fever.

Crooke hyaline change: Collection of light blue material in the ACTH-secreting cells of pituitary in hypercorticolism due to collection of intermediate filaments in the cytoplasm of these cells.

Fatty change: Small and large vacuoles based on amount of fat collection.

Foam cells: Macrophages filled with lipid—seen in atherosclerosis.

Foamy degeneration: Liver cell with bile accumulation.

Giant cells: These are formed by fusion of activated macrophages, e.g. in foreign bodies, HIV (HIV-infected macrophages. Seen in HIV encephalopathy, measels (*Warthin-Finkleday*), neoplasms (tumor giant cell), tuberculosis (*Langhans*), xanthoma (*touton*), sarcoidosis, Crohn's disease, etc.

Granulovacuolar degeneration: Autophagic vacuoles possibly due to protective segregation of early apoptotic alterations in the neuronal cytoplasm seen in Alzheimer's disease.

Hirano bodies: Intracellular eosinophilic, rod-shaped collection of actin and related proteins seen in the neurons (nerve cells) in the hippocampus of people with some neurodegenerative disorders, e.g. Alzheimer's disease, Creutzfeldt-Jacob disease.

Hydropic (vacuolar): With more than mild intracellular water collection (see cloudy swelling).

Intranuclear inclusions in CMV: Seen in brain cells in CMV encephalitis.

Lewy bodies: Pinkish circularly layered structures in the cytoplasm of neurons in cerebral cortex in Parkinson's disease and Alzheimer's diseases.

Mallory's body: Eosinophilic cytoplasmic inclusion in liver cells in alcoholic liver disease—made of prekeratin intermediate filaments.

Negri bodies: Seen in cytoplasm of nerve cells in brain in rabies.

Neurofibrillary tangles in Alzheimer's disease: Collection of microtubules-associated protein and abnormal tau protein in the cytoplasm of the nerve cells (neurons).

Neuronophagia: These are microglial cells in brain which have phagocytosed neurons seen with microglial nodules in viral encephalitis.

Owl-like cell: Macrophage as giant cell with two nuclei having large nucleoli appearing as two eyes of an owl. Seen in: Hodgkin's diseases as Reed-Sternberg giant cell, rheumatic carditis in Aschoff body as Aschoff cell.

Rod cells: Elongated microglial cells in brain in GPI (general paralysis of insane) in CNS tertiary syphilis.

Russel bodies: Newly made immunoglobulin in RER of plasma cells—seen as round-eosinophilic hyaline (glassy).

Appendix 4

Some of the Changes in the Tissues and Organs in Various Disorders

Amyloid angiopathy: Beta amyloid deposit in blood vessel walls in Alzheimer's diseases.

Aschoff body: Granuloma with central fibrinoid necrosis surrounded by mononuclear cells with some Aschoff and Anitschkow cells in rheumatic carditis.

Atherosclerotic plaque: Macrophages and smooth muscle cells filled with cholesterol seen in atherosclerosis.

Brown induration of lung: Edema and hemosiderin deposition in lungs in CCF making the lungs brown and firm.

Brown tumor of hyperparathyroidism: Brown-colored mass in bone due to hemorrhage, with collection of osteoclasts, and giant cells in hyperparathyroidism.

Charcot-Leyden crystals: Somewhat diamond-shaped crystals made of eosinophil proteins seen in lungs in asthma.

Cardiac cirrhosis: Fibrosis in liver due to CCF. Not true cirrhosis because there is no generalized disruption of liver architecture nor there are regenerating liver nodules which are necessary for the definition of cirrhosis.

Corpora amylacea: Proteinaceous, thick material in lumen of prostate gland and processes of astrocyte in old age.

Cor bovimum: Grossly, big flabby heart in syphilis (like a cow's big heart).

Curschman spirals: Mucus plugs with twisted exfoliated bronchial epithelium in asthma.

Dystrophic calcification: Calcium deposition in damaged/dead tissue seen in blood vessels, and other tissues (cardiac valves, kidney, stomach wall).

Hyaline arteriolosclerosis: Pinkish homogenous deposits in the walls of arterioles seen in mild hypertension, diabetes mellitus, ageing.

Hyperplastic arteriolosclerosis: Increased smooth mucles in circular layers seen in the wall of arterioles in malignant hypertension.

Heart failure cells: Macrophages with hemosiderin in lung alveoli in CCF.

Nutmeg liver: Nutmeg-like appearance due to congestion around central veins with nearby pale liver cells in CCF.

Gamna-gandy bodies: Fibrotic areas with iron and calcium deposits seen in congestive splenomegaly.

Hemorrhage in mamillary bodies of hypothalamus: Seen in Wernicke encephalopathy in vitamin B_1 deficiency due to capillary endothelial proliferation with increased vascular permeability.

Keyser-Fleischer ring: Greenish-brownish copper deposition in the periphery of cornea in Wilson's diseases.

Leucocytoclastic angitis: Fragmentation of neutrophils in the wall of BVs in microscopic polyarteritis.

Myelin ovoids: EM appearance in axonal degeneration.

Myelin vacuolation and degeneration: Seen in lateral dorsal columns of white matter of spinal cord in subacute combined degeneration of spinal cord in vitamin B_{12} deficiency.

Onion bulbs: Segmental demyelination: EM appearance of nerve showing circular deposition of collagen alternating with Schwann cell processes due to demyelination and remyelination in primary myeline neuropathic diseases such as Guillain-Barre syndrome.

Senile plaques: Central amyloid core surrounded by twisted degenerated nerve cell process in Alzheimer's disease.

Xanthomas: Collection of lipid-filled macrophages in subepithelial connective tissue or in tendons.

Appendix 5 Some of the Structural Changes in Various Neoplasms

Antoni-A tissue: Tissue with thickly packed spindle cells seen in schwannoma.

Antoni-B tissue: Tissue with loose myxoid structure in schwannoma.

Call-Exner body: Collection of dark-colored material among granulosa cells in normal ovarian follicles—similar structure also seen in granulosa-theca cell tumor of ovary.

Herringbone pattern: Cells arranged in pattern of herring fish bone seen in fibrosarcoma.

Paget's cell: Cancer cell with clear zone around the nucleus seen in a type of cancer of breast (Paget's disease) and of vulva.

Psammoma bodies: Calcified granules in circular layered configuration seen in:

1. Meningioma
2. Papillary carcinoma of thyroid
3. Serous cystadenoma of ovary.

Rosenthal fibres: Bright eosinophilic fibres in pilocytic astrocytomas.

Rosettes: In certain neoplasms, the neoplastic cells are arranged like a small flower. There are 2 type of rosettes:

1. *True rosettes:* When the neoplastic cells surrounding a clear space, e.g. in ependymoma (*ependymal true rosettes*), retinoblastoma (*Flexner-Wintersteiner true rosette*).
2. *Pseudorosettes:* When the neoplastic cells do not surround a central lumen, but surround a blood vessel, e.g. perivascular pseudorosettes in ependymoma or fibrillar extensions of the cells, e.g. *Homer-Wright pseudorosettes* seen in neuroblastoma or medulloblastoma.

Schiller-Duvall body (glomeruloid body): Structure appearing like glomerulus having cystic spaces with central blood vessel inside surrounded by immature epithelial cells seen in yolk sac tumor (endodermal sinus tumor) of ovary.

Starry-sky appearance in Burkitt's lymphoma.

Storiform pattern: In dermatofibrosarcoma, malignant fibrous histiocytoma, the neoplastic cells are arranged in a spiral form.

Verocay bodies: Small group of nerve fibrils with adjacent palisaded nuclei seen in shwannoma.

Resources

1. Juan Rosai: *Ackerman's Surgical Pathology,* 7th ed.: CV Mosby Company, 1996.
2. *Atlas of Tumor Pathology—Series of Fascicles,* 2nd series: American Registry of Pathology.
3. Burton DR, Rennke HG: *Renal Pathophysiology—The Essentials*: Williams and Wilkins, 1994.
4. Clements MHS: *Pathology: Pretest Self-Assessment and Review,* 7th ed.: McGraw-Hill, Inc. 1993.
5. Dacie and Lewis: *Practical Haematology,* 9th ed.: Churchill Livingstone.
6. Damjanov Ivan: *High-Yield Pathology,* 2nd ed.: Lippincott William and Wilkins, 2005.
7. *Dorland's Illustrated Medical Dictionary*, 29th ed.: WB Saunders Company, 2000.
8. Gelehrter TD, Collins FS: *Principles of Medical Genetics*: William and Wilkins, 1990.
9. Guyton AC, Hall JE: *Textbook of Medical Physiology,* 10th ed.: Saunders, 2000.
10. *Harrison's Principles of Internal Medicine*: McGraw-Hill Book Company.
11. Kissane JM: *Andersons's Pathology,* 9th ed.: 1 and 2: CV Mosby Co., 1990.
12. Garg K, Bedi I, Kaul M: *A Textbook of Histology,* 3rd ed.: CBSPD, 1999.
13. Kumar P, Clark M: *Kumar and Clark Clinical Medicine,* 6th ed.: Elsevier Saunders, 2005.
14. Kumar V, Cotran RS, Robins SL: *Robbins Basic Pathology,* 7th ed.: WB Saunders Co., 2003.
15. McPhee SJ, Ganong WF: *Pathophysiology of Disease—An Introduction to Clinical Medicine,* 5th ed.: Lange Medical Books/McGraw-Hill, 2006.
16. Norman S, Brostoff J, James K: *Introducing Immunology,* 2nd ed.: Mosby, 1993.
17. Miller FN: *Pathology: Review for New National Boards,* 1st ed.: J&S Publishing Co. Inc.,1996.
18. Schneider AS, Szanto PA: *Board Review Series, Pathology*: Williams and Wilkins, 1993.
19. Staines N, Brostoff J, James K: *Introducing Immunology,* 2nd ed.: Mosby, 1993.
20. *Sternberg's Diagnostic Surgical Pathology,* 3rd ed.: Lippincott Williams and Wilkins, 1999.

21. American Family Physician; many issues.
22. New England Journal of Medicine; many issues.
23. Internet: Several.

Index